Adrenal and endocrine tumors in children

Cancer Treatment and Research

WILLIAM L. MCGUIRE, *series editor*

R.B. Livingston, ed., Lung Cancer 1, 1981, ISBN 90-247-2394-9.
G. Bennett Humphrey, Louis P. Dehner, Gerald B, Grindey and Ronald T, Acton, eds., Pediatric Oncology 1, 1981, ISBN 90-247-2408-2.
Jerome J. DeCosse and Paul Sherlock, eds., Gastrointestinal Cancer 1, 1981, ISBN 90-247-2461-9.
John M. Bennett, ed., Lymphomas 1, including Hodgkin's Disease, 1981, ISBN 90-247-2479-1.
C.D. Bloomfield, ed., Adult Leukemias 1, 1982, ISBN 90-247-2478-3.
David F. Paulson, ed., Genitourinary Cancer 1, 1982, ISBN 90-247-2480-5.
F.M. Muggia, ed., Cancer Chemotherapy 1, 1982, ISBN 90-247-2713-8.
G. Bennett Humphrey and Gerald B. Grindey, eds., Pancreatic Tumors in Children, 1983, ISBN 90-247-2702-2.
John J. Costanzi, ed., Malignant Melanoma 1, 1983, ISBN 90-247-2706-5.
C.T. Griffiths and A.F. Fuller, eds., Gynecologic Oncology. 1983, ISBN 0-89838-555-5.
F. Anthony, Greco ed., Biology and Management of Lung Cancer. 1983, ISBN 0-89838-554-7.
Michael D., Walker, ed., Oncology of the Nervous System. ISBN 0-89838-567-9.
Donald J. Higby, ed., Supportive Care in Cancer Therapy. ISBN 0-89838-569-5.
Ronald B. Herberman, ed., Basic and Clinical Immunology. ISBN 0-89838-579-2.
Laurence H. Baker, ed., Soft Tissue Sarcomas. ISBN 0-89838-584-9.
John M. Bennett, ed., Controversies in the Management of Lymphomas. ISBN 0-89838-586-5

Adrenal and Endocrine Tumors in Children

Adrenal Cortical Carcinoma and Multiple Endocrine Neoplasia

edited by

G. BENNETT HUMPHREY

Oklahoma Children's Memorial Hospital and University of Oklahoma Health Sciences Center

GERALD B. GRINDEY

Lilly Research Laboratories

LOUIS P. DEHNER

University of Minnesota Medical School

RONALD T. ACTON

University of Alabama in Birmingham

THEODORE J. PYSHER

Oklahoma Children's Memorial Hospital and University of Oklahoma Health Sciences Center

1984 **MARTINUS NIJHOFF PUBLISHERS**
a member of the KLUWER ACADEMIC PUBLISHERS GROUP
BOSTON / THE HAGUE / DORDRECHT / LANCASTER

Distributors

for the United States and Canada: Kluwer Boston, Inc., 190 Old Derby Street, Hingham, MA 02043, USA
for all other countries: Kluwer Academic Publishers Group, Distribution Center, P.O.Box 322, 3300 AH Dordrecht, The Netherlands

Library of Congress Cataloging in Publication Data CIP

Main entry under title:

Adrenal and endocrine tumors in children.

(Cancer treatment and research ; v.)
Includes index.
1. Adrenal glands--Cancer--Addresses, essays, lectures. 2. Endocrine glands--Cancer--Addresses, essays, lectures. 3. Tumors in children--Addresses, essays, lectures. 4. Multiple tumors--Addresses, essays, lectures. I. Humphrey, G. Bennett (George Bennett), 1934- . II. Series. [DNLM: 1. Neoplasms--In infancy and childhood--Periodicals. W1 CA693 v. 2]
RC280.A3A36 1983 618.92'99445 83-11446
ISBN 978-94-011-8173-0 ISBN 978-94-011-8815-9 (eBook)
DOI 10.1007/978-94-011-8815-9

Contents

Section 2

Editors

G.B. Humphrey, M.D., Ph.D.
University of Oklahoma Health Sciences Center
Department of Pediatrics, Hematology-Oncology
Oklahoma Children's Memorial Hospital
P.O. Box 26307
Oklahoma City, OK 73126, USA

Dr. Gerald Grindey
Lilly Research Laboratories
Department M-305
307 E. McCarty Street
Indianapolis, IN 46285, USA

Dr. Louis P. Dehner
Department of Laboratory Medicine and Pathology
Box 609, Mayo Memorial Building
University of Minnesota Medical School
Minneapolis, MN 55455, USA

Ronald T. Acton, Ph.D.
University of Alabama in Birmingham
Diabetes Research Hospital, Room 817
1808 7th Avenue, South
Birmingham, AL 35233, USA

Dr. Theodore J. Pysher
University of Oklahoma Health Sciences Center
Department of Pathology
Oklahoma Children's Memorial Hospital
P.O. Box 26307
Oklahoma City, OK 73126, USA

Preface

'Adrenal and Endocrine Tumors in Children' is the third volume in the series, 'Cancer Treatment and Research' devoted to pediatric oncology. Like its predecessors, it is organized into two sections. The first section again deals with issues of basic research germane to the understanding of childhood malignancies. In volume 3, the scope of the first section has been broadened to include a review that is epidemiologically oriented and a second review that is psychologically oriented.

In the second part, major pediatric oncology units in Japan, Australia, Europe and the Americas have been invited to report their experience with adrenal cortical carcinomas and the presentation of the multiple endocrine neoplasia syndromes in children. In addition to these institutional reports of case material, there are reviews on genetics, pathology, and a diagnostic evaluation of children. The overview chapter on adrenal cortical carcinoma includes recommendations for radiotherapy from Dr. D'Angio and for chemotherapy from Dr. Philip Schein. Individuals using these recommended therapies are encouraged to report their results to the editors. The information will then be made available to others on request.

List of Contributors

ACTON, Dr. Ronald, Diabetes Research Hospital, Room 817, 1808 7th Ave. South, Birmingham, AL 35233, USA.

BAUM, Edward S., M.D., Division of Hematology/Oncology, Northwestern University Medical School, Children's Memorial Hospital, 2300 Children's Plaza, Chicago, IL 60614, USA.

BENZ, Dr. Chris C., Dept. of Medicine, Yale University School of Medicine, New Haven, CT 06510, USA.

BOWERMAN, Richard A., M.D., Dept. of Radiology, University of Michigan Medical Center, Ann Arbor, MI 48109, USA.

BROUGH, A. Joseph, M.D., Dept. of Laboratory Medicine, Children's Hospital of Michigan, 3901 Beaubien Blvd., Detroit, MI 48201, USA.

BURRIS, Dr. Terry E., Fellow, Dean McGee Eye Institute, 608 Stanton L. Young, Oklahoma City, OK 73104, USA.

CADMAN, Dr. Ed. C., Depts. of Medicine and Pharmacology, Yale University School of Medicine, New Haven, CT 06510, USA.

CAILLOU, B., M.D., Institut Gustave-Roussy, Villejuif, France.

CANGIR, Ayten, M.D., M.D. Anderson Hospital and Tumor Institute, University of Texas Cancer Center, Dept. of Pediatrics, 6723 Bertner Avenue, Houston, TX 77030, USA.

CARNEY, J. Aidan, M.D., Ph.D., Dept. of Surgical Pathology, Mayo Clinic and Foundation, Rochester, MN 55905, USA.

CHAN, Helen S.L., M.B., Hospital for Sick Children, 555 University Avenue, Toronto, Ontario, Canada M5G 1X8.

CHAUSSAIN, Dr. J.L., Endocrinology Dept., Hôpital Saint Vincent de Paul, Paris, France.

CHEVALIER, Louise, M.D., F.R.C.P.(C), Montreal Children's Hospital, 2300 Tupper Street, Montreal, Quebec, Canada H3H 1P3.

CHO, Kyung J., M.D., Dept. of Radiology, University of Michigan Medical Center, Ann Arbor, MI 48109, USA.

CONROY, Dr. Peter J., Dept. of Radiology, University of Rochester Medical

Center, Experimental Therapeutics Division, Cancer Center, 601 Elmwood Avenue, Rochester, NY 14642, USA.

CRIST, Dr. William M., University of Alabama, Children's Hospital, 1600 7th Avenue South, Birmingham, AL 35233, USA.

CUSHING, Barbara, M.D., Dept. of Pediatrics, Children's Hospital of Michigan, 3901 Beaubien Blvd., Detroit, MI 48201, USA.

D'ANGIO, Giulio J., M.D., Children's Cancer Research Center, Children's Hospital of Philadelphia, 34th & Civic Center Blvd., Philadelphia, PA 19104, USA.

DEHNER, Louis P., M.D., Dept. of Laboratory Medicine and Pathology, Box 609, Mayo Memorial Bldg., University of Minnesota Medical School, Minneapolis, MN 55455, USA.

ELLIOTT, Charles H., Ph.D., University of Oklahoma Health Sciences Center, Psychiatry & Behavioral Sciences, 616 NE 15, Oklahoma City, OK 73190, USA.

FIDLER, Dr. Isaiah J., Cancer Metastasis and Treatment Laboratory, NCI Frederick Cancer Research Center, Frederick, MD 21701, USA.

FRANCIOSI, Ralph A., M.D., Dept. of Pathology, Children's Health Center and Hospital, Minneapolis, MN 55404, USA.

GERARD-MARCHANT, Dr. Remy, Dept. of Pathology, Institut Gustave-Roussy, Villejuif, France.

GRANT, Dr. Steven, Dept. of Medicine, Columbia University School of Medicine, New York, NY 10012, USA.

GROSS, Milton D., M.D., Division of Nuclear Medicine, Dept. of Internal Medicine, University of Michigan Medical Center, Veterans Administration, 2215 Fuller Road, Ann Arbor, MI 48105, USA.

GUBLER, Dr. J.P., Institut Gustave-Roussy, Villejuif, France.

HANNA, Dr. Nabil, Cancer Metastasis and Treatment Laboratory, NCI Frederick Cancer Research Center, Frederick, MD 21701, USA.

HEYN, Ruth M., M.D., University of Michigan, Mott Children's Hospital, 1405 E. Ann Street, Ann Arbor, MI 48109, USA.

HOLCOMBE, John H., M.D., University of Oklahoma Health Sciences Center, Dept. of Pediatrics, Oklahoma Children's Memorial Hospital, 940 NE 13 Street, Oklahoma City, OK 73190, USA.

HUMPHREY, G. Bennett, M.D., Ph.D., University of Oklahoma Health Sciences Center, Dept. of Pediatrics, Oklahoma Children's Memorial Hospital, 940 NE 13 Street, Oklahoma City, OK 73190, USA.

HUTCHINSON, Raymond J., M.D., University of Michigan, Mott Children's Hospital, 1405 E. Ann Street, Ann Arbor, MI 48109, USA.

JAFFE, Norman, M.D., M.D. Anderson Hospital and Tumor Institute, University of Texas Cancer Center, Dept. of Pediatrics, 6723 Bertrer Avenue, Houston, TX 77030, USA.

JAY, Susan M., Ph.D., Psychosocial Program, Hematology-Oncology, Children's Hospital of Los Angeles, 4650 Sunset Blvd., Los Angeles, CA 90027, USA.

REBECCA T. Kirkland, M.D., Baylor College of Medicine, Dept. of Pediatrics, Section of Pediatric Endocrinology, 6621 Fannin St., Houston, TX 77030, USA.

LEFEVRE, Dr. M., Institut Gustave-Roussy, Villejuif, France.

LEMERLE, Jean, M.D., Chief, Dept. of Pediatrics, Institut Gustave-Roussy, Villejuif, France.

MALONE, Dr. Glen E., Dept. of Epidemiology, University of Alabama, University Station, Birmingham, AL 35294, USA.

MEADOWS, Anna T., M.D., Children's Cancer Research Center, Children's Hospital of Philadelphia, 34th & Civic Center Blvd., Philadelphia, PA 19104, USA.

MILLER, John D., M.D., F.R.C.P.(C), Children's Hospital Medical Center, Elland and Bethesda Ave., Cincinnati, OH 45229, USA.

MORGAN, Elaine R., M.D., Division of Hematology/Oncology, Northwestern University Medical School, Children's Memorial Hospital, 2300 Children's Plaza, Chicago, IL 60614, USA.

MORI, Kurt W., M.D., Dept. of Radiology, University of Michigan Medical Center, Ann Arbor, MI 48109, USA.

PARMENTIER, C., M.D., Institut Gustave-Roussy, Villejuif, France.

POLLACK, Dr. Vincent A., Pharmacology Department, Pfizer Central Research, Groton, CT 06340, USA.

PYSHER, Theodore J., M.D., University of Oklahoma Health Sciences Center, Dept. of Pathology, Oklahoma Children's Memorial Hospital, 940 NE 13 Street, Oklahoma City, OK 73190, USA.

RANEY, R. Beverly, Jr., M.D., Division of Oncology, Children's Hospital of Philadelphia, 34th & Civic Center Blvd. Philadelphia, PA 19104, USA.

ROSEMAN, Dr. Jeffrey, Dept. of Epidemiology, University of Alabama, University Station, Birmingham, AL 35294, USA.

ROUGIER, Ph., M.D., Institut Gustave-Roussy, Villejuif, France.

ROWSEY, Dr. J. James, Dean McGee Eye Institute, 608 Stanton L. Young, Oklahoma City, OK 73104, USA.

SCHEIN, Philip S., M.D., Vincent T. Lombardi Cancer Research Center, Georgetown University Medical Center, 3800 Reservoir Road, NW, Washington, DC 20007, USA.

SCHIMKE, R. Neil, M.D., F.A.C.P., Director, Division of Metabolism, Endocrinology, and Genetics, University of Kansas College of Health Sciences, 39th and Rainbow Blvd., Kansas City, KS 66103, USA.

SIEMANN, Dr. Dietmar W., University of Rochester Medical Center, School of Medicine and Dentistry, Dept. of Radiation Biology and Biophysics,

Experimental Therapeutics Division, Cancer Center, 601 Elmwood Avenue, Rochester, NY 14642, USA.

STERNBACH, Marion S., M.D., F.R.C.P.(C), Canadian Red Cross Society, 95 Wellesley Street East, Toronto, Ontario, Canada M4Y 1H6.

STERNLICHT, Dr. Himan, Dept. of Pharmacology, Case Western Reserve University, Cleveland, OH 44106, USA.

SUTHERLAND, Dr. Robert M., University of Rochester Medical Center, School of Medicine and Dentistry, Dept. of Radiation Biology and Biophysics, Experimental Therapeutics Division, Cancer Center, 601 Elmwood Avenue, Rochester, NY 14642, USA.

TUNELL, William P., M.D., University of Oklahoma College of Medicine, Oklahoma Children's Memorial Hospital, P.O. Box 26307, Oklahoma City, OK 73126, USA.

WEATHERBY, R. Paul, Jr., M.D., Dept. of Surgical Pathology, Mayo Clinic and Foundation, Rochester, MN 55905, USA.

WEST, Patrice M., B.S., Division of Hematology/Oncology, Northwestern University Medical School, Children's Memorial Hospital, 2300 Children's Plaza, Chicago, IL 60614, USA.

WILSON, Stuart D., M.D., Division of Surgery, Medical College of Wisconsin, 8700 West Wisconsin Avenue, Milwaukee, WI 53226, USA.

1. The Use of Young Nude Mice to Study Metastasis of Human Neoplasms[1]

NABIL HANNA, VINCENT A. POLLACK and ISAIAH J. FIDLER

1. INTRODUCTION

Understanding the pathobiological processes of cancer metastasis is fundamental to the development of successful cancer therapies. The process of metastasis involves a series of sequential events in which malignant cells are released from the primary tumor and reach distant sites where they proliferate to form new tumor foci. Metastasis begins with the local invasion of the surrounding host tissue by cells from the primary tumor. Tumors that grow in the major body cavities can shed cells which seed the mucosal and/or serosal surfaces of other organs and develop into secondary growths. The more common route of tumor spread involves invasion and penetration of tumor cells into blood vessels and/or the lymphatic system [1–4]. Release of tumor emboli is accelerated by intermittent changes in venous pressure, by turbulent blood flow, and by movement or manipulation of the neoplasms during routine examination, biopsy or surgery [1–5].

The presence of tumor cells in the circulation is not sufficient, in of itself, to produce metastasis. Most tumor cells entering the circulation are rapidly destroyed [6, 7]. Some nonspecific trapping and arrest of circulating tumor cells in the microcirculation occur as a result of mechanical factors, but again, these alone do not explain the patterns of metastasis. Data from studies using radiolabeled tumor cells show that, although circulating tumor cells arrest in many organs, metastases are found only in some [6]. Other properties of neoplastic cells determine the sites of metastases; for example, cells of murine tumors that normally metastasize to the lung also produce

[1] Research sponsored by the National Cancer Institute, DHHS, under Contract No. N01-CO-75380 with Litton Bionetics, Inc. The contents of this publication do not necessarily reflect the views or policies of the Department of Health and Human Services, nor does mention of trade names, commercial products, or organizations imply endorsement by the U.S. Government.

G. Bennett Humphrey et al. (eds), Adrenal and Endocrine Tumors in Children.

metastases in lung tissue transplanted ectopically (in the thigh muscle) but not in explants of other organs [8–10]. Initial cell arrest in a particular organ is influenced, in part, by the surface membrane properties of the tumor cells [11].

After arrest and implantation in the vessel wall, tumor cells must exit from the vessel into the surrounding tissue(s). Extravasation of malignant cells is believed to involve mechanisms similar to those responsible for the initial invasion of blood vessels. Successful extravasation and limited proliferation of malignant cells produce small colonies of tumor cells that surround blood vessels [12]. Further growth of these lesions requires the ingrowth of new blood vessels to provide adequate nutrition to support cell proliferation [12]. Release of angiogenic factors from host cells (such as lymphocytes) as a consequence of interaction with metastatic cells [13], together with release of cell growth-stimulating factors by host platelets [14], may create a situation in which normal host homeostatic mechanisms contribute to the success of metastasis.

Animal models have proven invaluable in the elucidation of host and tumor properties involved in tumor metastasis, and the utilization of such models may enhance considerably our knowledge of the biology, as well as contribute to the development of successful therapy, of metastatic disease [15–17]. To date, however, adequate animal models for studies of human neoplasia in general, and metastasis in particular, have been lacking. In this chapter, we review the advantages and limitations of the athymic nude mouse model for studies of cancer metastasis. We also propose a procedure by which the young nude mouse could serve as a model to ascertain the metastatic potential of human neoplasms and perhaps as a vehicle to isolate the metastatic subpopulations of cells residing within a malignant human tumor.

2. GROWTH OF HUMAN TUMORS IN NUDE MICE

After Rygaard and Poulsen [18] observed that xenogeneic human tumors could grow progressively when transplanted into immunodeficient athymic nude mice, intensive efforts were made to use these mice as an *in vivo* animal model for studying the biology of human neoplasms [19–23]. However, it was found that not all human tumors can be readily transplanted into the subcutaneous (s.c.) tissue of nude mice, and that many factors influence the rate of success of such a transplantation. A great deal of emphasis has been given to studies on the various properties of tumors that may determine whether or not they will grow progressively upon transplantation. These studies found that human melanomas, epidermoid carcinomas and sarcomas can be successfully transplanted and passaged in nude mice [23–26]. In contrast, carcinomas of the breast [26, 27] and prostate [28] and other hormone-secreting and hormone-dependent tumors [28, 29] are more difficult to establish as progressively growing tumors following s.c. implantation into nude mice. Special manipulations of the host are required to facilitate the growth of lymphomas and leukemias. Several investigators reported that most human lymphomas grow in nude mice only when injected intracranially [30, 31]. Recent reports, however, indicate that normal lymphoblastoid cell lines lacking markers of malignancy are also tumorigenic when inoculated into the brains of nude mice. This suggests that tumor growth after intracranial heterotransplantation in nude mice cannot be used as a test for the malignant transformation of established cell lines [32].

Shimosata *et al.* [25] reported that only 24% of 91 human tumors implanted into BAMB/c nude mice grew progressively. Among the 48 carcinomas implanted, transplantability of lung carcinomas was highest (10/21), followed by gastric (2/14) and breast (1/13) carcinomas. Sebesteny *et al.* [33] established transplantable tumors from 3 of 19 primary human breast carcinomas, and Rae-Venter and Reid [34] reported that only 4 of 32 malignant breast tumors implanted s.c. into female BALB/c nude mice were established as permanent transplantable tumor lines. In contrast, the percent of successful human malignant melanoma transplants in nude mice is impressive. Sordat *et al.* [35] successfully transplanted 11 of 14 primary or metastatic melanomas. Povlsen [36] on the other hand, failed to establish primary melanomas (0/13) in nude mice but succeeded in transplanting 10 of 13 samples from melanoma metastases. Similarly, Fodstad *et al.* [37] succeeded in establishing six human malignant melanoma tumors, which originated from cutaneous metastases.

The *in vivo* transplantability into nude mice of cultured cell lines derived from various types of human tumors has been evaluated extensively by Fogh *et al.* [38] who described the tumorigenic properties of more than 196 tumor cell lines transplanted to nude mice. Giovanella *et al.* [23, 39] reported that, although fresh specimens from surgically resected human tumors could be transplanted successfully into nude mice, such tumors grew slowly and did not metastasize. In contrast, malignant cells growing in culture expressed the malignant properties of invasiveness and even metastasis. These authors [23] and others [40–42] found that under similar experimental protocols nontumorigenic cells were not rejected by nude mice but also did not produce tumors. These observations suggested that the nude mouse somehow is able to differentiate between normal and transformed cells. A more attractive possibility, however, is that there are general differences in the behavior of nontumorigenic and tumorigenic cells [41, 42] which account for this observation and that the nude mouse is only incidental.

In addition to the influence of tumor cell properties on the success or failure of xenograft transplantation in nude mice, host-related factors are of paramount importance [43]. For example, Kameya *et al.* [44] reported that more than 95% of heterotransplanted gastric adenocarcinomas were implanted successfully in specific-pathogen-free (SPF) nude mice. In contrast, when the tumors were implanted into nude mice housed in conventional facilities, only 35% of the implanted tumors grew. Kyriazis *et al.* [45] reported that, unlike SPF mice, nude mice infected with mouse hepatitis virus were resistant to transplantation of two human carcinoma cell lines. Our own experience with a limited number of human melanoma cell lines and fresh specimens of colon carcinomas indicate that the percent takes and progressive growth of these tumors were accelerated in BALB/c nude mice as compared with age-matched outbred NIH/Swiss nude recipients (see below).

3. CELLULAR CHARACTERISTICS OF HUMAN TUMORS GROWN IN NUDE MICE

In order for the nude mouse to serve as an *in vivo* model for the study of xenogeneic human neoplasms, it is essential that the transplanted tumors preserve their cellular and biological characteristics. Most reports indicate that human tumors grown in nude mice maintain their karyotype [22, 39], morphological, histological and cytological appearance [18, 22, 24, 36, 44] and production of specific enzymes [21, 22], antigens [21, 22, 46] and hormones [21, 25, 44, 46]. Kanzaki *et al.* [47] observed that human melanoma cells, of epitheliod or spindle-shaped morphology, are quite pleomorphic when grown in culture. Even after prolonged maintenance *in vitro*, they revert to their original morphology upon transplantation into nude mice. Similarly, Fogh and Hajdu [48] reported the degree of differentiation of human tumors grown in nude mice correlated with that of the original tumors and not with that of cell lines established in culture. In a few instances, differences between human tumors explanted from nude mice and the original tumors were observed. In lymphomas transplanted intracranially, enrichment for cytogenically aberrant cells was noted [32]. Tompkins *et al.* [49] reported that human colon tumor cells xenografted into nude mice demonstrated increased tumorigenicity upon subsequent passages. The acquisition of xenotropic murine C-type viruses by human tumors grown in NIH/Swiss nude mice, which has been described [30, 50], could account for this phenomenon. Although the exact biologic activity of these viruses is not fully known, it is possible that infection of human lymphoma cells by murine xenotropic viruses could enhance their growth potential [30].

4. THE RESISTANCE OF RECIPIENT NUDE MICE AGAINST TRANSPLANTED TUMORS

Although the athymic nude mouse lacks functional mature T-lymphocytes, it should not be considered as a totally immunodeficient animal. Nude mice show almost a normal IgM-antibody response to T-independent antigens [51] and high titers of natural natibodies that can react with tumor cells [52]. Tumoricidal macrophages can be isolated from untreated nude mice [53, 54] and macrophage activity can be enhanced by stimulation of the mice with bacterial adjuvants such as BCG and *C. parvum* [54]. Moreover, nude mice exhibit a consistently high level of natural killer (NK) cell activity [55]. All these T-independent effector mechanisms could play a significant role in host-tumor interaction and undoubtedly contribute to the natural resistance of nude mice against transplanted neoplasms. There is strong evidence for the *in vivo* role of host defense mechanisms in limiting tumor growth. First, further immunosuppression of nude mice or the use of newborn recipients enhances the rate of successful tumor take, growth rate and occasionally invasiveness and metastasis of implanted xenogeneic human tumors [35, 43, 56–59]. For example, of 10 lymphoblastoid cell lines studied by Ohsugi *et al.* [58], 6 were transplanted successfully into nude mice which had been pretreated with antilymphocyte serum (ALS). All 10 lines also grew progressively in x-irradiated recipients. Similarly, Watanabe *et al.* [59] reported that the transplantability of lymphoid cell lines increased from 0% in untreated nude recipients to 38.5% after whole body X-irradiation. At the same time, the rate of successful transplantation of fresh leukemia and lymphoma tumor cells (24 cases) was only 29%. The limited success of heterotransplantation following X-irradiation of recipient mice can be explained in part by the finding of Bonmassar *et al.* [60] that a radioresistant defense mechanism in nude mice acts against lymphoma cells that express Hh antigens. In addition, a recent report by Minato *et al.* [61] demonstrated that cell lines known to be highly tumorigenic in nude mouse were rejected when persistently infected with a variety of RNA viruses. Unlike the parent cell lines, the virus-infected cells were susceptible to NK cell-mediated cytotoxicity *in vitro*. Collectively then, these studies illustrate that both tumor properties and host factors influence the outcome of transplantation of human tumors into nude mice.

5. TUMOR INVASION AND METASTASIS IN NUDE MICE

The usefulness of the nude mouse for studies of cancer metastasis has been limited because most allogeneic and/or xenogeneic neoplasms, although malignant in their original hosts, rarely metastasize following transplantation into nude mice [18, 22, 62]. As stated in the Introduction, the outcome of metastasis depends on a constant interplay between the metastatic tumor cells and their hosts. The relative contributions of these various factors may vary among different tumor systems. This could account for the conflicting findings reported from different laboratories regarding metastasis in nude mice [18, 39, 63]. Giovanella *et al.* [23, 39] observed metastases in lymph nodes and occasionally in lungs following inoculation of human melanoma cultured cell lines into s.c. tissue of nude mice. In contrast, Povlsen *et al.* [36] observed that several human tumors including malignant melanoma did not produce metastases. Sharkey and Fogh [64] found lymph node and lung metastases in only 14/1,045 nude mice (1.3%) implanted with 106 malignant human tumor cell lines; in this study, breast cancer cell lines metastasized with higher frequency than all other tumors. Microscopic pulmonary metastases were observed by Zamecnik and Long [65] in 4/36 nude mice with progressively growing s.c. tumors derived from Hodgkin's lymphoma cells grown *in vitro.* Shimosato *et al.* [25] reported that, of 91 surgically excised human tumors transplanted in nude mice, only one transplanted hepatocellular carcinoma produced lymph node metastases. High incidence of metastasis to the lymph nodes, ovaries and cerebrum of transplanted human neuroblastoma was reported by Hata *et al.* [66].

The site of tumor implantation into nude mice can influence subsequent metastasis. Kyriazis *et al.* [67] trasnplanted human tumor cell lines derived from larynx or colon carcinomas into s.c. or intraperitoneal (i.p.) sites of BALB/c nude mice. Only after i.p., and not s.c., growth did the tumor cells invade the intraabdominal organs and metastasize to lymph nodes and lung. Similarly, spleen and liver metastases in nude mice were found by Takahashi *et al.* [68] after i.p. injection of adenocarcinoma of the stomach.

Although the use of ALS-treated and x-irradiated immunosuppressed nude mice can increase the success of transplantation [43, 56, 58, 59], of 10 malignant human lymphoblastoid cell lines studied, no gross or histologic evidence of local or distant metastases was observed [58]. On the other hand, Sordat *et al.* [35] reported that human solid tumors and/or established lymphoid and/or myelogenous cell lines injected into newborn, but not adult, nude mice were invasive and frequently produced metastases in the lungs and kidneys. Similar results were obtained when the K-562 myeloid cell line was injected s.c. or intravenously (i.v.) into newborn nude mice [57]. At first, the resistance of T-cell-deficient mice to tumor growth and metastasis was considered as evidence in support of the immunostimulation theory of tumor growth [69]; but the susceptibility of immunosuppressed or newborn nude mice to tumor growth and metastasis strongly suggests that an active defense which is independent of the thymus could protect nude mice against cancer metastasis.

6. THE *IN VIVO* ROLE OF NK CELLS IN CONTROL OF HEMATOGENEOUSLY DISSEMINATED TUMOR CELLS

Unlike the cells within a solid tumor mass, the progenitors of metastatic foci usually circulate as single cells or small clump of cells and are, therefore, highly accessible and more vulnerable to the destructive effects of immune and nonimmune defense host mechanisms [70]. Moreover, while in the circulation, tumor cells are exposed to highly destructive forces that might not be present in the primary tumor mass [15–17]. Fidler *et al.* [71] and Skov *et al.* [72] reported that i.v. injection of metastatic murine tumor cells into adult nude mice produced only a few lung colonies, whereas the injection of an identical number of tumor cells into normal syngeneic recipients yielded a high number of pulmonary metastases. Growth at the s.c. tissue, however, was unaltered. Lozzio *et al.* [73] reported that leukemia cells could be detected in the blood of tumor-bearing nude mice in the absence of detectable metastases.

It has been well established that a majority of circulating tumor cells die and do not establish metastasis [15–17, 74–76]. Tumor cell death in the circulation could be due to mechanical factors and host defense mechanism(s). Our recent studies suggest that NK cells (whose level of activity is high in nude mice) are particularily efficient in destroying circulating tumor cells.

Recent reports from our laboratory [77, 78] and others [79] strongly suggest that NK cells can destroy circulating tumor cells. A close correlation between the levels of NK cell activity and the incidence of experimental metastases has been demonstrated [77, 78, 80, 81]. The incidence of metastasis was higher in recipients that exhibited low NK cell activity and vice versa. Furthermore, the *in vivo* depletion of NK cells in syngeneic mice by pretreatment with cyclophosphamide (Cy) enhanced pulmonary and extrapulmonary metastases.

We also compared the metastatic potential of metastatic and nonmetastatic tumors in 3- and 10-week-old syngeneic mice. The data showed that enhancement of lung tumor colonies in 3-week-old mice receiving i.v. injections of progressor metastatic tumors correlated with both low NK cell activity and increased tumor cell survival in the lungs. These favorable *in vivo* conditions apparently allowed progressor tumor cells with low metastatic capacity (as determined in normal adult mice) to develop into secondary tumor foci as a consequence of minimal host intervention. The increased metastasis seen in the younger mice could not be attributed to a deficiency in T-cell-immune response, because 3-week-old mice were as efficient as 10-week-old normal animals in rejecting an s.c. inoculation of immunogenic regressor tumors. The high incidence of artificial metastasis in

3-week-old mice was not due to a more efficient trapping mechanism of tumor cells in the microvasculature of the lungs but rather to enhanced survival of trapped cells. These data agree with recent reports demonstrating an inverse correlation between the levels of NK cells and the survival of circulating tumor cells [77–79]. Evidence that the increased metastatic incidence in 3-week-old mice is related partly to low natural cytotoxicity was also provided by the experiments in which boosting of NK activity by administration of agents such as poly I:C, *C. parvum*, or statolon 16–24 hours before tumor cell challenge reduced metastasis in 3-week-old mice to levels observed in adult (10-week-old) mice. These drugs were effective only when administered 16–24 hours before (but not after) tumor cell injection. This indicated that activation occurred quickly and that the effector cells were functional during a short period following tumor cell injection (12–24 hours). These results agree with our findings that reconstitution of Cy-treated mice with spleen lymphoid cells is beneficial only if the treatment takes place before tumor cell injection. Thus, in both systems, host destruction of tumor cells coincided with the presence of tumor cells in the circulation. Extravasation into organ parenchyma occurs by 6–12 hours [15, 16] and tumor cells can then escape destruction by the transferred cytotoxic cells. Finally, direct evidence that NK cells are responsible for inhibiting experimental tumor metastasis *in vivo* was provided by adoptive transfer experiments in which the reconstitutive antimetastatic activity of normal spleen cells transferred to Cy-treated recipients was abolished by pretreatment with specific anti-NK1.2 antibodies and complement. This treatment was shown by *in vitro* assays to deplete or inactivate NK selectively [111].

These studies demonstrate that NK cells are effective in host defense against circulating tumor cells and can interfere with the hematogenous tumor spread and the subsequent development of distant organ metastases.

7. THE EXPRESSION OF THE METASTATIC POTENTIAL OF ALLOGENEIC AND XENOGENEIC TUMORS IN YOUNG NUDE MICE WITH LOW LEVELS OF NK CELL ACTIVITY

The finding that enhanced incidence of tumor metastases in 3-week-old syngeneic mice correlated with low NK cell activity initiated an investigation for a similar correlation between age dependence of NK cell expression and the incidence of allogeneic and xenogeneic tumor metastases in nude mice. The NK-mediated cytotoxicity of spleen cells obtained from 2- to 3-week-old and 6- to 8-week-old nude mice was assessed *in vitro* against NK-sensitive fibrosarcoma target cells. The results of such experiments clearly indicated that only low levels of natural killing could be detected with cells harvested from spleens of 2- or 3-week-old donors. In contrast, mice older than 6 weeks of age consistently exhibited high NK cell activity [55, 78]. As in normal mice [78], the low NK cell cytotoxicity observed in young nude mice could be boosted readily by interferon inducers and bacterial adjuvants injected 24 hours before the test.

The i.v. injection of metastatic allogeneic murine melanoma and fibrosarcomas and xenogeneic rat chemically induced adenocarcinomas into 3-week-old, but not 6- to 8-week-old, nude mice resulted in the formation of large numbers of lung tumor colonies. Again, the successful metastasis of allogeneic and xenogeneic tumors in young nude mice correlated with their low levels of NK cell activity. The *in vivo* activation of NK cells by the injection of interferon inducers prior to tumor inoculation rendered the 3-week-old nude mice resistant to metastases development [78, 88]. Although all tumors grew s.c., only metastatic neoplasms formed pulmonary metastatic foci following i.v. inoculation into young nude mice.

The term 'experimental' metastases refers to tumor foci produced by the i.v. injection of cells. Direct injection of tumor cells into the circulation eliminates the need for initial detachment of cells from the primary neoplasm and invasion of blood vessels. However, all the subsequent steps in the metastatic process must occur for i.v.-injected cells to establish a metastasis. Elimination of the initial steps in the process introduces the risk that noninvasive tumor cells might form metastases when injected i.v., but might be unable to metastasize spontaneously when implanted s.c. or intramuscularly. This question has been addressed by Kripke *et al.* [82] who studied the metastatic behavior of 21 clones of the UV-2237 fibrosarcoma syngeneic to the C3H mouse using three different assays: (1) formation of experimental metastases after i.v. injection; (2) formation of experimental metastases after implantation s.c.; and (3) survival time of animals injected i.v. When the clones were ranked in order of increasing metastatic behavior, a strong correlation was found among all three tests for 20 of 21 clones. This indicates that the formation of experimental metastases by i.v.-injected tumor cells is a valid assay of cellular metastatic potential and parallels results obtained in more tedious and time-consuming assays of spontaneous metastatic activity.

The validity and applicability of the nude mouse model for ascertaining the metastatic potential of tumor cells were determined by the fact that the metastatic patterns of allogeneic and xenogeneic tumors were strikingly similar following injection into syngeneic hosts or young nude mice. All metastatic neoplasms, irrespective of their degree of antigenicity, produced lung tumor colonies in young nude mice, whereas nonmetastatic tumors did not. Moreover, the quantitative differences in formation of experimental metastases among a variety of well-established mouse tumor cell lines and clones with different metastatic behavior in their original hosts were maintained in the young nude recipients.

Because of the close correlation between high levels of NK cell activity and resistance of nude mice against experimental tumor metastasis, it is evident that genetic and perhaps environmental factors that could influence NK cell activity could also affect metastatic incidence. Our recent work supports this hypothesis. The i.v. injection of metastatic animal and/or human tumor cells into young BALB/c nude mice produced many more pulmonary metastases than the same inoculum injected into age- and sex-matched NIH/S nude recipients. The level of NK cell activity in BALB/c nude mice was much lower than that of their NIH/S nude counterparts. Moreover, for a given strain of nude mice, the housing conditions influenced both NK cell activity and the incidence of tumor metastases. Thus, nude mice raised under pathogen-free conditions in barrier or isolator facilities had more metastases than age-matched littermates housed under conventional conditions. Infections with mouse hepatitis virus, for example, enhanced NK-cell activity and thus rendered young nude mice resistant to experimental metastasis [78].

8. THE IMPLICATIONS OF TUMOR HETEROGENEITY TO STUDIES OF TRANSPLANTATIONS AND METASTASIS

Pathologists have long been aware that a tumor often exhibits a different morphological appearance in different zones. Therefore, the benign or malignant nature of a neoplasm can be definitively determined only when multiple samples from different areas of the tumor have been examined [83]. It has now become apparent that these zonal differences are not restricted to morphology alone, but can also apply to other biological characteristics of the tumor cells; for example, cells isolated from different parts of a chemically induced murine fibrosarcoma had varying antigenic properties [84]. Cells obtained from either different parts of other primary murine tumors [85, 86] or clones [87] were shown to have different *in vitro* sensitivities to several chemotherapeutic agents. In addition, tumor fragments transplanted individually propagated the morphological appearance of their site of origin from within a primary tumor [88], and it has been suggested that the repeated transfer of such fragments might lead to a restriction, or obliteration, of phenotypic diversity [89].

To maintain the biological diversity of the tumors, serial transfers must be done with suspensions of cells from all zones of the neoplasm. Small tumor fragments are frequently inadequate to establish definitive diagnoses [83], may not represent the correct populations for establishing the cross-protective nature of tumors [84, 90] and may not allow the determination of tumor susceptibility to chemotherapeutic agents [85–87, 89]. Investigations into the nature of metastatic tumor cells and their susceptibility to therapeutic agents must take these findings into consideration.

9. FUTURE PROSPECTIVES

Recent studies have demonstrated that many rodent and human neoplasms consist of subpopulations of cells with different growth rates, karyotypes, antigenicity, immunogenicity, susceptibility to cytotoxic drugs, and potential for invasion and metastasis [15, 17, 70]. In some rodent tumor systems, metastases result from the survival and growth of specialized subpopulations of cells that preexist within the parental tumor [15, 17, 91, 92]. Because not all cells in the primary neoplasm possess all of the properties necessary to complete the highly selective process of metastasis, methods should be designed that would allow isolation and identification of tumorigenic cells capable of invasion and metastasis. Tumor variants have been isolated by several methods. One method is to select cells *in vitro* for specific properties such as detachment from a monolayer [93], resistance to lysis by syngeneic lymphocytes [94], and resistance to lectin-mediated toxicity [95] and then to determine whether such procedures also select for cells with different metastatic behavior *in vivo*. A second method is establish *in vitro* numerous clones or lines from parent tumors. By this approach, the behavior *in vivo* and *in vitro* of such clones can be studied [91, 92]. Another approach performed recently with various neoplasms involves the isolation and propagation of variant lines from individual metastatic tumor foci. In such diverse murine tumor systems as melanoma [96], fibrosarcoma [97], 3-methylcholanthrene-induced sarcoma [98], lymphosarcoma [99], Lewis lung carcinoma [100], and lymphoma [101, 012], variants with different metastatic potentials have been selected. By similar experimental procedures, tumor cell lines with preferential growth in the lungs [96], liver [108], and brain [104, 105] have also been isolated.

We now wish to determine whether the young nude mouse (BALB/c background) could be used as a model to answer two specific questions. The first deals with the use of such a recipient in order to distinguish between metastatic and nonmetastatic human neoplasms. The second question deals with the use of young nude mouse as a vehicle for the isolation of metastatic cells that populate a malignant human tumor.

The presence within the primary tumor of subpopulations of cells with differing metastatic capabilities has profound implications for the way in which research is done to identify the cellular properties responsible for metastasis [17] and for the testing of potential agents for treating metastatic disease. Both human and animal neoplasms contain subpopulations of cells with differing sensitivities to cytotoxic drugs [85–87, 106, 107]. Differences in the response of primary and metastatic lesions to therapeutic agents is well documented in clinical practice [107–110] and metastatic cells showing increased resistance to chemotherapeutic agents have been selected in experimental animal tumors [109, 110]. Studies that examine the drug sensitivity of 'primary tumors' may be inadequate for screening agents for their anti-metastatic activity. Assays in which a drug or combination of drugs is found to limit growth of a tumor (injected at a 'primary site', i.e., s.c.) to 50% of that in untreated controls may only reveal the presence of a subpopulation(s) of drug-sensitive cells and need not offer any insight into the pharmacologic susceptibility of the tumor cell subpopulations that will give rise to metastases.

The successful metastasis of allogeneic and xenogeneic tumors in young made mice offers a unique opportunity to use the nude mouse as a vehicle for the selection and isolation of metastatic tumor cells from heterogeneous human primary neoplasms. Evidence supporting the validity of this *in vivo* model has been provided by our recent studies on the selection of several subpopulations of cells from the human melanoma cell line A375. In these

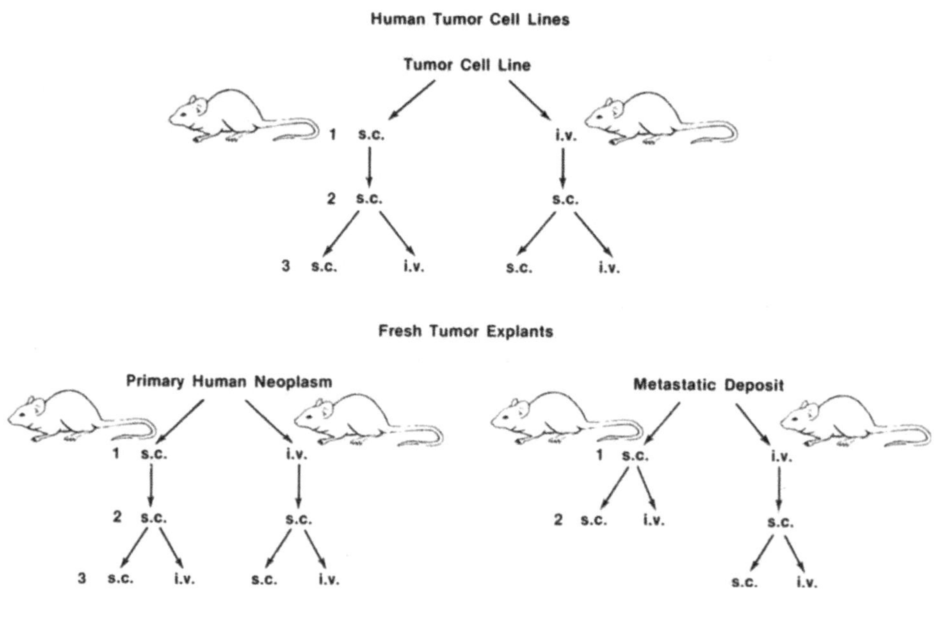

Figure 1

studies (see Chart 1) cells of the parental tumor were injected either s.c. or i.v. into 3-week-old nude mice. Several weeks thereafter, tumors growing in the s.c. tissue and individual (very few) lung metastases were harvested aseptically and dissociated with 0.2% of collagenase type I. The cells were then reinjected into the s.c. tissue of new nude mice to expand the populations. Three weeks later, large tumors growing s.c. which result from a s.c. to s.c. passage or lung to s.c. passage were again enzymatically dissociated. Cell suspensions were injected s.c. and i.v. into groups of young 3-week-old nude mice. The cells from the parent A375 tumor that was passaged s.c. to s.c. produced only a few lung nodules, demonstrating that the s.c. transfer did not enrich for metastasis. In contrast, cells harvested from s.c. tumors produced by the injection of cells harvested from pulmonary metastases produced 50 times more lung tumor colonies than the s.c. to s.c. transferred tumor cells. We interpret these results to indicate that the observed enhanced metastatic potential is a result of a selective process and not of mere adaptation to growth in the nude mouse.

In conclusion, we hope that young nude mouse may provide a potentially valuable tool for ascertaining the metastatic potential of surgically excised human primary tumors and for the testing of therapeutic agents designed to eradicate metastatic cells.

ACKNOWLEDGEMENT

We wish to thank Elynor Sass and Kelly Bivens for their editorial assistance.

REFERENCES

1. Zeidman I: Metastasis: A review of recent advances, Cancer Res 17:157–162, 1957.
2. Fisher B, Fisher ER: The interrelationship of hematogenous and lymphatic tumor cell dissemination. Surg Gynecol Obstet 122:791–798, 1966.
3. Fisher ER, Fisher B: Recent observations on concepts of metastasis. Arch Pathol 83:321–324, 1977.
4. del Regato JA: Pathways of mestastatic spread of malignant tumors. Semin Oncol 4:33–38, 1977.
5. Hoover HC Jr, Ketcham AS: Effect of fine-needle biopsy, incisional biopsy, and palpation on experimental metastasis formation. Surg Forum 27:110–112, 1976.
6. Fidler IJ: Metastasis: Quantitative analysis of distribution and fate of tumor emboli labeled with ^{125}I-5-iodo-2′-deoxyuridine. J Natl Cancer Inst 45:773–782, 1970.
7. Butler TP, Gullino PM: Quantitation of cell shedding into efferent blood of mammary adenocarcinoma. Cancer Res 35:512–517, 1975.
8. Kinsey DL: An experimental study of preferential metastasis. Cancer 13:674–676, 1960.
9. Sugarbaker EV, Cohen AM, Ketcham, AS: Do metastases metastasize? Ann Surg 174:161–166, 1971.

10. Hart IR, Fidler IJ: Role of organ selectivity in the determination of metastatic patterns of the B16 melanoma. Cancer Res 40:2281–2287, 1980.
11. Poste G, Nicolson GL: Modification of the arrest of poorly metastatic tumor cells in the microcirculation after treatment with plasma membrane vesicles from highly metastatic cells. Proc Natl Acad Sci USA 77:399–403, 1980.
12. Folkman J: Tumor angiogenesis. Adv Cancer Res 19:331–358, 1974.
13. Auerbach T, Kubai L, Sidky Y: Angiogenesis induction by tumors, embryonic tissues and lymphocytes. Cancer Res 36:3435–3440, 1976.
14. Eastment CT, Sirbasku DA: Human platelet lysate contains growth factor activities for established cell lines derived from various tissues of several species. *In Vitro* 16:694–701, 1980.
15. Fidler IJ: Tumor heterogeneity and the biology of cancer invasion and metastasis. Cancer Res 38:2651–2660, 1978.
16. Fidler IJ: General considerations for studies of experimental cancer metastasis. In: Methods in Cancer Research, Bush H, (ed), New York, Academic Press, 1978, p 399–439.
17. Poste G, Fidler IJ: The pathogenesis of cancer metastasis. Nature 283:139–146, 1980.
18. Rygaard J, Povlsen CO: Heterotransplantation of human malignant tumor to nude mice. Acta Pathol Microbiol Scand, [A] 77:758–760, 1969.
19. Kindred B: Nude mice in immunobiology. Prog Allergy 26:137–238, 1979.
20. Fogh J, Giovanella BC (eds): The Nude Mouse in Experimental and Clinical Research, New York, Academic Press, 1978.
21. Nomura T, Ohsawa N, Tamaoki N, Fujiwara K (eds): Proceedings of the Second International Workshop on Nude Mice. Tokyo, University of Tokyo Press, 1977.
22. Povlsen CO, Fialkow PJ, Klein E, Klein G, Rygaard J, Wiener F: Growth and antigenic properties of a biopsy-derived Burkitt's lymphoma in thymus-less (nude) mice. Int J Cancer 11:30–39, 1973.
23. Giovanella BC, Stehlin JS, Williams LJ Jr: Heterotransplantation of human malignant tumors in 'nude' thymusless mice. II. Malignant tumors induced by injection of cell cultures derived from human solid tumors. J Natl Cancer Inst 52:921–927, 1974.
24. Povlsen CO, Rygaard J: Heterotransplantation of adenocarcinomas of the colon and rectum in the mouse mutant nude. A study of nine consecutive transplantations. Acta Pathol Microbiol Scand [A] 79:159–169, 1971.
25. Shimosato Y, Kameya T, Nagai K, Hirohaski S, Koide T, Hayashi H, Normura T: Transplantation of human tumors in nude mice. J Natl Cancer Inst 56:1251–1260, 1976.
26. Kuga N, Yoshida K, Seido T, Oboshi S, Koide T, Shimosato Y, Nomura T: Heterotransplantation of cultured human cancer cells and human cancer tissues into nude mice. Gann 66:547–560, 1975.
27. Outzen HC, Custer RP: Growth of human normal and neoplastic mammary tissues in the cleared mammary fat pad of the nude mouse. J Natl Cancer Inst 55:1461–1463, 1975.
28. Reid LC, Shin SI: Transplantation of heterologous endocrine tumor cells in nude mice. In: The nude mouse in experimental and clinical research, Fogh J, Giovanella B (eds). New York, Academic Press Inc, 1978, p 313–351.
29. Kameya T, Shimosato Y, Hayashi H, Tsumuraya T: Growth and differentiation of hormone producing human tumors in nude mice. In: Proceeding of the second national workshop on nude mice, Nomura T, Ohsawa N, Tamaoki N, Fujiware K (eds), Tokyo, University of Tokyo, 1977, p 405–412.
30. Epstein AL, Herman MM, Kim H, Dorfman RF, Kaplan HS: Biology of the human malignant lymphomas III. Intracranial heterotransplantation in the nude, athymic mouse. Cancer 37:2158–2176, 1976.
31. Giovanella B Nilsson K, Zech L, Yim O, Klein G, Stehlin JS: Growth of diploid Epstein-

Barr virus-carrying human lymphoblastoid cell lines heterotransplanted into nude mice under immunologically priviledged conditions. Int J Cancer 24:103–113, 1979.
32. Schaadt M, Kirchner H, Fonatsch C, Diehl V: Intracranial heterotransplantation of human hematopoietic cells in nude mice. Int J Cancer 23:751–761, 1979.
33. Sebesteny A, Taylor-Papadimitriu J, Ceriani R, Millis R, Schmitt C, Trevan D: Primary human breast carcinomas transplantable in the nude mouse. J Natl Cancer Inst 63:1331–1333, 1979.
34. Rae-Venter B, Reid LM: Growth of human breast carcinomas in nude mice and subsequent establishment in tissue culture. Cancer Res 40:95–100, 1980.
35. Sordat B, Merenda C, Carrel S: Invasive growth and dissemination of human solid tumors and malignant cell lines grafted subcutaneously to newborn nude mice, Nomura T, Ohsawa N, Tamaoki N, Fujiwara K (eds), Tokyo, University of Tokyo Press, 1977, p 313–326.
36. Povlsen CO: Heterotransplantation of human malignant melanomas to the mouse mutant nude. Acta Pathol Microbiol Scand [A] 84:9–16, 1976.
37. Fodstad Ø, Aass N, Pihl A: Response to chemotherapy of human malignant melanoma xenografts in athymic, nude mice. Int J Cancer 25:453–458, 1980.
38. Fogh J, Fogh JM, Orfeo T: One hundred and twenty-seven cultured human tumor cell lines producing tumors in nude mice. J Natl Cancer Inst 59:221–226, 1977.
39. Giovanella BC, Yim SO, Morgan AC, Stehlin JS, Williams LJ: Metastases of human melanomas transplanted in 'nude' mice. J Natl Cancer Inst 50:1051–1053, 1973.
40. Rygaard J: Immunobiology of the mouse mutant 'nude'. Acta Pathol Microbiol Scand [A] 77:761–762, 1969.
41. Stiles CD, Desmond W, Chuman LM, Sata G, Saier MH: Growth control of heterologous tissue culture cells in the congenitally athymic nude mouse. Cancer Res 36:1353–1360, 1976.
42. Stiles CD, Desmond W, Chuman LM, Sata G, Saier MH, Jr.: Relationship of cell growth behavior *in vitro* to tumorigenicity in athymic nude mice. Cancer Res 36:3300–3305, 1976.
43. Reid LM, Holland J, Jones C, Wolf B, Sato G: Some of the variables affecting the success of transplantation of human tumors into the athymic nude mouse. In: Proceedings of the symposium on the use of athymic (nude) mice in cancer research, Houchens DP, Ovejera AA (eds). New York, Gustav Fischer Verlag, 1978, p 107–121.
44. Kameya T, Shimosato Y, Tumuraya M, Ohsawa N, Nomura T: Human gastric choriocarcinoma serially transplanted in nude mice. J Natl Cancer Inst 56:325–329, 1976.
45. Kyriazis A, DiPersio L, Michael JG, Pesce AJ: Influence of the mouse hepatitis virus (MHV) infection on the growth of human tumors in the athymic mouse.. Int J Cancer 23:402–409, 1979.
46. Miwa M, Hirohashi S, Shimosato Y, Mukojima T, Ohkura H, Sakura H, Kawachi T, Sugimura T: Coproduction of carcinoembryonic antigen and α-fetoprotein in transplantable human colon cancer in nude mice. In: Proceedings of the second international workshop on nude mice. Nomura T, Ohsawa N, Tamaoki N, Fujiwara K (eds), Tokyo, University of Tokyo Press, 1977, p 435–441.
47. Kanzaki T, Hashimoto K, Bath DW: Heterotransplantation of human malignant melanoma cell lines in athymic nude mice. J Natl Cancer Inst 62:1151–1158, 1979.
48. Fogh J, Hajdu SI: The nude mouse as a diagnostic tool in human tumor cell research. J Cell Biol 67:117–122, 1975.
49. Tomphins MB, Rama Rao GV, Tomphins WAF: Increased tumorigenicity and resistance to antibody lysis of human colon tumor cells xenografted in congenitally athymic mice. Cancer Res 39:2160–2165, 1979.
50. Price PJ, Arnstein P, Suk WA, Vernon ML, Huebner RJ: Type 'C' RNA viruses of the

NIH 'nude' mouse. J Natl Cancer Instt 55:1231–1232, 1975.
51. Manning JK, Reed ND, Jutila JW: Antibody response to Escherichia coli lipopolysaccharide and type III pneumococcal polysaccharide by congenitally thymusless (nude) mice. J Immunol 108:1470–1476, 1972.
52. Martin WJ, Martin SE: Naturally occurring cytotoxic anti-tumor antibodies in sera of congenitally athymic (nude) mice. Nature 249:564–565, 1974.
53. Meltzer MS: Tumoricidal responses *in vitro* of peritoneal macrophages from conventionally housed and germ-free nude mice. Cell Immunol 22:176–181, 1976.
54. Johnson WJ, Balish E: Macrophage function in germ-free, athymic (nu/nu), and conventional-flora (nu/+) mice. J Reticuloendothel Soc 28:55–66, 1980.
55. Herberman RB, Ninn ME, Laurin Dh: Natural cytotoxic reactivity of mouse lymphoid cells against syngeneic and allogeneic tumors. I. Distribution of reactivity and specificity. Int J Cancer 16:216–229, 1975.
56. Gershwin ME, Ikeda RM, Erickson K Owens R: Enhancement of heterotransplanted human tumor graft survival in nude mice treated with antilymphocytic serum and in congenitally athymic-asplenic (lasat) mice. J Natl Cancer Inst 61:245–248, 1978.
57. Lozzio BB, Machado EA, Lair SV, Lozzlo CB: Reproducible metastatic growth of K-562 human myeologenous leukemia cells in nude mice. J Natl Cancer Inst 63:295–298, 1980.
58. Ohsugi Y, Gershwin ME, Owens RB, Nelson-Rees WA: Tumorigenicity of human malignant lymphoblasts: Comparative study with unmanipulated nude mice, antilymphocyte serum-treated nude mice, and x-irradiated nude mice. J Natl Cancer Inst 65:715–718, 1980.
59. Watanabe S, Shimosato Y, Kuroki M, Sato Y, Nakajima T: Transplantability of human lymphoid cell line, lymphoma, and leukemia in splenectomized and/or irradiated nude mice. Cancer Res 40:2588–2595, 1980.
60. Bonmassar E, Campanile F, Houchens D, Crino L, Goldin A: Impaired growth of a radiation-induced lymphoma in intact or lethally irradiated allogeneic athymic (nude) mice. Transplantation 20:343–346, 1975.
61. Minato N, Bloom BR, Jones C, Holland J, Reid LM: Mechanism of rejection of virus persistently infected tumor cells by athymic nude mice. J Exp Med 149:1117–1133, 1979.
62. Ozello L, Sordat B, Merenda C, Carrel S, Hulimann J, Mach JP: Transplantation of a human mammary carcinoma cell line (BT 20) into nude mice. J Natl Cancer Inst. 52:1669–1672, 1974.
63. Giovanella BC, Yim SO, Stehlin JS, Williams LJ: Development of invasive tumors in the 'nude' mouse after injection of cultured human melanoma cells. J Natl Cancer Inst 18:1531–1533, 1972.
64. Sharkey FE, Fogh J: Metastasis of human tumors in athymic nude mice. Int J Cancer 24:733–738, 1979.
65. Zamecnik PC, Long JC: Growth of cultured cells from patients with Hodgkin's disease and transplantation into nude mice. Proc Natl Acad Sci USA 74:754–758, 1977.
66. Hata J, Ueyama Y, Tamaoki N, Furukawa T, Morita K: Human neuroblastoma serially transplanted in nude mice and metastases. Cancer 42:468–473, 1978.
67. Kyriazis AP, DiPersio L, Michael GJ, Pesce AJ, Stinnett JD: Growth patterns and metastatic behavior of human tumors growing in athymic mice. Cancer Res 38:3186–3190, 1978.
68. Takahashi S, Konishi Y, Nakatani K, Inui S, Kojima K, Shiratori T: Conversion of a poorly differentiated human adenocarcinoma to ascites form with invasion and metastasis in nude mice: Brief Communication. J Natl Cancer Inst 60:925–929, 1978.

69. Prehn RT, Lappé M: An immunostimulation theory of tumor development. Transplant Rev 7:26–51, 1971.
70. Fidler IJ, Gersten DM, Hart IR: The biology of cancer invasion and metastasis. Adv Cancer Res 28:149–250, 1978.
71. Fidler IJ, Caines S, Dolan Z: Survival of hematogenously disseminated allogeneic tumor cells in athymic nude mice. Transplantation 22:208–212, 1976.
72. Skov CB, Holland JM, Perkins EH: Development of fewer tumor colonies in lungs of athymic nude mice after intravenous injection of tumor cells. J Natl Cancer Inst 56:193–195, 1976.
73. Lozzio BB, Lozzio CB, Machado EA: Human myelogenous (Ph′+) leukemia cell line: Transplantation into athymic mice. J Natl Cancer Inst 56:627–629, 1978.
74. Liotta LA, Kleinerman J, Saidel GM: Quantitative relationships of intravascular tumor cells, tumor vessels and pulmonary metastases following tumor implantation. Cancer Res 34:997–1004, 1974.
75. Liotta LA, Kleinerman J, Saidel GM: The significance of hematogenous tumor cell clumps in the metastatic process. Cancer Res 36:889–894, 1976.
76. Fidler IJ: The relationship of embolic homogeneity, number, size and viability to the incidence of experimental metastasis. Eur J Cancer 9:223–227, 1973.
77. Hanna N, Fidler IJ: The role of natural killer cells in the destruction of circulating tumor emboli. J Natl Cancer Inst 65:801–809, 1980.
78. Hanna N: Expression of metastatic potential of tumor cells in young nude mice is correlated with low levels of natural killer cell-mediated cytotoxicity. Int J Cancer 26:675–680, 1980.
79. Riccardi C, Puccetti P, Santoni A, Herberman RB: Rapid *in vivo* assay of mouse natural killer cell activity. J Natl Cancer Inst 63:1041–1045, 1979.
80. Talmadge JE, Meyers KM, Prieur DJ, Starkey JR: Role of NK cells in tumor growth and metastasis in beige mice. Nature 284:622–624, 1980.
81. Hanna N, Fidler IJ: Expression of metastatic potential of allogenic and xenogeneic in young nude mice. Cancer Res 41:438–444, 1981.
82. Kripke ML, Gruys E, Fidler IJ: Metastatic heterogeneity of cells from an ultraviolet light-induced murine fibrosarcoma of recent origin. Cancer Res 38:2962–2967, 1978.
83. Willis RA: The spread of tumors in the human body. London, Butterworth, 1972.
84. Prehn RT: Analysis of antigenic heterogeneity within individual 3-methylcholanthrene-induced mouse sarcomas. J Natl Cancer Inst 45:1039–1045, 1970.
85. Biorklund A, Hakansson L, Stenstam B, Trope C, Akerman M: Heterogeneity of non-Hodgkin's lymphomas as regards sensitivity to cytostatic drugs. An *in vitro* study. Eur J Cancer 16:647–654, 1980.
86. Hakansson L, Trope C: On the presence within tumors of clones that differ in sensitivity to cytostatic drugs. Acta Pathol Microbiol Scand [A] 82:35–40, 1974.
87. Heppner GH, Dexter DL, DeNucci T, Miller FR, Calabresi P: Heterogeneity in drug sensitivity among tumor cell subpopulations of a single mammary tumor. Cancer Res 38:3758–3763, 1978.
88. Henderson JS, Rous P: The plating of tumor components on the subcutaneous expanses of young mice. Findings with benign and malignant epidermal growths and with mammary carcinomas. J Exp Med 115:1211–1230, 1962.
89. Trope C: Different susceptibilities of tumor cell subpopulations to cytotoxic agents. In: Design of Models for Testing Cancer Therapeutic Agents, Fidler IJ, White RJ (eds), New York, Van Nostrand, in press.
90. Kerbel RS: Implications of immunological heterogeneity of tumors. Nature 280:358–360, 1979.

91. Kripke ML, Gruys E, Fidler IJ: Metastatic heterogeneity of cells from an ultraviolet light-induced murine fibrosarcoma of recent origin. Cancer Res 38:2962–2967, 1978.
92. Fidler IJ, Kripke ML: Metastasis results from preexisting variant cells within a malignant tumor. Science 197:893–895, 1977.
93. Briles EB, Kornfeld S: Isolation and metastatic properties of detachment variants of B16 melanoma cells. J Natl Cancer Inst 60:1217–1222, 1978.
94. Fidler IJ, Gersten DM, Budmen MB: Characterization *in vivo* and *in vitro* of tumor cells selected for resistance to syngeneic lymphocyte-mediated cytotoxicity. Cancer Res 36:3160–3165, 1976.
95. Tao TW, Burger MM: Nonmetastasizing variants selected from metastasizing melanoma cells. Nature 270:437–438, 1977.
96. Fidler IJ: Selection of successive tumor lines for metastasis. Nature 242:148–149, 1973.
97. Suzuki N, Withers HR, Koehler MW: Heterogeneity and variability of artificial lung colony-forming ability among clones from mouse fibrosarcoma. J Natl Cancer Inst 60:179–183, 1978.
98. Kerbel RS, Twiddy RR, Robertson DM: Induction of a tumor with greatly increased metastatic growth potential by injection of cells from a low-metastatic H-2 heterozygous tumor cell line into an H-2 incompatible parental strain. Int J Cancer 22:583–594, 1978.
99. Brunson KW, Nicolson GL: Selection and biologic properties of malignant variants of a murine lymphosarcoma. JNCI 61:1499–1503, 1978.
100. Fogel M, Gorelik E, Segal S, Feldman M: Differences in cell surface antigens of tumor metastases and those of the local tumor. JNCI 62:585–588, 1979.
101. Killion JJ, Kollmorgen GM: Isolation of immunogenic tumor cells by cell-affinity chromatography. Nature 259:673–676, 1976.
102. Schirrmacher V, Shantz G, Glauer K, Komitowsky D, Zimmerman HP, Lohmann-Matthes ML: Tumor metastases and cell-mediated immunity in a model system in DBA/2 mice. I. Tumor invasiveness *in vitro* and metastasis formation *in vivo*. Int J Cancer 23:233–244, 1979.
103. Tao TW, Matter A, Vogel K, Burger MM: Liver-colonizing melanoma cells selected from B16 melanoma. Int J Cancer 23:854–857, 1979.
104. Brunson KW, Beattie G, Nicolson GL: Selection and altered properties of brain-colonising metastatic melanoma. Nature 272:543–545, 1978.
105. Raz A, Hart IR: Murine melanoma: A model for intracranial metastasis. Br J Cancer 42:331–341, 1980.
106. Lotan R: Different susceptibilities of human melanoma and breast carcinoma cell lines to retinoic acid-induced growth inhibition. Cancer Res 39:1014–1019, 1979.
107. Fugmann RA, Anderson JC, Stolfi RL, Martin DS: Comparison of adjuvant chemotherapeutic activity against primary and metastatic spontaneous murine tumors. Cancer Res 37:496–500, 1977.
108. Schabel FM Jr: Concepts for systemic treatment of micrometastases. Cancer 35:15–24, 1975.
109. Trope C, Hakansson L, Dencker H: Heterogeneity of human adenocarcinomas of the colon and the stomach as regards sensitivity to cytostatic drugs. Neoplasma 22:423–430, 1975.
110. Trope C: Different sensitivity to cytostatic drugs of primary tumor and metastasis of the Lewis carcinoma. Neoplasma 22:171–180, 1975.
111. Hanna N, Burton RC: Definitive evidence that natural killer (NK) cells inhibit experimental tumor metastasis *in vivo*. J Immunol 127:1754–1758, 1981.

2. Potentials and Limitations for the Use of Radiation Sensitizers of Resistant Hypoxic Cells in Tumors

ROBERT M. SUTHERLAND, DIETMAR W. SIEMANN and PETER J. CONROY

1. INTRODUCTION

Abnormal vascularization often associated with tumor growth may result in the presence of significant numbers of radiation resistant hypoxic cells in some solid tumors, thereby limiting the effectiveness of radiotherapy in cancer treatment. Sufficiently low levels of oxygen have been well-documented as causing radiation resistance of mammalian cells in culture and in tumors in animals. There is also a significant amount of data available suggesting the presence of hypoxic resistant cells in human tumors. Hypoxic cells in tumors are not abnormally oxygenated because of the large diffusion distances from blood vessels and intervening consumption of oxygen by other tumor cells. One area of major research emphasis in the past ten years has been the search for compounds which sensitize hypoxic cells to ionizing radiation but are not readily consumed by the tumor cells and with pharmacological properties which result in sensitizing concentrations in regions of hypoxic cells in poorly vascularized tumor tissue.

Radiation sensitizing compounds have been called oxygen mimetic agents since many of the most effective sensitizers contain nitro groups which make them highly electron affinic like oxygen. Although several classes of nitro compounds possess this property including nitrofurans and nitrobenzenes, the agents which currently are most promising for clinical use because of combination of favorable radiation sensitizing and pharmacological/physiological properties are the nitroimidazoles (Figure 1). In addition to the effects of these agents as radiation sensitizers, that is, increasing cell kill when present at the time of irradiation, the nitroimidazoles also possess other properties which must be considered in evaluating their clinical usefulness. Over extended exposure periods both *in vitro* and *in vivo* these agents can also kill hypoxic cells in the absence of irradiation. A possibly related effect is the reduction of the shoulder of radiation survival curves

G. Bennett Humphrey et al. (eds), Adrenal and Endocrine Tumors in Children.

METRONIDAZOLE (NSC 69587)
[1(2-hydroxyethyl)-2-methyl-5-nitroimidazole]

MISONIDAZOLE (NSC 261037)
[1(2-nitro-1-imidazoyl)-3-methoxy-2-propanol]

Figure 1. Nitroimidazole radiation sensitizers which are currently being evaluated clinically.

caused by preincubation of hypoxic cells with the drug for several hours before irradiation. In addition recent experiments both *in vitro* and *in vivo* have demonstrated marked enhancement of effects of several different cancer chemotherapy agents when used in combination with sensitizers in the absence of irradiation. A major limitation for the clinical use of sensitizers is the toxicity, which, in addition to nausea and vomiting, takes the form of peripheral sensory neuropathies which may also be associated with central manifestations. This chapter will consider radiosensitization, hypoxic cell cytotoxicity, enhancement of chemotherapeutic agent toxicity and neurotoxicity of nitroimidazoles and attempt to delineate the potentials and limitations for the clinical use of these drugs and to review the information available on mechanisms of these effects.

2. RADIATION SENSITIZATION

It has been long known that oxygen has a strong influence on the sensitivity of mammalian cells to radiation. As early as 1934 Crabtree and Cramer [1] demonstrated that the degree of cell killing *in vitro* was dependent upon the degree of oxygenation at the time of irradiation. This sensitization subsequently was shown to be directly related to the cellular oxygen tension such that with increasing oxygen concentration, radiation sensitivity usually reaches a plateau at a partial pressure of oxygen of ~20–30 mm Hg [2]. Further increases in oxygen concentration have little additional effect. Figure 2 illustrates the characteristics of radiation survival curves of mammalian cells and the influence of oxygen on radiation sensitivity. These survival curves obtained under anoxic (absence of oxygen) or aerobic conditions can be defined in terms of their terminal slopes and extrapolation numbers. The slopes of the curves usually are expressed by a term called the D_0 which is defined as the dose required to reduce the survival to 37 percent along the exponential portion of the curves. Oxygen generally is regarded as changing only the slope (D_0) but not the shoulder or threshold regions of these curves (extrapolation number) and consequently has been termed a dose-modifying agent. The degree of dose modification, estimated from the ratio of the D_0

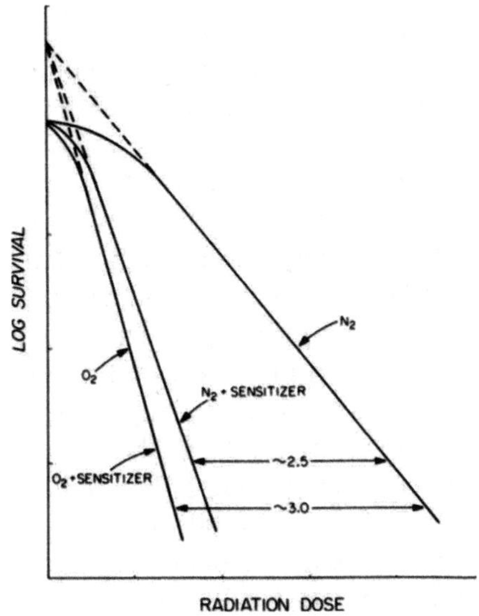

Figure 2. Typical mammalian cell radiation survival curves illustrating effects of oxygen and sensitizers. The oxygen enhancement ratio (OER) = 3.0 and the sensitizer enhancement ratio (ER) = 2.5.

values of the anoxic and aerobic clonogenic cell survival curves, is called the oxygen enhancement ratio (OER). In a variety of different mammalian cell lines the OER has been found to have a maximum value of ~3.0 [3–6]. This means that in order to obtain the same level of cell killing under anoxic conditions as in air, radiation doses nearly 3 times as large are required. As a consequence larger radiation doses would be required to eradicate successfully a tumor possessing oxygen deficient or hypoxic cells than one that did not.

Most animal tumors have been shown to possess various proportions of hypoxic cells [6, 7] and recent evidence strongly suggests that hypoxic cells play an important role in the management of at least some human tumors by radiotherapy [8, 9]. Since hypoxic cells are resistant to radiation damage due to their inherent lack of oxygen, one approach to reducing the hypoxic cell problem is to attempt to improve the level of tumor oxygenation through the inhalation of high oxygen content gases during the irradiation. Although recent results from the combined trials organized by the Medical Research Council in England have suggested that hyperbaric oxygen may improve local control rates at some tumor sites, many other clinical studies have been inconclusive (for review see [9]).

One of the major drawbacks of using oxygen to sensitize hypoxic cells is that oxygen is rapidly metabolized by all tissues. Consequently there has been considerable interest in developing chemical agents which could (1) mimic oxygen's ability to sensitize hypoxic cells, (2) be able to diffuse through poorly vascularized cell masses and (3) be only minimally or not all metabolized by well-oxygenated cells. In 1971 Adams *et al.* [10] showed that certain electron affinic compounds were radiation sensitizers under anoxic conditions without affecting the radiation sensitivity of well-oxygenated cells. *In vitro* radiosensitization by nitroimidazoles was demonstrated using metronidazole (METRO) and subsequently misonidazole (MISO) in a variety of mammalian cells [11–16]. Figure 2 illustrates that these so-called oxygen mimetic nitro-containing radiosensitizers produce effects similar to those observed with oxygen when present during the irradiation. As is also shown in this figure these radiation sensitizing compounds are active only on hypoxic cells and do not sensitize cells in the presence of adequate oxygen concentrations [10, 13, 14]. However, although these agents are considered to be dose modifying they usually do not possess the full sensitizing ability of oxygen. Generally sensitizer enhancement ratios, determined from the slopes of the survival curves of cells irradiated under nitrogen in the presence or absence of the sensitizer, are in the range of 2.1 to 2.7 [14]. The radiation sensitizing effect of these compounds does not require temperatures above ice bath temperatures for most cell systems [17]. In addition it has been shown that in order to observe the full sensitizing effect these agents need only be present for very short periods of time after their addition to hypoxic cells [18]. These findings imply that sensitizer metabolism is not involved in the dose modifying effect.

Sensitizers are thought to act mainly be fixing radiation damage in the cells, probably on target DNA molecules. The sensitizer compound may form adducts where the ionizing radiation has produced free radicals because of electron affinic properties [17, 19]. Although the mechanism of action of the radiosensitizers has not been completely delineated, evidence for the involvement of the electron affinic properties of these compounds in the radiation sensitizer mechanism is very strong since compounds of higher electron affinity in general are better radiosensitizers [12, 14, 20–22].

Although *in vitro* experiments have shown cell sensitization by a variety of compounds [10, 22–26] most of these were found to either sensitize not at all *in vivo* or only at drug doses near the lethal range [27–30]. However, two compounds, METRO and in particular MISO, have within the last few years been shown to be effective against a wide range of animal tumors (for review see [31, 32]). Figure 3 illustrates schematically the effect of one of these sensitizers on tumor control by large single doses of radiation. The curves show that the addition of such an agent to the radiation therapy can reduce significantly the dose required to cure 50 percent of the animals of their tumors. Using endpoints such as *in situ* tumor control, *in situ* tumor growth delay or *in vivo* to *in vitro* clonogenic cell survival, the effects of

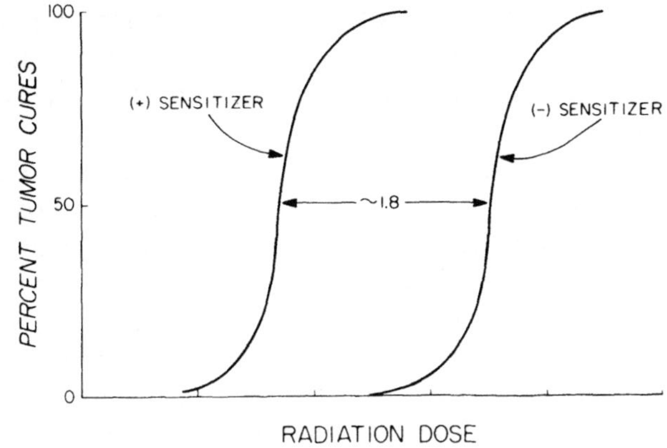

Figure 3. Typical tumor control probability curve showing improved cure rates when misonidazole is combined with radiation (ER = 1.8).

METRO and MISO on tumor response to radiation have been extensively studied (for review see [33] and [34]). In a variety of tumor systems these nitroimidazole compounds have given sensitizer enhancement ratios of ~1.3–2.1 when air-breathing animals are treated with large radiation and sensitizer doses [7, 30, 35–40]. Although most mouse studies have utilized large subcutaneous or intramuscular tumors, the sensitizing effects of these compounds in the treatment of microscopic tumor deposits also have been evaluated [41–44]. In general such studies have indicated that the sensitizers, although effective over a range of tumor sizes, usually showed reduced enhancement ratios in the smaller tumors likely because these tumors contained a lower proportion of severely hypoxic cells.

When nitroimidazoles and irradiation are combined most normal tissues evaluated in animals have indicated little or no enhanced damage [36, 44–46] with the possible exceptions of cartilage [47] and esophagus [48]. In man the dose limiting toxicity of these compounds however is neurotoxicity and consequently considerable efforts have been spent recently to develop suitable assay systems for evaluating this toxicity (see Section 5 on neurotoxicity for detailed discussion).

In addition to the dose limiting neurotoxicity of the nitroimidazoles, animal studies also have demonstrated that in a fractionated radiation dose regimen there is a decrease in the sensitizing ability of these compounds both in murine tumor models [30, 32, 33, 38–40, 49–52] and in the human tumor xenografts [53]. This result probably is a consequence of both the reduction in size of the radiation and sensitizer doses and the rapid reoxygenation which can occur in some tumors between subsequent radiation doses. Nevertheless, despite the decrease in sensitizing ability with fractionation and the dose-limiting neurotoxicity, preliminary reports of studies carried out in humans appear promising and consequently the nitroimidazole compounds METRO and MISO are currently being used as radiation sensitizers in Phase I-II and Phase III clinical trials [54–67].

Yet, clearly, METRO and MISO are not the optimum radiation sensitizers and extensive research to develop better and less neurotoxic compounds is presently in progress. Recently these investigations have led to promising new findings with the natural metabolites of MISO including the O-desmethylation product, Ro-05-9963 as well as with other more hydrophilic 2-nitromidazole amides such as the SR-2508 and SR-2555 compounds produced at the Stanford Research Institute. These agents do not penetrate the lipid layers in the nervous system as readily [68] yet seem to have sensitizing abilities as effective as MISO [69]. It appears that these or other newer compounds hold considerable promise for the future.

3. PREFERENTIAL HYPOXIC CELL CYTOTOXICITY

Although studies with several different nitro compounds have been reported, we will outline here results obtained mainly with the nitroimidazoles and especially the agent misonidazole (MISO). In addition to acting as radiation sensitizers, nitroimidazoles are preferentially toxic to hypoxic cells even in the absence of irradiation if present for sufficient periods of time (Figure 4) [70–73]. After much longer exposure periods, cell killing also occurs under oxic conditions. This hypoxic cytotoxicity, unlike the radiosensitization, is temperature dependent. Hypoxic cytotoxicity is inhibited at 0 °C [72, 74] and is enhanced significantly by moderate hyperthermia [75–78]. In addition to temperature, factors such as drug exposure time, pH, cell

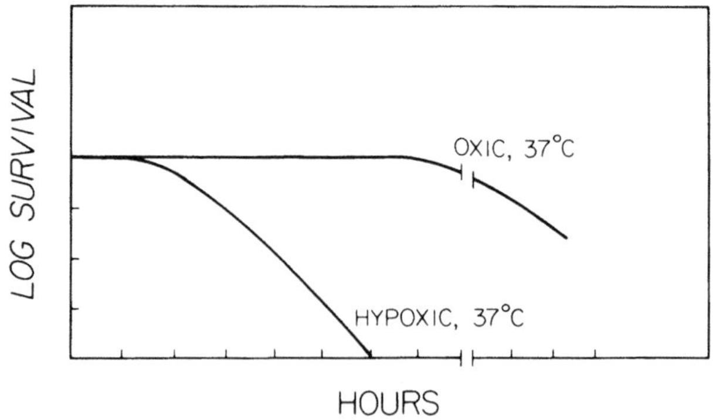

Figure 4. Typical toxicity curves for exposure of cells to sensitizers including misonidazole for extended periods under hypoxic and oxic conditions.

type, serum and medium constituents greatly affect the cell killing produced under hypoxic conditions [71, 72, 74–76, 79–81]. Taken together these data strongly suggest that metabolism of the drug is required to produce hypoxic cytotoxicity.

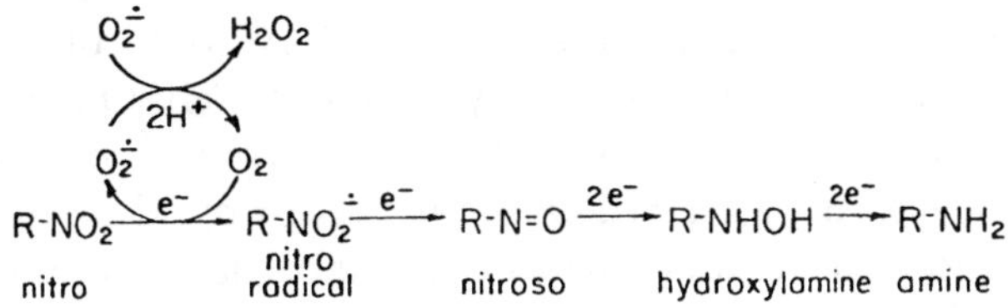

Figure 5. Possible metabolic pathways for nitro-heterocyclic compounds such as many radiation sensitizers. Under hypoxic conditions nitroreductases catalyse the reduction of the nitro group.

The probable metabolic pathways under oxic or hypoxic conditions are outlined in Figure 5. Hypoxic cell cytotoxicity probably requires the action of nitro-reductases which are inhibited by the presence of oxygen. Under oxygenated conditions very reactive superoxide radicals as well as other toxic substances will be produced when very high concentrations of drugs are used over long exposure periods [82–86]. There has been considerable interest in the hypoxic cell cytotoxicity because it may be exploitable clinically since under normal conditions only tumors would be expected to contain sufficient quantities of hypoxic cells thus, producing preferential toxicity for tumor relative to normal tissues. As indicated in Figure 5 there are several possible mechanisms by which the toxic effects may occur. Hypoxic drug metabolism may produce reactive intermediates or terminal stable products which may react with critical cellular targets. Furthermore, this metabolism may unbalance the redox state of the cell and lead indirectly to toxic effects.

Aminoimidazole derivatives have been identified in hypoxic but not aerobic cells [87]. This confirms the potential relevance of the metabolic pathway proposed in Figure 5. Other reactive intermediates of this pathway have been formed by various chemical reduction procedures [85, 88, 89]. There is no strong evidence at the moment for any specific final stable product in this pathway producing the cytotoxicity. Investigations are underway in several laboratories of possible involvement of reactive intermediates in the pathway and/or of the biochemical imbalance produced to the redox state of the cells.

A variety of cellular effects of MISO or its products have been examined which may relate to these mechanisms. Chemical reduction products of misonidazole have been shown to bind to cellular macromolecules including

DNA and to result in more cell killing than MISO alone when incubated with cells *in vitro* [88–91]. Products which damage DNA are also produced from intracellular MISO metabolism [88, 92–94]. Strong correlations among rate of metabolic reduction, redox potential of nitroheterocycles including nitroimidazoles and various endpoints such as DNA damage and synthesis, mutagenicity, survival and growth have been observed [94]. The redox state of the cell also is definitely altered by MISO [95]. Lower levels of protein and nonprotein sulfhydryls under hypoxic conditions were obtained after incubation with MISO. Depletion of pyridine nucleotides such as NADPH and NADH may also occur since flavoprotein requiring enzymes are implicated in the reduction of nitro-compounds. These include xanthine oxidase, aldehyde oxidase, NADPH-cytochrome c reductase and mitrochondrial flavo-enzymes [82, 84, 96]. Evidence for the biochemical interference mechanism related to redox balance of the cell is provided by other studies such as 5-thio-D-glucose which inhibits glucose metabolism and transport and produces preferential toxicity to hypoxic cells [97]. Either of these mechanisms, that is, reactive or stable product damage to important target molecules or imbalance of redox biochemistry of the cell may be involved in the mechanism of hypoxic cell toxicity either separately or together under certain circumstances, depending upon the metabolic state and microenvironment of the cell within the tumor.

Accumulation and repair of any sublethal DNA damage could be influenced by either of these mechanisms. Sublethal damage by reactions with target molecules and modification of the ability to repair that damage is implicated by studies where it was shown that hypoxic preincubations at normal temperatures resulted in altered sensitivity to secondary exposure to agents such as radiation [98], heat and chemotherapeutic drugs [99]. Short incubations before irradiation only modified the slopes of the survival curves whereas incubation for periods of 3 hours at 37 °C removed the shoulder or the region related to sublethal damage of the radiation survival curves (see Figure 2). The ability to modify this sublethal damage depends upon the concentration and the duration of pre-irradiation treatment and is maximal at the point where decrease of cell survival begins to occur on the slope of the survival curve. Apparently this effect requires only that the pretreatment be under hypoxic conditions; subsequent exposure to the second agent may be under aerobic conditions and the same effect is found [81]. This pretreatment effect also occurs to subsequent exposures to hyperthermia (41°–43 °C) and chemotherapeutic agents such as cis-platinum, mustine and melphelan [99]. It is likely that this so-called pretreatment sensitization is related mechanistically to the hypoxic cell preferential toxicity.

In addition to producing cell killing, nitro-compounds may alter significantly the oxygen consumption rate of cells [82]. Generally nitro-compounds produce immediate inhibition or stimulation of cellular oxygen consumption. MISO, however, has essentially no immediate effect on oxygen consumption and inhibition of consumption only begins to occur under conditions of long exposure where toxicity also results [100]. Other studies related to the redox state of the cell have demonstrated that oxidizing and reducing agents may modify the degree of hypoxic toxicity obtained with misonidazole. In 1978 Josephy *et al.* [101] reported that ascorbate enhanced the toxicity of MISO in mammalian cell cultures. Thiol-containing compounds have been demonstrated to reduce hypoxic cytotoxicity, for example, cysteamine [75, 102] D-penicillamine [79] and reduced glutathione, cysteine and mercaptoethanol [102]. There is some evidence that this protective effect may also occur under aerobic conditions [79]. The relationship of the metabolic state of the cell and its reducing capacity and of oxygen concentrations has been studied by Taylor and Rauth [100, 103]. Protection by reduced glutathione and cysteamine and enhancement by ascorbate of hypoxic cell toxicity in Chinese hamster ovary and HeLa cells were accompanied by changes in drug metabolism as shown by radiochromatograms of cell extracts obtained after treatment with ^{14}C-labelled MISO. No drug metabolism was found under aerobic conditions. It was also shown that very low oxygen concentrations, less than about 2×10^{-7} M O_2, are inhibitory to the hypoxic cytotoxic effect of MISO [100]. An interesting model for the metabolism mediated toxicity of MISO and the roles which sulfhydryls and oxygen may play has been presented by Taylor and Rauth [103].

Preferential hypoxic cell toxicity has also been demonstrated in the more complex multicell spheroid *in vitro* tumor model [70, 104–108] indicating that drug penetration, at least for MISO, is not limiting and that the microenvironmental conditions related to such factors as hypoxia and pH are appropriate. In fact it appears that the toxicity in spheroids is greater than would be expected for the degree of hypoxia [70, 104–108]. Either the toxic products of hypoxic drug metabolism diffuse to and kill nearby oxic cells or the combination of microenvironmental conditions and cellular metabolic states produced conditions which enhance cytotoxicity despite significant levels of oxygen.

Cytotoxicity in different tumor types varies significantly and cannot be correlated with the fraction of radiobiologically hypoxic cells in the tumors. Marked cytotoxicity has been demonstrated using clonogenic assays and histology in the EMT6 mammary tumor [109, 110] while little cytotoxicity has been found in the KHT fibrosarcoma at similar drug concentrations [111]. *In vivo* cytotoxicity of hypoxic tumor cells has been recently reviewed by Rauth *et al.* [111]. Because of the observed differences in sensitivity of different mouse tumor models, and other factors such as pharmacokinetics and *in vivo* tumor microphysiology which might influence oxygen concentrations and cellular redox states, it is difficult to predict the role hypoxic cell toxicity may play in the clinical situation.

4. MODIFICATION OF CHEMOTOXICITY BY SENSITIZERS

There recently has been considerable interest in combining radiation sensitizing compounds with chemotherapeutic agents because studies in multicellular spheroids and animal tumors have indicated that (1) hypoxic cells in tumors may be resistant to some conventional anti-tumor agents [70, 112–114], (2) it is often difficult to achieve appreciable drug concentrations in the hypoxic regions of spheroids and tumors [114] and (3) hypoxic cells may be spared from proliferation dependent chemotherapeutic agents because these cells often are not cycling [115, 116].

Thus, since hypoxic cells may limit the effectiveness of conventional chemotherapy, experimental studies have been initiated to evaluate protocols combining anti-tumor drugs with agents which are preferentially toxic to hypoxic cells. One group of compounds which may fulfill this role are the nitroimidazoles which readily penetrate into the hypoxic regions of tumors [117] and have been shown to be preferentially cytotoxic to hypoxic cells (see previous section of this chapter). Using multicell spheroids Sutherland *et al.* [114] have shown that pretreatment with MISO before adriamycin can effectively reduce the clonogenic cell survival and result in apparent supra-additivity [108]. Treatments *in vivo* with combinations of chemotherapeutic agents, primarily alkylating agents, and radiation sensitizers, usually MISO, also have demonstrated enhanced cytotoxicity in a number of different tumor systems [118–124]. At present maximum tumoricidal effect appear to occur when the agents are administered close to each other in time. Although most investigations have utilized large nitroimidazole doses, studies employing substantially reduced doses of the sensitizer have proven effective at least with some chemotherapeutic agents in some tumor systems [123]. To date anti-tumor agents adriamycin, cyclophosphamide, L-phenylalmine mustard (L-PAM) and 1-(2-chloroethyl-3-cyclohexyl-1-nitrosourea) (CCNU) appear to show the most promise when combined with MISO but much more experimentation to determine therapeutic effectiveness is required.

As in any evaluation of a combination of different agents, the assessment of normal tissue toxicity following the administration of a chemotherapeutic agent and radiation sensitizer is of utmost importance. *In vivo* studies have indicated that compared to what is observed for the anti-tumor agent alone the addition of MISO to a chemotherapeutic agent can enhance animal weight loss and deaths, reduce bone marrow and gut stem cell numbers, and decrease peripheral white blood cell counts [118–124]. Although some studies suggest that the enhancement of the toxicity may be greater in the tumor than in the normal tissue(s), at present considerable uncertainty remains concerning whether an enhanced therapeutic result can be achieved through such a combination.

Currently little is known about the mechanism responsible for the enhanced cell killing associated with combinations of some chemotherapeutic agents and radiation sensitizers. However several possibilities which may be of importance *in vivo* are: (1) independent action of the agents against different subpopulations in the tumor (i.e. the anti-tumor agent acting against well-oxygenated cells while the sensitizer is preferentially toxic to hypoxic cells), (2) the interference by the sensitizer with repair of damage resulting from the chemotherapeutic agent, (3) altered pharmacokinetics of either agent or both and (4) interaction between the agents resulting in an enhanced tumor response.

The evaluation of studies combining radiosensitizers and chemotherapeutic agents represents a new and exciting area of research for the use of chemical radiation sensitizers which requires further evaluation. In particular it will be necessary to determine the potential enhancement of damage in critical normal tissues. Nevertheless it appears that such combinations of agents may lead to improved cancer therapy.

5. NEUROTOXICITY

5.1. Clinical studies

Several Phase I and II trials have demonstrated that the clinical effectiveness of MISO and METRO is considerably reduced by the incidence of dose limiting side effects such as convulsions after large single doses and the development of peripheral neuropathy, ototoxicity and encephalopathies following smaller multiple doses of these compounds [54–63, 125–132]. A reduction in the size of the administered dose of MISO (or other sensitizer) prior to irradiation in a fractionated schedule is disadvantageous since animal studies have shown that the degree of sensitization likely to be achieved is directly proportional to the concentration of sensitizer present in the tumor at the time of irradiation [32, 39, 133, 134]. Depending on the size of the tumor hypoxic fraction and the degree of reoxygenation following radiation therapy, an obvious therapeutic gain can be made if larger amounts of sensitizer can be given at more frequent intervals without unacceptable neurotoxic side effects. We wish to briefly review the clinical experiences with MISO and METRO related to the dose-limiting toxicities of these compounds in humans. We will also examine the data available from experimental animal models in order to assist in the selection of more effective radiosensitizers for clinical use with improved potential therapeutic gain. Ideally, the drug candidate for this purpose should be (a) equal or superior to MISO in sensitizing efficiency at equimolar doses and (b) 5–10 times less neurotoxic.

Preliminary studies with MISO given orally in single doses of 1–4 g to normal human volunteers did not indicate any toxic side effects [135]. However, the Phase I/II studies have reported contraindicative side effects such as convulsions at high doses and peripheral sensory polyneuropathies in cancer patients receiving lower multiple doses of MISO [55, 57, 60–62, 65–67, 125, 126, 130, 132]. The most troublesome toxic manifestation of MISO neurotoxicity is peripheral sensory polyneuropathy of the hands and feet with mild to moderate paresthesias and loss of vibration sensitivity. Most of the neuropathies occurred as the total administered dose exceeded 10 g/m^2. None of the neuropathies progressed when drug administration stopped, although some lasted for several weeks and occasionally months. In the RTOG Phase I MISO studies, the overall incidence of peripheral neuropathies (grades I and II) was 49 percent in 99 patients evaluable for toxicity. Nine patients (~10 percent) developed central toxicity. Dose schedules were revised downwards in the RTOG (and other) Phase II trials to establish a maximum tolerated dose of 10.5–12 g/m^2 in 3 weeks or 13–15 g/m^2 in 6 weeks, irrespective of the dose fractionation of MISO [58, 60, 61, 127, 130, 132]. The overall incidence of peripheral neuropathies among 324 available patients in the RTOG Phase II MISO trials was 23 percent; overall central neurotoxicity was 9.0 percent, while the incidence of severe (Grade III or IV) central toxicity was reduced to 1.5 percent. The incidence and severity of peripheral neuropathy is primarily related to the total dose of MISO administered. It also appears that patients who have received the greatest exposure dose (product of half-life and serum plateau level of the drug) may be most at risk [58, 127]. Some evidence suggests that those patients who received concomitant administration or phenytoin (Dilantin) with MISO showed reduced incidence of neurotoxicity [65, 130]. Phenytoin shortens the half life (and therefore the exposure dose) of MISO in man [65, 130] and rodents [137], presumably by microsomal enzyme induction. This leads to increased metabolism of MISO to the o-desmethylated product, desmethylmisonidazole (Ro-05-9963). The latter is less lipophilic than the parent compound and is more readily excreted into urine. The peak tumor levels (MISO and desmethylmisonidazole) are unaffected.

The clinical observations of peripheral neuropathy due to MISO are consistent with distal axonal degeneration [55, 57, 66, 125] and are similar to those observed for METRO which is 2–3 times less toxic [128, 131, 138–140]. Primary demyelination has not been observed.

The clinical data on the CNS toxicity of MISO are difficult to evaluate. It is clear the CNS toxicity can occur with large total doses ($>15\ g/m^2$) of MISO. However, encephalopathies and convulsions have been observed in a few patients who received less that $10\ g/m^2$ [125]. The other toxicities that have been reported with MISO are gastrointestinal toxicity (nausea with mild to moderate vomiting), possible allergic reaction (skin rashes, fever and hypotension in a few patients) and ototoxicity (high frequency hearing loss and transient tinnitus) in the majority of patients with peripheral neuropathy [62, 141, 142]. None of the Phase I and II studies with MISO reported liver, bone marrow, renal or other organ toxicities.

Although the Phase I and II clinical trials with MISO have yielded equivocal results with regard to improvements in local tumor control rates, considerable experience has been gained in terms of the pharmacology and toxicity of the compound. Phase III randomized clinical trials with MISO are underway in the USA and several other countries on patients with high grade astrocytomas, head and neck carcinomas, bladder and cervical cancers.

5.2. Animal studies

5.2.1. Electrophysiology. The early reports that acute [143] or chronic administration [144] of MISO to mice results in decreased conduction velocity in peripheral nerves have not been confirmed by other investigators [145–147]. MISO induced peripheral neurotoxicity has been evaluated in rats by analysis of high frequency nerve train evoked response recorded from the ventral tail nerve [148]. At relatively high doses, the MISO treated rats showed small, though significant, changes in nerve train latency and amplitude before exhibiting signs of clinical toxicity. The small size of the effect could limit its potential clinical value. In general, these electrophysiological studies of MISO peripheral neurotoxicity in rodents have yielded equivocal results. Little or no change in peripheral nerve conduction velocity or refractory time were found following chronic administration of MISO to monkeys [149] although significant changes in vibration sensitivity were observed at late times.

5.2.2. Histopathology. MISO administration to mice induces a peripheral lesion after 3 weeks with a total administered dose of $13.5\ g/m^2$ or an exposure of 57–74 mM $\times$ hrs, which is similar to the doses causing neuropathy in humans [146]. In general, the deleterious changes produced by MISO treatment consisted of distal axonal degeneration of a Wallerian type, myelin sheath degeneration and vacuolation which was most severe in peripheral intramusculature (e.g. interosseous) nerve branches. In addition, marked edematous damages were seen in the dorsal root ganglia. These observations have been confirmed [150–152]. Pathologically, the overall topography of CNS lesions and hemorrhagic necrosis produced by MISO (and the related fluorinated nitroimidazole, Ro-07-0741) in mouse closely resembles the pattern observed in thiamine deficient rats [153, 154]. In both disorders, the lateral and superior vestibular nuclei and cochlear nuclei are most vulnerable and the cerebellar roof nuclei may be involved [155]. In both disorders the topography of the lesions is specific and selective, with neighboring regions remaining normal. The same picture was presented by Griffin [156, 157] for MISO in the rat where in addition to the spongy changes and scattered petechia described above, the major distinctive feature was the prominent involvement of the superior olives. Involvement of this structure has not been described in thiamine deficient rats. Purkinje cell loss has been described in dogs treated with MISO or METRO [158]. In monkeys, abnormalities have been observed on the vestibular nuclei [159]. Little data are available on specific CNS lesions following MISO treatment in humans. It is unlikely that there will be a close correlation between lesion topography in the rodent models and potential lesions in humans at high doses. One common feature is that high frequency hearing losses (ototoxicity) occur both in rodents [160, 161] and in humans exposed to MISO [62, 141, 142]. This suggests some involvement of the cochlear nucleus, auditory tracts or cochlear hair cells.

5.2.3. Symptoms. The clinical symptoms of MISO neurotoxicity in the mouse [146, 147, 160] and the rat [156, 157] are fairly similar and include lethargy, the abrupt onset of anorexia and weight loss, the loss of righting reflexes, brain stem dysfunction and dystonic posturing of the tail. In general, severe symptoms are preceeded by marked weight losses (typically 25 percent). In comparison with rodents, brain stem dysfunction has not been observed clinically as a toxic manifestation of MISO. In the small percentage of patients who exhibit central toxicity with MISO, typical symptoms include confusion, lethargy, seizures and rarely, focal findings ([125] and Phillips, personal communication, 1980).

5.2.4. Assays and comparative neurotoxicity. In general terms, the types of assay systems developed to evaluate nitromidazole neurotoxicity in experimental animals (chiefly rodents) can be divided into 2 groups: (i) functional and (ii) biochemical. The first functional assay for MISO neurotoxicity in the mouse was reported by Conroy *et al.* [146]. The rotarod performance test employed in this and subsequent studies [69, 147, 150, 151, 160] is based on the methods developed by Dunham and Miya [162] and Kaplan and Murphy [163]. It is a quantitative and objective test of the ability of an animal to maintain locomotor coordination and balance on a rotating rod which increases in speed linearly over a fixed time. The relative neurotoxicity for different nitroimidazoles on the basis of administered dose (and verified by clinical scoring and histology) for MISO, Ro-05-9963, Ro-07-0741, SR 2508, SR 2555 and METRO was 1.0, 0.5, 3.5, 0.2, <0.15 and 0.3 respectively. SR 2508 and SR 2555 were the least neurotoxic agents studied. The results agree with the clinical ranking order of neurotoxicity where known. The rotarod performance test is an indirect measure of neurotoxicity since both sensory and motor deficit are involved in the endpoint. A more direct measurement of sensory deficit in mice exposed to nitroimidazole sensitizers has been developed [160, 161]. The method involves the assessment of the ototoxic potential of sensitizers by measurement of modulation of the startle reflex in mice. High frequency hearing loss and transient tinnitus are clinical covariates of peripheral neuropathy in humans treated with MISO [62, 141, 142]. In mice, high frequency hearing loss (16 or 32 KHz) can be demonstrated for several sensitizers before the appearance of severe clinical symptoms or weight loss. Relative ototoxicity for MISO, Ro-05-9963, Ro-07-0741, SR-2508, SR-2555 and METRO was 1.0, 0.46, 3.3, 0.2, ~0.1 and 0.25 respectively. These data are in good agreement with the ranking given by the rotarod performance test. Figure 6 is a schematic illustration of relative neurotoxicity for several sensitizers in the mouse based on the data cited above. Panel A plots the data as a function of total administered dose and panel B as a function of brain exposure dose. On the basis of cumulative brain exposure dose (approx. 300–400 mM × hrs), MISO, Ro-05-9963, SR 2508 and SR 2555 are equally neurotoxic. Ro-07-0741 has a similar electron affinity (−390 mv) but is 2–3 times more toxic. The reason for this is unknown and may be related to the presence of a fluorine substituent in the side chain. METRO is 2–3 × less neurotoxic per exposure dose and is also less electron affinic (−480 mv). The difference between a ranking based on administered does (g/m^2) and brain exposure dose (mM × hrs) is related to differences in the lipophilicity and bioavailability of these sensitizers. Panel C shows relative neurotoxicity as a function of lipophilicity. It is clear that for sensitizers of equal electron affinity, less lipophilic compounds are less neurotoxic (i.e. they penetrate the blood-brain barrier and perineurium less well than more lipophilic agents).

Biochemical methods for detecting neurotoxicity have been recently reviewed by Dewar and Moffett [164]. Peripheral nerve degeneration induced by several neurotoxins correlates with increases in lysosomal enzyme (β-glucuronidase, acid phosphatase) activity in rats [163–165]. Changes in these lysosomal enzyme activities have been measured by quantitative cytochemistry in the peripheral nerves of mice treated with MISO [166, 167]. MISO administration resulted in considerable increases (100–160 percent) in β-glucuronidase and acid phosphatase enzyme activities in the sciatic

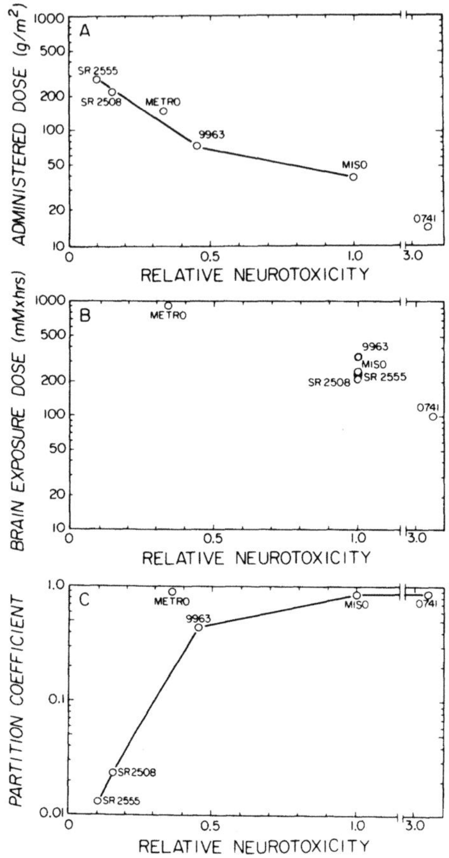

Figure 6. Relative neurotoxicity of different nitroimidazole radiation sensitizers as related to administered dose (A), measured exposure dose (B), and octanol: water partition coefficient of the sensitizers (C).

nerves of mice. These increases reached a maximum at 3–4 weeks and returned to normal by 8 weeks. These lysosomal enzyme changes were greater in the distal than the proximal portion of the nerve and are qualitatively similar to those seen in Wallerian degeneration [168]. In terms of overall sensitivity, this assay could detect lysosomal changes produced by MISO administration at clinically relevant doses [167]. Similarly, increased enzyme activity has been detected biochemically in homogenates of the peripheral nerves of rats following MISO treatment [169]. Several attempts to confirm this effect in homogenates of the peripheral nerves of mice treated with MISO have not proven successful ([160, 170], Brown, personal communication, 1980). This may indicate some species difference in the response of mice to MISO compared to rats. Acetylcholinesterase and cholinesterase activities both *in vitro* [171] and *in vivo* [172] remain unchanged following MISO treatment, even under conditions where the drug was present in considerable excess of that obtained clinically.

5.2.5. Potential Mechanism(s) of Neurotoxicity. The mechanism(s) of nitromidazole neurotoxicity are unknown. There are several potential mechanisms based largely on what is currently known about the anaerobic and aerobic toxicity of radiation sensitizers and their metabolism *in vitro* and *in vivo* (see preceding section of this chapter). They include the following:

(1) binding of nitro-reduced metabolites to macromolecules [87, 88];
(2) inhibition of pyruvate oxidation to acetyl coenzyme A [173];
(3) inhibition of glycolytic pathways including the hexose monophosphate shunt [82];
(4) increased oxidation of neurotransmitters [174];
(5) reactions of O_2-derived radicals formed from the oxidation of nitro reductases with cell macromolecules [100];
(6) disturbances in cellular redox balance and impaired capacity to repair damage produced by radical initiated damage to membranes [160].

Although it cannot be excluded from consideration, it is felt that if there is any connection between nitromidazole toxicity towards nerve tissue *in vivo* and the cytotoxicity of these compounds towards mammalian cells *in vitro*, then mechanism(s) put forward to explain the cytotoxicity of sensitizers through the production of reduced metabolites under hypoxic conditions are less likely to account for neurotoxicity than mechanisms which involve aerobic cytotoxicity, changes in glycolysis and the overall redox balance of cells. The data in the literature indicate that the oxygen inhibition of nitroreductases presumed responsible for the production of reduced intermediates (nitroso-, hydroxylamine, amine) from nitroaromatic compounds occurs at an oxygen level at least one order of magnitude less than that likely to occur in nerve tissue. Studies to better understand the mechanism(s) of nitroimidazole neurotoxicity are being undertaken in several laboratories at present in order to provide improved methods of protection from this dose-limiting toxicity.

6. SUMMARY AND CONCLUSION

Experience to date with MISO has clearly demonstrated the ability of these drugs to sensitize hypoxic radiation resistant tumor cells both in cell and spheroid cultures and in many different types of animal tumors. Most aerobic tissues do not appear to be sensitized when these drugs are combined with radiation. These effects have been confirmed in humans. Nevertheless, early results from clinical trials indicate that these two sensitizers are not likely to significantly improve most tumor responses in the clinic. This is mainly because of dose-limiting neurotoxicity and pharmacological properties.

Despite the limitations with these particular sensitizers, intensive research in this field over the past decade involving close interaction between laboratory scientists and clinical oncologists has rapidly expanded our knowledge so that at this time there is considerable optimism that, of the many new sensitizers which have been synthesized, agents will be found which will prove to be even more clinically effective as radiation sensitizers and with less toxicity.

As often occurs in research, another new and exciting area of investigation has resulted from the discovery that certain radiation sensitizers can also enhance the response of tumor cells to specific cancer chemotherapy agents. This recent development of a potentially new class of drug which might be effective in combination with other drugs as well as with radiation has stimulated considerable basic research into the characteristics of hypoxic tumor cells, their contribution to drug resistance in tumors, mechanisms and effectiveness of the interaction of sensitizers with different classes of drugs, and responses of tumors and normal tissues in animals. Results of these studies and further clinical evaluation of new sensitizers hold great promise for future significant impact of these combined modalities on cancer therapy.

ACKNOWLEDGEMENTS

The authors would like to gratefully acknowledge support from NIH Grants CA-20329, CA-11051, CA-11191 and NS-16147.

REFERENCES

1. Crabtree HG, Cramer W: Action of radium on cancer cells; some factors determining susceptibility of cancer cells to radium. Eleventh scientific report on the investigation of the Imperial Cancer Research Fund: 89–101, 1934.
2. Churchill-Davidson I: The oxygen effect in radiotherapy. Oncologia 20:18–29, 1966.
3. Dewey DL: Effect of oxygen and nitric oxide on radiosensitivity of human cells in tissue culture. Nature 186:780–782, 1960.
4. Elkind MM, Whitmore GF: The Radiobiology of Cultured Mammalian Cells. Gordon and Breach, New York, 1967.
5. Andrews JR: The Radiobiology of Human Cancer Radiotherapy. 2nd edition, Baltimore, University Park Press, 1978.
6. Hall EJ: Radiobiology for the Radiologist. 2nd ed., Harper and Row, Hagerstown, Md., 1978.
7. Denekamp J: Testing of hypoxic cell radiosensitizers *in vivo*. Cancer Clin Trials 3:139–

148, 1980.
8. Bush RS, Jenkin RDT, Allt WEC, Beale FA, Beau H, Dembo AJ, Pringle JF: Definitive evidence for hypoxic cells influencing cure in cancer therapy. Br J Cancer 37 (Suppl. III): 302–206, 1978.
9. Dische S: Hyperbaric oxygen: The Medical Research Council trials and their clinical significance. Br J Radiol 51:888–894, 1979.
10. Adams GE, Asquith JD, Dewey DL, Foster JL, Michael DB, Willson RL: Electron-affinic sensitization II. p-Nitroacetophenone: a radiosensitizer for anoxic bacteria and mammalian cells. Int J Radiat Biol 19:575–585, 1971.
11. Foster JL, Willson RL: Radiosensitization of anoxic cells by metronidazole. Br J Radiol 46:234–235, 1973.
12. Asquith JC, Watts ME, Patel K, Smithen CE, Adams GE: Electron-affinic sensitization. V. Sensitization of hepoxic bacteria and mammalian cells *in vitro* by some nitroimidazoles and nitropyrazoles. Radiat. Res., 60:108–118, 1974.
13. Hall EJ, Roizin-Towle L, Theus RB, August LS: Radiobiological properties of high energy cyclotron-produced neutrons used for radiotherapy. Radiology 117:173–178, 1975.
14. Adams GE, Flockhart IR, Smithen CE, Stratford IJ, Wardman P, Watts ME: Electron-affinic sensitization. VII. A correlation between structures, one-electron reduction potentials and efficiencies of nitroimidazoles as hypoxic cell radiosensitizers. Radiat Res 67:9–20, 1976.
15. Whitmore GF, Gulyas S, Varghese AJ: Sensitizing and toxicity properties of misonidazole and its derivatives. Br J Cancer 37 (Suppl III):115–119, 1978.
16. Chapman JD, Urtasun RC, Blakely EA, Smith KC, Tobias CA: Hypoxic cell sensitizers and heavy charged-particle radiations. Br J Cancer 37 (Suppl III):184–188, 1978.
17. Chapman JD, Dugle DL, Reuvers AP, Meeker BE, Borsa J: Studies on the radiosensitizing effect of oxygen in chinese hamster cells. Int J Radiat Biol 26:383–390, 1974.
18. Whillans DW, Hunt JW: Rapid mixing studies of the mechanisms of chemical radiosensitization and protection in mammalian cells. Br J Cancer 37 (Suppl III):38–41, 1978.
19. Chapman JD, Reuvers AP, Borsa J, Greenstock CL: Chemical radioprotection and radiosensitization of mammalian cells growing *in vitro*. Radiat Res 56:291–302, 1973.
20. Adams GE, Dewey DL: Hydrated electrons and radiobiological sensitization. Biochem Biophys Res Comm 12:473–477, 1963.
21. Adams GE: Chemical radiosensitization of hypoxic cells. Br Med Bulletin 29:48–53, 1973.
22. Adams GE, Clarke ED, Flockhart IR, Jacobs RS, Shemi DS, Stratford IJ, Wardman P, Watts ME, Parrick J, Wallace RG, Smithen CE: Structure-activity relationships in the development of hypoxic cell radiosensitizers. I. Sensitizing efficiency. Int J Radiat Biol 35:133–150, 1979.
23. Chapman JD, Reuvers AP, Borsa J, Petkau A, McCalla DR: Nitrofurans as radiosensitizers of hypoxic mammalian cells. Cancer Res 32:2616–2624, 1972.
24. Chapman JD, Reuvers AP, Borsa J: Effectiveness of nitrofuran derivatives in sensitizing hypoxic mammalian cells to X-rays. Br J Radiol 46:623–630, 1973.
25. Parker L, Skarsgard LD, Emmerson PT: Sensitization of anoxic mammalian cells to X-rays by triacetoneamine-N-oxyl; survival and toxicity studies. Radiat Res 38:493–500, 1969.
26. Adams GE, Asquith JC, Watts ME, Smithen CE: Radiosensitization of hypoxic cells *in vitro*: a water soluble derivative of paranitroacetophenone. Nature 239:23–24, 1972.
27. Hewitt HB, Blake ER: Studies of the toxicity and radiosensitizing activity of triacetoneamine-N-oxyl in mice. Br J Radiol 43:91–96, 1970.
28. Denekamp J, Michael BD: Preferential sensitization of hypoxic cells to radiation *in vivo*.

Nature 239:21–23, 1972.
29. Whitmore GF: The potential for radiation sensitizers and possible strategy for use. Laryngoscope, LXXXV:1145–1154, 1975.
30. Rauth AM, Kaufman K, Thomson JE: *In vivo* testing of hypoxic cell radiosensitizers. In: Radiation Research Biomedical, Chemical and Physical Perspectives. Proceedings of the 5th International Congress of Radiation Research. Eds. Nygaard OF, Adler HI, and Sinclair WK, New York, San Francisco, London, Academic Press, Inc., 761–772, 1975.
31. Adams GE: Hypoxic cell sensitizers for radio-therapy. In: Cancer. A Comprehensive Treatise, FF Becker, ed., Vol. 6, Plenum Press, N.Y., 181–224, 1977.
32. Fowler JF, Denekamp J: A review of hypoxic cell radiosensitization in experimental tumours. J Pharmacol Ther 7:413–444, 1979.
33. Fowler JF, Adams GE, Denekamp J: Radiosensitizers of hypoxic cells in solid tumors. Cancer Treat Rev 3:227–256, 1976.
34. Denekamp J, Hirst GD, Stewart FA, Terry NHA: Is tumour radiosensitization by misonidazole a general phenomenon? Br J Cancer 41:1–9, 1980.
35. Begg AC, Sheldon PW, Foster JL: Demonstration of radiosensitization of hypoxic cells in solid tumours by metronidazole. Br J Radiol 47:399–404, 1974.
36. Stone HB, Withers HR: Tumor and normal tissue response to metronidazole and irradiation in mice. Radiology 113:441–444, 1974.
37. Brown JM: Selective radiosensitization of the hypoxic cells of mouse tumors with the nitroimidazoles metronidazole and Ro-07-0582. Radiat Res 64:633–647, 1975.
38. Sheldon PW, Hill SA: Further investigations on the effects of the hypoxic-cell radiosensitizer, Ro-07-0582, on local control of a mouse tumour. Br J Cancer 36:198–205, 1977.
39. Hill RP, Bush RS: The effect of misonidazole in combination with radiation dose fractionation. Br J Cancer 37 (Suppl III):255–258, 1978.
40. Suit HD, Brown JM: Relative efficacy of high-pressure oxygen and misonidazole to reduce TCD_{50} of a mouse mammary carcinoma. Br J Radiol 52:159–160, 1979.
41. Brown JM: Cytotoxic effects of the hypoxic cell radiosensitizer Ro-07-0582 to tumor cells *in vivo.* Radiat Res 72:469–486, 1977.
42. Stanley JA, Peckham MJ, Steel GG: Influence of tumour size on radiosensitization by misonidazole. Br J Cancer 37 (Suppl. III):220–224, 1978.
43. Davies BMA, Watling DC: An *in vivo* investigation of the radiosensitization of metastases by nitroimidazoles. Int J Radiat Oncol Biol Phys 4:809–819, 1978.
44. Siemann DW, Kochanski, K: Combinations of radiation and misonidazole in a murine lung tumor model. Radiat Res 86:381–391, 1981.
45. Yuhas JM, Yurconic M, Kligerman MM, West G, Peterson, DF: Combined use of radioprotective and radiosensitizing drugs in experimental radiotherapy. Radiat Res 70:433–443, 1977.
46. Hendry JH: Sensitization of hypoxic normal tissue. Br J Cancer, 37 (Suppl. III):232–234, 1978.
47. Gonzales DG, Breur K: Dose-modifying effect of misonidazole on the radiation response of growing cartilage in mice. Br J Cancer 37 (Suppl. III):235–236, 1978.
48. Hornsey S, Field SB: The effect of single and fractionated doses of X-rays and neutrons on the oesophagus. Eur J Cancer 15:491–498, 1979.
49. Sheldon PW, Fowler JF: Radiosensitization by misonidazole (Ro-07-0582) of fractionated X-rays in a murine tumour. Br J Cancer, 37 (Suppl. III):242–245, 1978.
50. Fowler JF, Sheldon PW, Denekamp J, Field SD: Optimum fractionation of the C3H mouse mammary carcinoma using X-rays, the hypoxic cell radiosensitizer Ro-07-0582, or fast neutrons. Int J Radiat Oncol Biol Phys 1:579–592, 1976.
51. Denekamp J, Harris SR: The response of a transplantable tumor to fractionated irradia-

tion. 1. X-rays and the hypoxic cell radiosensitizer Ro-07-0582. Radiat Res 66:66–75, 1976.
52. Denekamp J Stewart FA: Sensitization of mouse tumours using fractionated X-irradiation. Br J Cancer 37 (Suppl. III):259–263, 1978.
53. Rofstad EK, Brustad T: Radiosensitizing effect of misonidazole in athymic nude mice. Br J Radiol 52:393–397, 1979.
54. Urtasum RC, Band P, Chapman JD, Feldstein JL, Mielke B, Fryer CG: Radiation and high dose metronidazole in supratentorial gliomas. N Eng J Med 294:1364–1367, 1976.
55. Urtasun RC, Band PR, Chapman JD, Rabin H, Wilson AF, Fryer CG.: Clinical phase I study of the hypoxic cell radiosensitizer Ro-07-0582, a 2-nitroimidazole derivative. Radiology 22:801–804, 1977.
56. Deutsch G, Foster JL, McFadzean JA, Parnell M: Human studies with high dose metronidazole: a non-toxic radiosensitizer of hypoxic cells. Br J Cancer 31:75–80, 1975.
57. Dische S, Saunders MI, Lee ME, Adams GE, Flockhart IR: Clinical testing of the radiosensitizer Ro-07-0582: experience with multiple doses. Br J Cancer 35:568–579, 1977.
58. Dische S: Misonidazole in the clinic at Mount Vernon. Cancer Clin Trials 3:175–178, 1980.
59. Gray AJ, Dische S, Adams GE, Flockhart IR, Foster JL: Clinical testing of the radiosensitizer Ro-07-0582. Dose tolerance, serum and tumor concentration. Clin Radiol 27:151–157, 1976.
60. Wasserman TH, Phillips TG, Johnson RJ, Gomer CJ, Lawrence AG, Sadee W, Marques RA, Levin TA, Van Raaltie G: Initial clinical and pharmacological evaluation of misonidazole (Ro-07-0582), a hypoxic cell radiosensitizer. Int J Radiat Oncol Biol Phys 5:775–786, 1979.
61. Wasserman TH, Stetz J, Phillips TL: Clinical trials of misonidazole in the United States. In: Radiation Sensitizers, their use in the Clinical Management of Cancer. Brady LW, (Ed.), Masson Publishing, USA, Inc. N.Y., 387–396, 1980.
62. Kogelnik HD: Clinical experience wiht misonidazole. High dose fractions versus daily low fractions. Cancer Clin Trials 3:179–186, 1980.
63. Thomlinson RH, Dische S, Gray AJ, Errington LM: Clinical testing of the radiosensitizer Ro-07-0582. III. Response of tumours. Clin Radiol 27:167–174, 1976.
64. Ash DV, Peckham MJ, Steel GG: The quantitative response of human tumours to radiation and misonidazole. Br J Cancer 40:883–889, 1979.
65. Bleehan NM: The Cambridge glioma trial of misonidazole and radiation therapy with associated pharmacokinetic studies, Cancer Clin Trials 3:267–273, 1980.
66. Jentzsch K, Karchar KH, Kogelnik HD, Maida E, Mannoli B, Wessely P, Zambauer F, Nitsche V: Initial clinical experience with the radiosensitizing nitroimidazole Ro-07-0582. Strahlenterapie, 153:825–531, 1977.
67. Wiltshire CR, Workman P, Watson JV, Bleehan NM: Clinical studies with misonidazole. Br J Cancer 37 (Suppl. III):286–289, 1978.
68. Brown JM, Workman P: Partition coefficient as a guide to the development of radiosensitizers which are less toxic than misonidazole. Radiat Res 82:171–190, 1980.
69. Brown JM, Yu NY, Brown DM, Lee WW: SR-2508 and SR-2555: 2-nitroimidazole amides which appear superior to misonidazole as radiosensitizers for clinical use. Int J Radiat Oncol Biol Phys 7:695–703, 1981.
70. Sutherland RM: Selective chemotherapy of noncycling cells in an *in vitro* tumor model. Cancer Res 34:3501–3503, 1974.
71. Hall EJ, Roizin-Towle L: Hypoxic sensitizers: Radiobiological studies at the cellular level. Radiobiology 117:453–457, 1975.
72. Mohindra RC, Rauth AM: Increased cell killing by metronidazole and nitrofurazone of

hypoxic compared to aerobic mammalian cells. Cancer Res 36:930–936, 1976.
73. Moore BA, Palcic B, Skarsgard LD: Radiosensitizing and toxic effects of the 2-nitroimidazole Ro-07-0582 in hypoxic mammalian cells. Radiat Res 67:459–473, 1976.
74. Sridhar R, Koch C, Sutherland R: Cytotoxicity of two mitroimidazole radiosensitizers in an *in vitro* tumor model. Int J Radiat Oncol Biol Phys 1:1149–1157, 1976.
75. Hall EJ, Astor M, Geard C, Biaglow J: Cytotoxicity of Ro-07-0582: Enhancement by hyperthermia and protection by cysteamine. Br J Cancer 35:809–815, 1977.
76. Stratford IJ, Adams GE: Effect of hyperthermia on differential cytotocity of a hypoxic cell radiosensitizer, Ro-07-0582, on mammalian cells *in vitro*. Br J Cancer 35:307–313, 1977.
77. Sutherland R, MacFarlane W: Cytotoxicity of radiosensitizers in multicel spheroids: Combination treatment with hyperthermia. Br J Cancer 37:Suppl. III, 168–172, 1978.
78. Sridhar R, Sutherland R: Hyperthermic potentiation of cytotoxicity of Ro-07-0582 in multicell spheroids. Int J Radiat Oncol Biol Phys 2:531–535, 1977.
79. Stratford IJ, Gray P: Some factors affecting the specific toxicity of misonidazole towards hypoxic mammalian cells. Br J Cancer 37:Suppl. III, 129–131, 1978.
80. Taylor YC, Rauth AM: Differences in the toxicity and metabolism of the 2-nitroimidazole misonidazole (Ro-07-0582) in HeLa and Chinese hamster ovary cells. Cancer Res 38:2745–3752, 1978.
81. Whitmore CF, Gulyas S: The lethal and sublethal effects of misonidazole under hypoxic conditions. In: Radiation Sensitizers: Their Use in the Clinical Management of Cancer. Brady L. (Ed.) Masson Publishing USA, Inc., N.Y., Chap. 15, pp. 99–106, 1980.
82. Biaglow JE: The effect of hypoxic cell radiosensitizing drugs on cellular oxygen utilization. Pharmac Ther 10:283–299, 1980.
83. Koch C, Biaglow JE: Toxicity, radiation sensitivity modification, and metabolic effects of dehydroascorbate and ascorbate in mammalian cells. J Cell Physiol 94:299–306, 1978.
84. Mason RP, Holtzman J: The role of catalytic superoxide formation in the O_2 inhibition of nitroreductase. Biochem Biophys Res Commun 67:1267–1274, 1975.
85. Wardman P, Clarke ED: Oxygen inhibition of nitroreductase: Electron transfer from nitro radical-anions to oxygen. Biochem Biophys Res Comm 69:942–949, 1976.
86. Sealy RC, Swartz HM, Olive PL: Electron spin resonance spin trapping. Detection of superoxide formation during aerobic microsomal reduction of nitro compounds. Biochem. Biophys. Res. Commun 82:680–684, 1978.
87. Varghese AJ, Gulyas S, Mohindra JK: Hypoxia dependent reduction of 1-(2-nitro-1-imidazolyl)-3-methoxy-2-propanol by Chinese hamster ovary cells and KHT tumor cells *in vitro* and *in vivo*. Cancer Res 36:3761–3765, 1976.
88. Varghese AJ, Whitmore GF: Binding to cellular macromolecules as a possible mechanism for the cytotoxicity of misonidazole. Cancer Res 40:2165–2169, 1980.
89. Varghese AJ, Whitmore GF: Binding of nitroreduction products of misonidazole to nucleic acids and protein. Cancer Clinical Trials 3:43–46, 1980.
90. Knight RC, Rowley DA, Skolimowski I, Edwards DI: Mechanism of action of nitroimidazole antimicrobial and antitumour radiosensitizing drugs. Effects of reduced misonidazole on DNA. Int J Radiat Biol 36:367–375, 1979.
91. Rowley DA, Knight RC, Skolimowski IM, Edwards DI: The relationship between misonidazole cytotoxicity and base composition of DNA. Biochem Pharm 29:2095-2098, 1980.
92. Whitmore GF, Gulyas S, Varghese AJ: Sensitizing and toxicity properties of misonidazole and its derivatives. Br J Cancer 37:Suppl. III, 115–119, 1978.
93. Palcic B, Skarsgard LD: Cytotoxicity of misonidazole and DNA damage in hypoxic mammalian cells. Br J Cancer 37:Suppl. III, 54–57, 1978.

94. Olive PL: Mechanisms of the *in vitro* toxicity of nitroheterocycles, including Flagyl and misonidazole. In: Radiation Sensitizers: Their Use in the Clinical Management of Cancer, Luther W. Brady (ed), New York, Masson Publishing, 1980, p. 39–44.
95. Varnes ME, Biaglow JE, Koch CJ, Koch EJ: Depletion of non-protein thiols of hypoxic cells by misonidazole and metronidazole. In: Radiation Sensitizers: Their Use in the Clinical Management of Cancer, Luther W. Brady (ed), New York, Masson Publishing, 1980, p. 121–126.
96. Ainsworth PJ, Channon M, Sridhar R, Gushulak B, Tustanoff ER: Effect of radiosensitizing agents on electron transport systems. Can J Biochem 56:457–461, 1978.
97. Song CW, Clement JJ, Levitt SH: Cytotoxic and radiosensitizing effects of 5-thio-D-glucose on hypoxic cells. Radiology 123:201–205, 1977.
98. Wong TW, Whitmore GF, Gulyas S: Studies on the toxicity and radiosensitizing ability of Ro-07-0582 under conditons of prolonged incubation. Radiat Res 75:541–555, 1978.
99. Stratford IJ, Adams GE, Horsman MR, Kandaiya S, Rajaratnam S, Smith E, Williamson C: The interaction of misonidazole with radiation, chemotherapeutic agents or heat. Cancer Clin Trials 3:231–236, 1980.
100. Taylor YC: Modifiers of the toxicity and metabolism of misonidazole, a hypoxic cell radiation sensitizer. Ph.D. Thesis, University of Toronto, 1980.
101. Josephy PD, Palcic B, Skarsgard LD: Ascorbate-enhanced cytotoxicity of misonidazole. Nature 271:370–372, 1978.
102. Koch CJ, Howell RL, Biaglow JE: Ascorbate anion potentiates cytotoxicity of nitro-aromatic compounds under hypoxic and anoxic conditions. Br J Cancer 39:321–329, 1979.
103. Taylor YC, Rauth AM: Sulphydryls, ascorbate and oxygen as modifiers of the toxicity and metabolism of misonidazole *in vitro*. Br J Cancer 41:892–900, 1980.
104. Sutherland RM: The multicellular spheroid system as a tumor model for studies of radiation sensitizers. Pharmac Ther 8:105–123, 1980.
105. Olive PL, Durand RE: Activation of radiosensitizers by hypoxic cells. Br J Cancer 37:Suppl. III, 124–128, 1978.
106. Sutherland RM, Durand RE: Radiation response of multicell spheroids-an *in vitro* tumor model. Current Topics in Radiat Res Quarterly 11:87–129, 1976.
107. Sutherland R, Richardson J, Koch C, Sridhar R: Radiation sensitization and cytotoxicity of metronidazole in an *in vitro* tumor model. Metronidazole: Proceedings Montreal, May 26-28, Exerpta Medica, 193–203, 1977.
108. Sutherland RM, Bareham BJ, Reich KA: Cytotoxicity of hypoxic cell sensitizers in multicell spheroids. Cancer Clinical Trials 3:73–83, 1980.
109. Brown JM: Cytotoxic effects of the hypoxic cell radiosensitizer Ro-07-0582 to tumor cell *in vivo*. Radiat Res 72:469–486, 1977.
110. Conroy PJ, Sutherland RM, Passalacqua W: Cytotoxicity of misonidazole *in vivo*: A comparison of large single doses with smaller doses and prolonged contact of the drug with tumor cells. Radiat Res 83:169–189, 1980.
111. Rauth AM, Paciga JE, Mohindra JK: *In vivo* studies of the cytotoxicity of hypoxic cell radiosensitizers. In: Radiation Sensitizers: Their Use in the Clinical Management of Cancer, Luther W. Brady (ed), New York, Masson Publishing, 1980, p. 207–214.
112. Hill RP, Stanley JA: The response of hypoxic B16 melanoma cells to *in vivo* treatment with chemotherapeutic agents. Cancer Res 35:1147–1153, 1975.
113. Hill RP: Combined nitrogen mustard-radiation studies with a mouse tumor. Int J Radiat Oncol Biol Phys 5:1611–1616, 1979.
114. Sutherland RM, Eddy HA, Bareham B, Reich K, Vanantwerp D: Resistance to adriamycin in multicellular spheroids. Int J Radiat Oncol Biol Phys 5:1225–1230, 1979.
115. Tannock IF: Population kinetics of carcinima cells, capillary endothelial cells, and fibro-

blasts in a transplanted mouse mammary tumour. Cancer Res 30:2470–2476, 1970.
116. Steel GG: Growth kinetics of tumours. Clarendon Press, Oxford, 1977.
117. Rauth AM, Chin J, Marchow L, Paciga J: Testing of hypoxic cell radiosensitzers *in vivo*. Br J Cancer 37 (Suppl. III):202–205, 1978.
118. Clement JJ, Gorman MS, Wodinsky I, Catane R, Johnson RK: Enhancement of antitumor activity of alkylating agents by the radiation sensitizer misonidazole. Cancer Res 40:4165–4172, 1980.
119. Rose CM, Miller JL, Peacock JH, Phelps TA, Stephens TC: Differential enhancement of melphalan cytotoxicity in tumor and normal tissue by misonidazole. Cancer Clin Trials, in press, 1980.
120. Tannock I: The *in vivo* interaction of anti-cancer drugs with misonidazole or metronidazole: cyclophosphamide and BCNU. Br J Cancer 42:871–880, 1980.
121. Tannock I: The *in vivo* interaction of anti-cancer drugs with misonidazole or metronidazole: methotrexate, 5-fluorouracil and adriamycin. Br J Cancer 42:861–870, 1980.
122. Mulcahy RT, Siemann DW, Sutherland RM: *In vivo* response of KHT sarcomas to combination chemotherapy with radiosensitizers and BCNU. Br J Cancer 43:93–99, 1981.
123. Siemann DW: *In vivo* combination of misonidazole and the chemotherapeutic agent CCNU. Br J Cancer, 43:361–377, 1981.
124. Law MP, Hirst DG, Brown JM: Enhancing effect of misonidazole on the response of the RIF-1 tumour to cyclophosphamide. Br J Cancer, in press, 1981.
125. Urtasun RC, Chapman JD, Feldstein JL, Band PR, Rabin HR, Wilson AF, Marynowski B, Starreveld E, Shnitka T: Peripheral neuropathy related to misonidazole: incidence and pathology. Br J Cancer, 37 (Suppl. III):271–275, 1978.
126. Dische S, Sanders MI, Anderson P, Urtasun RC, Karcher KH, Kogelnik HD, Bleehan HD, Bleehan NH, Phillips TL, Wasserman TH: The neurotoxicity of misonidazole: The pooling of data from 5 centers. Br J Radiol 51:1023–1024, 1978.
127. Dische S, Saunders MI, Flockhart IR, Lee ME, Anderson P: Misonidazole, a drug for trial in radiotherapy and oncology. Int J Radiat Oncol Biol Phys 5:851–860, 1979.
128. Frytak S, Moertal CG, Childs DS, Albers JW: Neurologic toxicity associated with high-dose metronidazole therapy. Ann Intern Med 88:361–362, 1978.
129. Saunders MI, Dische S, Anderson P, Flockhart IR: The neurotoxicity of misonidazole and its relationship to dose, half-life and concentration in the serum. Br J Cancer 37 (Suppl. III):268–270, 1978.
130. Wasserman TH, Phillips TL, Van Raaltee G., Urtasun RC, Parkington J, Kozio A, Schwade JG, Ganfji D, Strong JM: The neurotoxicity of misonidazole: potential modifying role of phenytoin sodium and dexamethasone. Br J Radiol 53:172–173, 1980.
131. Thomas GM, Rawth AM, Bush RS, Black BE, Cummings BJ: A toxicity study of daily dose metromidazole with pelvic irradiation. Cancer Clin Trials 3:223–230, 1980.
132. Kogelnik HD, Meyer HJ, Jentzsch K, Szepesi T, Karcher KH, Maida E, Mandi B, Wessely P, Zawnbauer F: Further clinical experiences of a phase I study with the hypoxic cell radiosensitizer misonidazole. Br J Cancer 37 (Suppl. III):281–285, 1978.
133. McNally NJ, Danekamp J, Sheldon PW, Flockhart IR, Stewart PA: Radiosensitivity by misonidazole (Ro-07-0582): the importance of timing and of tumor concentrations. Radiat Res:568–580, 1978.
134. Brown JM, Yu NY, Workman P: Pharmacokinetic considerations in testing hypoxic cell radiosensitizers. Br J Cancer 39:310–320, 1979.
135. Foster JL, Flockhart IR, Dische S, Gray AJ, Lenox-Smith I, Smithen CE: Serum concentration measurements in man of the radiosensitzer Ro-07-0582: some primary results. Br J Cancer 31:679–682, 1975.
136. Workman P, Bleehan NM, Wiltshire CR: Phenytoin shortens the half-life of the hypoxic

cell radiosensitizer misonidazole in man: implications for possible reduced toxicity. Br J Cancer 41:302–304, 1980.

137. Workman P: The effects of pretreatment with phenobarbitone or phenytoin on the pharmacokinetics and toxicity of misonidazole in mice. Br J Cancer 40:163:396–402, 1979.
138. Ramsay ID: Endocrine opthalmopathy, Br Med J 4:706–708, 1968.
139. Coxon A, Pallis CA: Metronidazole neuropathy. J Neurol Neurosurg Psychiatry 39:403–405, 1976.
140. Bradley WG, Karlsson IJ, Rassol CG: Metronidazole neuropathy. Br Med J 2:610–1977.
141. Cooper JS: Evaluation of ototoxicity in humans treated with misonidazole. In: Neurotoxicity of Hypoxic Cell Radiosensitizers, Proceedings of conference sponsored by Division of Cancer Treatment, NCI, NIH, Bethesda, Maryland, March, 1980.
142. Cooper JS, Fife KD, Borok TL, Waltzman SB: Detection of toxicity from the readiosensitizing drug misonidazole by serial audiograms. In: Radiation Sensitizers, Their Use in the Clinical Management of Cancer. Brady LW, (Ed). Masson Publishing, USA, Inc., N.Y., p. 490–494, 1980.
143. Hirst DE, Vojnovic B, Stratford IJ, Travis EL: The effect of the radiosensitizer misonidazole on motor nerve conduction velocity in the mouse. Br J Cancer 37 (Suppl. III) 237–281, 1978.
144. Hirst DE, Vojnovic B, Hobson B: Changes in nerve conduction velocity in the mouse after acute and chronic administration of nitroimidazoles. Br J Cancer 38:159–167, 1979.
145. Von Burg R, Conroy PJ, Passalacqua W: Peripheral electrophysiological parameters in mice treated with misonidazole. Br J Cancer 40:34–143, 1979.
146. Conroy PJ, VonBurg R, Passalacqua W, Penney DP, Sutherland RM: Misonidazole neurotoxicity in the mouse. Evaluation of functional, pharmacokinetic, electrophysiologic and morphologic parameters. Int J Radiat Oncol Biol Phys 5:983–991, 1979.
147. Conroy PJ, VonBurg R, Penney DP, Passalacqua W, Sutherland RM: Effect of acute and chronic misonidazole administration or peripheral-nerve electrophysiology in mice. Br J Cancer 41:523–527, 1980.
148. Edwards MS, Jewett DL, Bolger C, Phillips TL, Levin V: Diagnosis of misonidazole neurotoxicity by nerve train evoked responses. In: Neurotoxicity of Hypoxic Cell Radiosensitizers, Proceedings of conference sponsored by Division of Cancer Treatment, NCI, NIH, Bethesda, Maryland, March 1980.
149. Maurissen JPJ, Conroy PJ, Passalacqua W, VonBurg R, Weiss B, Sutherland RM. Somatosensory deficits in monkeys treated with misonidazole. Toxicol Appl Pharm 57:119–126, 1981.
150. Johnson RJR: Studies of the neuropathy produced by misonidazole and desmethylmisonidazole in mice. In: Neurotoxicity of Hypoxic Cell Radiosensitizers. Proceedings of Conference sponsored by Division of Cancer Treatment, NCI, NIH, Bethesda, Maryland, March 1980.
151. Subject JR, Chao CF, Johnson RJR, Drechsel R, Repasky E: Behavioral, ultrastructural and gel electrophoresis studies of misonidazole-induced neuropathy in mice. In: Radiation Sensitizers, Their use in the Clinical Management of Cancer. Brady LW (Ed.) Masson Publishing USA, Inc., N.Y., p. 478–484, 1980.
152. Conroy PJ, Shaw AB, McNeill TH, Passalacqua W, Sutherland RM. Radiation sensitizer neurotoxicity in the mouse. In: Radiation Sensitizers, Their use in the Clinical Management of Cancer. Brady LW (Ed.) Masson Publishing USA, Inc., N.Y., p. 397–410, 1980.
153. Rogulja PV, Kovac W, Schmid H: Metronidazole-encephalopathie der Ratte. Acta Neuropath. (Berl) 25:36–45, 1973.
154. Tellez I, Terry R: Fine structure of the early changes in the vestibular nuclei of the thiam-

ine deficient rat. Am J Path 52:777–794, 1968.
155. Chan-Palay V: Indoleamine neurons and their processes in the normal rat brain and in chronic diet-induced thiamine deficient animals. J Comp Neurol 176:567–594, 1977.
156. Griffin JW, Price DL, Kuethe DO, Goldberg AM: Neurotoxicology of misonidazole in rats. I. Neuropathology. Neurotoxicology 1:299–312, 1979.
157. Griffin JW: Neurotoxicity of misonidazole in rats. In: Neurotoxicity of Hypoxic Cell Radiosensitizers, Proceedings of Conference sponsored by Division of Cancer Treatment, NCI, NIH, Bethesda, Maryland, March 1980.
158. Scharer K: Selective Purkinje-Zellschadigungen nach orater Verabreichung grosser dosen von nitroimidazol-derivaten am und. Verhandlunger der Deutschen Geselschaft für Pathologie 56:407–410, 1972.
159. Parkes MW: cited in Gray AJ, Dische S, Adams GE, Glockhart IR, Foster JL: Clinical testing of the radiosensitizer Ro-07-0582. I. Dose tolerance, serum and tumor concentrations. Clin Radiol 27:151–157, 1976.
160. Conroy PJ, Shaw AB: Nitroimidazole neurotoxicity: quantitative evaluation by behavioral and biochemical methods in the mouse. Radiat Res 83:468, 1980.
161. Conroy PJ: Comparative neurotoxicity of radiation sensitizers in the mouse. Abs 3932 72nd Mtg Amer Assoc Cancer Res Washington, D.C., April 1981.
162. Dunham NW, Miya TS: A note on a simple apparatus for detecting neurological deficit in rats and mice. J Am Pharmacol Assoc 46:208–209, 1957.
163. Kaplan ML, Murphy SD: Effect of acrylamide on rotarod performance and sciatic nerve β-glucuronidase activity of rats. Toxicol Appl Pharm 22:259–268, 1972.
164. Dewar AJ, Moffet DJ: Biochemical methods for detecting neurotoxicity—a short review. Pharmac Ther 5:545–562, 1979.
165. Zimmer L, Johnson PC, Carter DE: A comparison of biochemical, pathological or behavioral methods for the assessment of the effectiveness of treatment for methylmercury poisoning in rats. Neurobehav Toxicol 2:323–330, 1980.
166. Clarke C, Dawson KB, Sheldon PW, Chaplin DJ, Stratford IJ, Adams OE: Quantitative cytochemical method for assessing the neurotoxicity of misonidazole. In: Radiation Sensitizers, their use in the clinical management of Cancer. Brady LW (Ed). Masson Publishing USA, Inc., N.Y., p. 245–249, 1980a.
167. Clarke C: The neurotoxicity of hypoxic cell radiosensitizers. In: Neurotoxicity of Hypoxic Cell Radiosensitizers, Proceedings of conference sponsored by Division of Cancer Treatment, NCI, NIH, Bethesda, Maryland, March, 1980b.
168. Hollinger DM, Rossiter RJ: Chemical studies of peripheral nerve during Wallerian degeneration. Biochem J 52:659–663, 1952.
169. Rose GP, Dewar AJ, Stratford IJ: A biochemical method for assessing the neurotoxic effects of hypoxic cell radiosensitizers: experience with misonidazole: Br J Cancer 42:890–899, 1980.
170. Shaw AB, Conroy PJ: Species difference in biochemical expression of misonidazole neurotoxicity. Abs 72, 20th Mtg Soc Toxicol San Siego, CA, March 1981.
171. VonBurg R, Conroy PJ: Evaluation of the anticholinesterase activity of metronidazole and misonidazole. Eur J Pharmacol 55:417–420, 1979.
172. Clarke C, Hobbiger F, Sheldon PW: Acetylcholinesterase and cholinesterase activities in the mouse cerebellum following misonidazole treatment. Eur J Pharm 69:209–211, 1981.
173. Mamoli B, Wessely P, Kogelnik HD, Muller M, Rathkolb O: Electroneurographic investigations of misonidazole polyneuropathy. Eur Neurol 18:405–414, 1979.
174. Sridhar R: Increased rates of oxygen consumption by catecholamines in the presence of aromatic nitro and nitroso compounds—implications for neurotoxicity and cytotoxicity. Radiat Res 83:466, 1980.

3. A Review of Evidence that the Feline Leukemia Virus (FeLV) might be causative in Childhood Acute Lymphocytic Leukemia (ALL)*

GLEN E. MALONE, JEFFREY ROSEMAN, WILLIAM M. CRIST and RONALD T. ACTON

INTRODUCTION

Approximately 40% of childhood cancer is acute leukemia and non-Hodgkin lymphoma [1, 2], and nearly 85% of all childhood leukemia in the United States and Europe is acute lymphocytic leukemia (ALL) [2, 3]. ALL is of worldwide distribution, and everywhere it tends to be predominantly a disease of children, with most patients being under ten years of age [3–7]. According to the Third National Cancer Survey [8], the average incidence rate in the United States for ALL in children ages 0–14 years is 2.4 per 100,000. In the United States there is no significant regional variation in the incidence of ALL. Nevertheless, the northern region has the lowest incidence rate (1.8/100,000), whereas the southern and western regions of the country share the highest incidence rate (2.9/100,000). The same survey showed a higher incidence rate (2.7/100,000) in males than in females (2.0/100,000) [8]. Most studies have reported a lower incidence of ALL in American blacks [8–11]. Childhood ALL has a peak incidence at about four years of age in white children [3, 8, 12]. Interestingly, American blacks have a different age of peak incidence, 10–14 years of age [8]. In the United States, it has been documented that the frequency of leukemia is more closely associated with socio-economic status than ethnic group [9]. As the socio-economic status increases, the frequency of ALL rises accordingly [13].

There have been a number of agents suggested as causing ALL. These include irradiation, specific genes, benzene, and viruses. This manuscript will review the evidence for the hypotheses concerning the etiology of ALL, with emphasis on the possible role of the Feline Leukemia Virus (FeLV).

* This investigation was supported by grants number CA09128 and CA-25408, awarded by the National Cancer Institute, DHEW.

G. Bennett Humphrey et al. (eds), Adrenal and Endocrine Tumors in Children.

Variations in clinical presentation and immunologic origins of the lymphoid cells involved and response to therapy make it apparent that ALL is a heterogenous group of diseases [14]. As shown in Table 1, several methods of biologic assessment of ALL cells have permitted classification into at least four distinct subgroups: T-cell, B-cell, pre B-cell, and non-B, non-T-cell ALL [5, 14–18]. Methods of cell lineage assessment of ALL include cytochemical stains such as acid phosphatase and esterase [19], and the use of monoclonal or heteroclonal antibodies against T- and B-cell antigens [20–23] or against common acute leukemia cell antigen (CALLA) [23]. Currently, rosette formation with sheep erythrocytes is the most widely used marker for human T-cells [19]. The presence of surface immunoglobulin (sIg) identifies B-lymphocytes and cytoplasmic immunoglobulin (cIg), pre B lymphoid cells [23]. Most pre B and non-B, non-T childhood ALL expresses CALLA [23]. Whereas, most cases of T-cell ALL lack this antigen.

Table 1. Methods of determining ALL phenotypes.

	Methods of biologic assessment of ALL phenotypes				
Phenotype	CALLA	E Rosetting	Anti-T monoclonal Abs	SIg	cIg
Non B, Non T	+/–	–	–	–	–
Pre B	+/–	–	–	–	+
B	–	–	–	+	–
T	–	+/–	+	–	–

B-cell ALL, which is rare (approximately 2 percent), has the poorest prognosis; T-cell ALL, which is more common (10–15 percent), also has a poor prognosis; and non B, non T-cell ALL, which is the most common (65 percent) has the best prognosis [14, 15, 17, 24–26]. Recent data suggest that children with pre-B-cell leukemia fare significantly worse than non-B, non-T-cell patients [27]. T-cell ALL often presents with a distinctive clinical syndrome. Such patients are often adolescent males with a high WBC (100,000/mm^3), an anterior mediastinal mass, and extramedullary disease [1].

Recent evidence supports the hypothesis that many cases of T-cell ALL in children represent advanced stages of T-cell non-Hodgkin lymphoma [28, 29]. However, a relatively large group of T-cell ALL is of early thymocyte derivation, as identified by monoclonal antibodies [28, 29, 30]. The early thymocyte T-cell phenotype is rare in the NHL presentation suggesting a tendency of this phenotype to involve marrow and blood early.

ETIOLOGY OF ALL

The etiology of ALL is basically unknown, although a number of host factors and environmental agents have been suggested as causal. Exposure to environmental factors such as irradiation and certain chemicals (particularly benzene) have been implicated in leukemogenesis. Ionizing radiation was one of the first environmental agents incriminated as a cause of leukemia [31, 32]. Studies by the Atomic Bomb Casualty Commission have shown that there is an increased risk of ALL with a single exposure of about 50 rads or more of radiation [33]. Survivors of the atomic bomb explosions at Hiroshima and Nagasaki were found to have developed an excessive amount of leukemia within a 2–6 year period after exposure [32, 34, 35]. March [36] and Ulrich [37] have reported leukemia among radiologists to be 8–10 times greater than in the general population. Within the last decade, leukemia has been observed as a complication of radiotherapy for Wilms' tumor [38]. Chronic benzene exposure has been shown to be leukemogenic in persons occupationally exposed [39, 40]. Manning and Carroll [41] published evidence which suggested that some cases of childhood leukemia might result from exposure to certain pharamacologic agents (i.e., antihistamines, phenylbutazone, chloramphenicol, aspirin) which are toxic to bone marrow in susceptible children.

Associations have been found between several genetic disorders and leukemia. ALL has been shown to occur with increased frequency and earlier in life in children with Down's syndrome [42]. Risk for leukemia is greatly increased in some recessively-transmitted chromosomal disorders, such as Bloom's syndrome [43] and Fanconi's anemia [44]. Patients with ataxia-telangiectasia, a disease with both chromosomal fragility and immunodeficiency, have a strong predisposition for the development of ALL [45]. The specific reasons for the increased risk in these genetic disorders remains unclear. It may reflect increased contact with an environmental agent or a decreased ability to respond to such a challenge.

In mice, the presence of an antigen coded for by a gene in the H-2 region of the Major Histocompatibility Complex (MHC) on chromosome 17 promotes leukemia resistance to infection with viruses known to cause ALL [46] in mice. The specific role of the H-2 linked loci in the resistance to murine leukemia is not known. Resistance, as well as susceptibility, is associated with various regions of the H-2 complex [47]. Meruelo [48] showed that resistance to radiation-induced leukemia virus infection in mice is associated with increased H-2 antigenic expression. His observations suggested that elevated H-2 antigen expression enhances the effectiveness of the mouse's immune responses to virus-infected cells.

Recent studies examining a specific association between ALL and gene products from the MHC in man, including the human leucocyte antigen (HLA) loci, have demonstrated abnormal distribution of certain HLA phenotypes in ALL cases. Specifically, HLA-A2 has been found significantly associated with increased risk for ALL [49–51]. However, conflicting results were presented by Grumet [52], who concluded from his studies that the HLA-A2 antigen was associated with better prognosis in affected persons, rather than an increased risk for the development of the disease. A9 has been reported decreased in ALL patients, and patients with this phenotype appear to have a better prognosis [49, 50, 53, 54]. Recently, patients with A9 have been shown to have a significant increase in early first remission duration [55]. Moreover, patients treated with transfer factor who had the A2B1 and/or A2B40 haplotypes survived longer than patients lacking these halotypes [56]. Michel *et al.*, in a small group of patients, found the duration of first remission and survival was longer for those free of DR3 [57], while Révész *et al.* [58] observed a significant association between the presence of DR3 and long remission. Recently Budowle *et al.* [59] observed a significant association of the BfF allele of properdin factor B, that is also coded by a gene at the MHC, with ALL. The relationship of MHC genes to ALL risk is interesting, since the MHC region in man is believed to be analogous to the H-2 region in mice, where the absence or presence of a gene(s) governs susceptibility or resistance to infection with viruses known to cause ALL [46].

For the remainder of this discussion, we will focus on the possible viral causes of ALL. One way by which researchers have attempted to demonstrate a contagious agent in disease etiology is to search for space-time clustering. Studies of clustering of childhood ALL have yielded equivocal results [60–67]. A number of separate 'epidemics' of leukemia have been reported [64–67]. Attempts have been made using a variety of statistical tests for identifying clustering in childhood leukemia. The studies which found some evidence for clustering were conducted by Knox in 1964; Meighan and Knox in 1965; Mainwaring in 1966; and Heath and Hasterlik in 1963. Studies conducted by Pike and Smith in 1974; Smith *et al.* in 1975; Till *et al.* in 1967; and Lock and Merrington in 1967 found no evidence of clustering. Also, there is controversy in the literature concerning the most appropriate statistical technique to use in identifying clusters [60, 61, 63, 68].

The absence of clustering, however, would not exclude the possible role of a transmissible agent, such as a virus, having involvement in disease etiology. The widespread prevalence of a potentially contagious agent, such as FeLV which probably has little variation over time and space, would be expected to yield very little evidence of disease clustering.

Viral etiology has been identified for leukemias in several animal species [69]. Within the last decade, horizontally-transmissible RNA viruses have been documented to cause various types of leukemia and lymphomas in cats [70–72], cattle [73–76], gibbons [77], rodents [78], and fowl [79]. A viral etiology for several human cancers, including some types of leukemias, has been suggested [80]. It is currently felt that a virus must possess a DNA stage for it to transform cells from a normal state to a malignant one [81]. RNA viruses having RNA-dependent DNA polymerase (reverse transcriptase) have the capability of producing virally coded DNA [81]. Baxt *et al.* [82] isolated reverse transcriptase (a hallmark of oncogenic viruses) from leukemic cells of many patients with acute leukemia. Other scientists have reported RNA-instructed DNA polymerase in a significant number of fresh acute human leukemic cells [83]. Gallo *et al.* [84] demonstrated that significant amounts of reverse transcriptase activity could be found in cells of ALL in man, but not in normal lymphocytes transformed to blasts by phytohemagglutination.

The Gross leukemia, radiation-induced leukemia viruses and the Friend virus are C-type RNA viruses (retroviruses) which can cause leukemia in mice. Induction of leukemia in rats by the Gross murine leukemia virus (GLV) is age-dependent, with leukemogenesis occurring only before and briefly after birth [78]. Data by Ioachim [78] showed that the transition from total susceptibility to complete resistance occurred at about two weeks of age. Furthermore, the fact has been well established that the murine type-C RNA virus must be inoculated into newborn or very young mice for successful leukemogenesis to occur [48].

There is evidence that a virus which predominantly infects one species can cause leukemia in a second species. Ioachim *et al.* [85] published data which indicated that lymphoid leukemia could be induced in rats of the same strain by murine GLV, which has been specific for lymphoid leukemia induction in mice. The ability of GLV to induce leukemia was definitely dependent on the age of the recipient. The leukemia induced in rats with murine GLV was lymphoid and almost always involved the thymus.

A viral etiology for an adult form of T-cell leukemia has now been supported [86–89]. As a result of research involving a protein termed T-cell growth factor [90], scientists have recently isolated a novel C-type retrovirus called human malignant T-cell leukemia virus [91, 92]. Cultured human malignant T-cells served as the source of the T-cell leukemia virus. Both epidemiological and biochemical evidence have shown the virus to be associated with adult T-cell leukemias and lymphomas [91, 92].

Many infectious diseases are transmitted between animals and man. The question of oncogenic viral transmission from animal to man has, therefore, been raised [4, 81]. Two animal viruses have been hypothesized as agents which could cause ALL in man, bovine leukemia virus (BLV) and feline leukemia virus. The evidence to support BLV as a cause is sparse. Donham *et al.* [93], presented data indicating an ecologic association of excess ALL in Iowa males, including age group 1–4 years, in rural counties with high populations of dairy cattle, particularly where dairy cattle are infected with BLV.

Drs. P. Gupta and J.F. Ferrer found in a recent study that the blood of cattle infected with BLV contained a factor that specifically blocks the expression of the genetic material of the virus [94]. They believed these results explained why BLV is present in infected cattle in a covert, non-productive manner, in complete contrast to the mechanism in which leukemia viruses of mice, cats, gibbons, and other animals react. The covert, non-productive manner in which BLV reacts in naturally infected cattle implies that while the virus is found within the infected cell in the form of BLV genome, the cell may not be synthesizing viral antigens and viral particles. The scientists noted that if human leukemia viruses do in fact exist, as well as other animal leukemia viruses then they may very well be controlled by a similar blocking factor. BLV, which causes leukemia in cattle and sheep, is often found in cow's milk [95] indicating that humans have an excellent probability of being exposed to BLV orally. Consumption of unpasteurized milk could serve as a source of exposure to the viruses.

A number of facts concerning the nature of feline leukemia and its epidemiological behavior suggest that FeLV should be considered a potential human oncogen [96, 97]. ALL in cats is caused by FeLV, and there are similarities between human and feline ALL in clinical findings, laboratory data, and response to treatment [71, 98]. The feline leukemia virus is a single-stranded, enveloped RNA virus, classed as an oncornavirus [99]. Immunological studies have supported the theory that FeLV-related genes were transmitted from a rodent to the cat ancestor within the last ten million years, based on the immunologic relationships seen between FeLV and endogenous rodent type C-viruses [100]. FeLV has three serotypes (A, B, and C) with A and B being the most commonly occurring types in pet cats [101]. It is a naturally-occurring oncoviral disease in cats which can be transmitted horizontally [70–72, 102, 103]. The virus is present in abundant quantities in many tissues and body fluids, mostly in the salivary glands, suggesting the possibility that the agent may be spread by bite, scratch or aerosolization [96, 103]. Saliva from infected cats can contain from 5×10^3 to 2×10^6 infectious FeLV per ml [104–106]. Epigenetically, FeLV is transmitted via the placenta or the milk [101]. Urine and feces of infected cats have been shown to contain large quantities of FeLV [107], thus indicating that contact with the secretions and excretions of FeLV infected cats can be a mode of transmission.

The estimated prevalence of FeLV infection among cats appears to depend upon the source of the cats and the type of test used. Some of the tests used to detect FeLV in cats include: indirect immunofluorescent antibody (IFA) test, enzyme-linked immunosorbent assay (ELISA) test, serum neutralizing (SN) antibody test, and feline oncornavirus associated cell membrane antigen (FOCMA) test.

IFA and the ELISA test are tests which detect the presence of the virus. The IFA test detects viral antigens in blood leukocytes and platelets, whereas the ELISA test detects viral antigens in serum or plasma. Using the IFA test, Ladiges *et al.* [108] found a 4.9% prevalence among pound-source cats. With the same diagnostic test, Hardy *et al.* [71, 101] found 0.7% of the cats from single cat households positive for FeLV, and nearly 28% of the cats in multiple cat households positive. Among stray cats, Hardy [109] found 0.9% of the cats positive for FeLV. Combining all three sources, the estimated prevalence of FeLV infection was 14.7%. As a more conservative estimate, based on the IFA test, the prevalence of FeLV infection among cats is about 1–5% [103, 108].

The other two tests used, SN and FOCMA, detect antibodies present against FeLV antigens. These tests estimate the frequency of exposure to FeLV, although not all exposed cats develop antibodies. Based on the SN antibody test, Hardy [101] found 18% of the tested cats had protective titers against FeLV infection. The FOCMA antibody test [109] revealed that nearly 8% of the tested stray cats had protective antibody titers, along with nearly 39% of the uninfected exposed cats. Only 25% of the infected healthy cats were FOCMA positive. During the lifetime of most domestic cats, approximately 15–30% will have mounted an immune response to FeLV.

ALL is the most common type of malignant neoplasm in the domestic cat, accounting for 8–10% of all fatal cat diseases seen in veterinary practice [96, 110, 111]. Lymphomas and aplastic leukemia in the cat are also known to be caused by FeLV [71–73]. Cats with leukemia have been shown to have viral particles which were formed by C-type viruses, 100 to 115 mU in diameter, that bud from the plasma or vacuolar cell membranes [99, 112, 113]. The majority of leukemias and virtually all the mediastinal lymphomas in the cat are of T-cell origin [114].

As with the GLV infectivity relationship in rats there is evidence that the newborn cat is most susceptible to FeLV [115, 116]. When the virus is transmitted to adult cats most cats never develop an overt clinical disease state, although they frequently develop antibodies to the virus [115]. Research by Essex *et al.* [117] indicated that a majority of household cats in the general population are not persistently infected with FeLV, although they do have low titers to feline oncornavirus-associated cell-membrane antigen (FOCMA), indicating that at some period within their lives they were infected with FeLV.

Following infection with FeLV, a susceptible cat may develop either a sufficient immunc response to result in only temperary viremia, or an inadequate immune response resulting in a persistent viremia. With the onset of a persistent viremia, the animal could (a) remain asymptomatic with no clinical disease and be a carrier or (b) be viremic for weeks or years before developing a clinical disease. In other words, cats with perceived good health have been shown to excrete FeLV [94, 101].

There is *in vitro* evidence that FeLV can be transmitted to man.Many investigators have reported that FeLV can be cultivated *in vitro* in human cell lines [96, 103, 113, 118]. One study showed, using human fibroblasts and human lymphoid cell lines, that T-cell lines appeared to be more sensitive to FeLV infection with the production of more virus than the autochthonous B-cells [119]. In addition, various FeLV-related antibodies have been found in people exposed to cats and leukemic cats, in particular [120, 121].

Sordillo *et al.* [122] reported using a number of immunological tests to determine if 230 patients with hematologic cancers or with sarcomas had antibodies to FeLV or FeLV induced antigens. They found no evidence of FeLV exposure with any of the test systems. Of the patients tested, 19.7% were children. No ALL subtypes in children, nor adults, were reported. The authors noted, however, that the negative results should be interpreted with caution in view of the research [123–125] which reveals that in cats with FeLV induced lymphosarcoma 30% will have no evidence of FeLV infection in the form of FeLV antigens, F OCMA antibodies, or FeLV SN antibodies.

A number of epidemiological studies have been done to assess the relationship between cat exposure and human cancers (see Table 2). Evidence has been obtained from epidemiological survey data that exposure to cats, particularly sick cats, is associated with some cases of leukemia in children [126, 127]. The most convincing study is by Bross and Gibson [126]. They examined 300 children with leukemia and a random sample of 831 children from the same geographical areas as controls. Among the children 1–14 years of age, the only statistically significant difference (5% level) between cases and controls occurred with exposure to cats. The overwhelming majority of the cases in the children were ALL. The relative risk for exposure to sick cats was more than double in the leukemic cases. The difference was significant at the one percent level.

In a similar study by Penrose [127], using all lymphoid tumors (N = 28), a twofold increase in exposure to cats was seen in the case households as compared to control households. The author discovered that the households of eight out of twenty-one children who had recently died of leukemia had kept cats (some of which were known to have been sick), in comparison to

Table 2. Epidemiological studies assessing cat exposure and human neoplasia.

Study	Index cases	Comparison group(s)	Cancer(s) of interest	Conclusions
Bross and Gibson [126]	300 children with leukemia	831 children without leukemia from same geographic area	Leukemia	Relative risk for exposure to ill or dead cats was more than double in leukemia cases (p<0.01).
Penrose [127]	28 children with lymphoid tumors	28 children with non-lymphoid tumors	Leukemia Lymphosarcoma Hodgkin Disease	Cases had a twofold increase in exposure to cats.
Bross *et al.* [128]	1400 Adults with leukemia	1370 Adults without leukemia from same geographic areas	Acute lymphatic leukemia; Chronic lymphatic leukemia; Acute myelocytic leukemia; Chronic myelocytic leukemia; Leukemia with incomplete description of type	The largest age and sex adjusted relative risk occurred in cases with ALL and the estimated relative risk for sick cat exposure was greatest (10.6) within the youngest age group [15–44].
Fasal *et al.* [129]	1723 White male California veterinarians	White male California Population of 1960	All cancers subclassified by leukemia	No significant difference between observed and expected deaths for all cancers, but S.M.R. for leukemia 148.9
Botts *et al.* [130]	390 white male Missouri veterinarians	U.S. white males (1960), Missouri white males, and Physician speciallists	All Cancers	No statitistically significant difference in the presence of cancer among the veterinarians as compared to the comparison group.

Table 2. Epidemiological studies assessing cat exposure and human neoplasia (*continued*).

Study	Index cases	Comparison group(s)	Cancer(s) of interest	Conclusions
Schnurrenberger *et al.* [131]	486 Illinois veterinarians	Illinois white male of 1950, 1960 and 1970. California veterinarians* Missouri veterinarians**	All cancers	No statistically significant difference in the frequency of cancer among the Illinois veterinarians as compared to the comparison groups.
Blair and Hayes [132]	1551 white male veterinarians	White males in the U.S. Population	All cancers subclassified by leukemia and Hodgkin disease categories	A significantly high proportion of deaths due to leukemia and Hodgkin's disease seen among clinical practice veterinarians.
Guthensohn *et al.* [133]	19,000 U.S. Veterinarians who died after age 46	U.S. Population and Physicians	Lymphoid tumors	Among the veterinarians an 80% increase in the occurrence of lymphoid tumors was seen.
Schneider [134]	675 households containing cats with confirmed cancer	675 households containing cats with non-neoplastic conditions	All cancers	No increased association of human cancer with feline lymphoma and little evidence of horizontal transmission of cancer from cats to man.

* From reference 129.
** From reference 130.

Table 2. Epidemiological studies assessing cat exposure and human neoplasia (*continued*).

Study	Index cases	Comparison group(s)	Cancer(s) of interest	Conclusions
Hanes *et al.* [135] Survey 1	301 cancer households	301 non-cancer households	Leukemia Lymphoma Sarcoma	An excess of total years exposure to cats in households with lymphoma and in leukemia households the total years of exposure to cats exceeded that of controls.
Survey 2	229 Cancer households	229 non-cancer households matched for age, sex, and duration of residence	Leukemia Lymphoma Sarcoma	No difference in exposure to cats and other pet animals was found between index households and matched control households; however 6 index cases reported infection caused by a cat scratch or bite vs. 0 controls.

five out of an equal number of normal paired control households [127]. None of the differences were statistically significant; however, the sample sizes in the survey were very small.

Bross *et al.* [128] also reported results of a study which explored the relationship between ill or dead cats and occurrence of leukemia in adults. The study [128] consisted of 1400 adults with leukemia and 1370 randomly selected controls from the same geographical area. Adult leukemia cases were obtained from tumor registry listings. They concluded that the degree of relationship depended on the type of leukemia. When the age and sex adjusted relative risks for the exposure to sick cats was calculated, the largest relative risk occurred in those with ALL as compared to those with chronic lymphatic, acute myelocytic, and chronic myelocytic leukemia. The estimated relative risk for sick cat exposure was greatest (10.57) within the youngest age group [15–44].

Several epidemiological studies have reportedly failed to identify any leukemia association with exposure to cats [129–131]; however, as will be shown, most of the negative studies either used only adult samples or mixed various types of cancers. In 1966, Fasal *et al.* [129] conducted a mortality study in white male veterinarians licensed in California between 1950 and 1962 to obtain evidence that cancer in man might be caused by agents transmissible to man from animals. The white male California population of 1960 was used as standard. The study did not demonstrate an increase in total cancer mortality for white male veterinarians. There was no significant difference between observed and expected deaths for any of the cancers analyzed, including leukemia; however the S.M.R. for leukemia was 148.9. The authors did not attempt to separate the different forms of leukemia (ALL versus CLL, etc.) within their study and no children were sampled. The authors did note, however, that since leukemia is a rare disease, a much larger study population would have been needed to make sure that no increased risk existed.

Studying the mortality experience of 390 white male Missouri veterinarians, Botts *et al.* [130] found no statistically significant difference in the presence of cancer among these persons as compared to controls. The authors did note the smallness of their sample size and the strong possibility that chronically ill and retired veterinarians could have been excluded from the study.

Similarly, a study conducted on 486 Illinois veterinarians by Schnurrenberger *et al.* [131] revealed no statistically significant difference in the occurrence of cancer among these veterinarians as compared to controls. As seen in the previous study, only adult males were studied along with small sample size for detecting a difference. The cause of this increased risk of lymphoid tumors in veterinarians could not be conclusively stated. Also, Blair and Hayes [132] found a significantly high proportion of deaths due to leukemia and Hodgkin disease among veterinarians primarily in clinical practice. However, the lymphatic type of leukemias among these individuals was less than the expected. Not all such studies have been negative. In another recent study, Guthensohn *et al.* [133] reported that Matanowski had found an 80% increase in the presence of lymphoid tumors among 19,000 veterinarians in the U.S. who died after age 46 as compared to the general U.S. population and physicians.

Schneider [134] carried out a retrospective case control study to determine within households with cancerous cats, if there was an increase in tumors in human beings, dogs and other cats. Case households were households containing cats with histologically confirmed cancer, submitted to the Alameda-Contra Costa Counties Animal Neoplasm Registry (ANR) during a five-year period. Control households were households that contained cats with non-neoplastic conditions submitted during the same period. Interviews were conducted on 675 cases and 675 control households. Schneider found no increased association of human cancer with feline lymphoma and concluded there was little evidence of horizontal transmission of cancer from cats to man. A variety of neoplasms in cats and man were included in the study. The investigator did not subclassify the various types of leukemias, and the sample size was probably not large enough to detect transmission of the virus from cats to man and the subsequent development of ALL, which, given the incidence of ALL (2.0/100,000), must be a rare event, even in the presence of a viremic cat.

Hanes *et al.* [135] conducted two household questionnaire surveys to ascertain the degree of family exposure to domestic cats, dogs and parakeets in selected human (index) cancer households and control households. Results of the first study suggested an excess of total years exposure to cats in households with lymphoma (8.0 in cases versus 4.1 in controls). Also, in the leukemia household, the total years of exposure to cats exceeded that of the controls (5.8 versus 5.1). However, the authors felt that within this survey failure to match control with index households for duration of residence at the present address led to a bias, which accounted for an excessive exposure to cats in families with lymphoma. In a second survey, each index household was compared to a selected control household, carefully matched for duration of residence, age and sex of the case. No difference in exposure to cats, dogs or parakeets was found between the index households and matched control households. The authors concluded that the cats were an unlikely causal factor for human cancers, as a whole. Nonetheless, results of the survey indicated specifically that leukemia and lymphomas households had more index cases than controls who reported an infection caused by a scratch or bite (6 versus 0). The authors, however, considered this outcome to be potentially biased because of a press release linking cats with cancers which appeared in local newspapers during the period in which the study was being conducted.

CONCLUSIONS

In conclusion, with regard to a causal relationship between FeLV and human ALL, most of the relevant literature supports the possibility. On the basis of this evidence, FeLV has been classified as a moderate risk (class 2) agent [136]. The experimental animal results clearly demonstrate that viruses can cause leukemias in several species [69, 73, 74, 77] and that FeLV, which can be spread horizontally in cats, causes leukemias in cats. A healthy FeLV positive cat may live for several years [96, 102]. Evidence suggests a carrier state, as well as a possible extended latency period [137]. Furthermore, there is evidence that some cats lack sufficient ability to respond immunologically to FeLV, and thus the virus, once established, is able to persist in the body of the host [138, 139]. The persistence or even the periodic presence of the FeLV in the infected household cat can certainly expose individuals having intimate contact with the cat to FeLV.

Essex [7] proposed the hypothesis which suggested that oncornaviruses (FeLV) could be responsible for some human lymphoreticular neoplasms. He cited as evidence to incriminate feline oncornaviruses as a possible cause of human lymphoreticular neoplasms: (1) feline oncornaviruses will induce tumors in several species, including subhuman primates; (2) field strains of FeLV will replicate in human cells; and, (3) feline sarcoma virus (FSV) will transform human cells.

Past epidemiological studies have produced conflicting results and conclusions concerning the relationship between cats and leukemia in humans. The studies of the immunological responsiveness to FeLV by cats and the relationship in rodents between the age of exposure to GLV and the likelihood of developing leukemia suggest that yoyng children (presumably after maternal antibodies have diminished) and immunosuppressed individuals would be at greatest risk for developing an infection with FeLV. The bimodal distribution of age of onset for ALL in man is consistent with different causes predominating at each mode. As a group, children are most likely to experience exposure to FeLV and to have short-term periods of immune depression as a result of exposure to childhood viral diseases and viral vaccines. The FeLV should act primarily during the childhood mode. Many epidemiological studies have obscured a possible childhood ALL and cat exposure relationship by mixing adult with childhood cases, by grouping together all lymphoreticular cancers, or by using samples sizes too small to detect the relationship. The majority of epidemiological evidence supporting a relationship between lymphoid cancer and cat exposure, particularly ill or dead cats, comes from studies of children and young adults, and primarily those with leukemia.

We have not been able to identify any epidemiological studies of the relationship between sick cat exposure and human ALL published since 1973. Since then, it has become possible to detect C-type viral particles in serum and immunologically to subcategorize ALL with regard to cell of origin. There is now considerable evidence that an adult form of T-cell leukemia has a viral cause. It is possible that FeLV induced leukemia in children is predominantly an acute luekemia of T-cell origin. An overwhelming majority of the malignancies caused by FeLV in cats are of the T-cell type. ALL of the T-cell type which develops in the cat has similar clinical findings, laboratory data and response to treatment as in human T-cell ALL. *In vitro,* T-cells appear more sensitive to FeLV than B-cells. Perhaps the possibility that T-cell malignant lymphomas in man are also caused by FeLV should be considered. The question of whether FeLV is the cause of T-cell malignancies in man can now be directly addressed. We are currently conducting a study where T-cell malignancy cases, cases with non-T-cell leukemias, and age-sex-matched normal controls are compared with respect to exposure to sick cats, and presence of C-type viral antigens/particles and anti-viral antibodies in the serum.

In summary, pertinent literature has provided evidence which supports the hypothesis that childhood ALL may be associated with cat exposure. Furthermore, based on increased knowledge concerning ALL in recent years, it appears to be appropriate to propose the sub-hypothesis that T-cell ALL, specifically, may be associated with cat exposure.

There is additional public health significance to addressing the question at this time. Vaccines for mass inoculation against FeLV in cats should be available in a few years. If it is demonstrated that FeLV is a cause of ALL, it would add enormous momentum to the implementation of such a program and hopefully a reduction in the incidence of childhood ALL.

REFERENCES

1. Castleberry RP: Current trends in childhood acute lymphocytic leukemia and non-Hodgkin's lymphoma. Al Jour Med Sci 18(3):243–248, 1981.
2. Borella L, Sen L, Dow LW, Casper JT: Cell differentiation antigens versus tumor related antigens in childhood acute lymphoblastic leukemia (ALL). Clinical significance of leukemia markers. Hematol Bluttrans 20:77–85, 1977.
3. Altman AJ, Schwartz AD: The Leukemias. Malignant Diseases of Infancy, Childhood and Adolescence (MPCP), Vol 19, 169, 1978.
4. The Lancet, Epidemiology of leukemia. Lancet 1(741):82-3, 1972.

5. Greaves MF, Janossy G, Roberts M, Rapson NT, Ellis RB, Chessels J, Lister TA, Catovsky D: Membrane phenotyping: Diagnosis, monitoring and classification of acute 'lymphoid' leukacmias. Hematol Bluttrans 20:61–75, 1977.
6. Merck Manual, 13th Edition, (eds. Berkow, R., et al.) Merck Sharp and Dohme Res. Lab.; Rahway, NJ, 325–329, 1977.
7. Essex M: Can feline oncornaviruses cause leukemia in man? Oncology 25:345–356, 1972.
8. Third National Cancer Survey: Incidence Data. National Cancer Institute Monograph 41, March, 1975. DHEW Publication No. (NIH) 75-787, USDHEW, Public Health Service, NIH, National Cancer Institute, Bethesda, MD.
9. MacMahon B, Koller EK: Ethnic differences in the incidence of leukemia. Blood 12:1–10, 1957.
10. Szklo M, Gordis L, Tonascia J, Kaplan E: The changing survivorship of white and black children with leukemia. Cancer 42:59–66, 1978.
11. Olisa EG, Chandra R, Jackson MA, Kennedy J, Williams AO: Malignant tumors in American black and Nigerian children: A comparative study. JNCI 55(2):281–284, 1975.
12. Robbins SL, Cotran RS: Leukemias, Pathologic Basis of Disease 2nd Ed., W.B. Saunders Co., Philadelphia, p. 779, 1979.
13. Githens JH, Elliot FE, Saunders LH: The relationship of socioeconomic factors to incidence of childhood leukemia. Public Health Reports 80(7):573–578, 1965.
14. Humphrey GB, Blackstock R, Filler J: Cell surface markers in acute lymphoblastic leukemia. Ann Clin Lab Sci 10(3):169–80, 1980.
15. Kumar S, Carr TF, Evans DI, Morris-Jones P, Hann IM: Prognostic significance of cell surface markers in childhood acute lymphoblastic leukemia. Clin Lab Haematol 1:121–128, 1979.
16. Aiuti F, Lacava V, Fiorilli M, Ciarla MV: Lymphocyte surface markers in lymphoproliferative disorders. Acta Haematol 50:275–283, 1973.
17. Chessells JM, Hardisty RM, Rapson NT, Greaves MF: Acute lymphoblastic leukemia in children: Classification and prognosis. Lancet 2(8052-53):1307–9, 1977.
18. Nadkarni JJ, Nadkarni JS, Advani SH: Surface markers in human lymphoid leukaemias. Ind J Cancer 15:43–47, 1978.
19. Huhn D, Thiel E, Rodt H: Classification of normal and malignant lymphatic cells using acid phosphatase and acid esterase. Klin Wochenschr 58:65–71, 1980.
20. Foon KA, Billing RJ, Terasaki PI: Dual B and T markers in acute and chronic lymphocytic leukemia. Blood (55)1:16–20, 1980.
21. Rodt H, Netzel B, Thiel E, Jager G, Huber D, Haas R, Gotze D, Thierfelders: Classification of leukemia cells with T and O ALL specific antisera. Hematology and Blood Trans 20:87–96, 1977.
22. Sallan SE, Chess L, Frei E III, O'Brien, Nathan DG, Strominger JL, Schlossman SF: Utility of B- and T-cell-specific antisera in the classification of human leukemias. In: Differentiation of Normal and Neoplastic Hematopoietic Cells (eds. Clarkson B, Marks PA, Till JE), p. 479–483, Cold Spring Harbor Laboratory, 1978.
23. Vogler LB, Crist WM, Sarrif AM, Pullen DJ, Bartolucci AA, Falletta JM, Dowell B, Humphrey GB, Blackstock R, van Eys J, Metzgar RS, Cooper MD: An analysis of clinical and laboratory features of acute lymphocytic leukemias with emphasis on 35 children with pre-B leukemia. Blood 58(1):135–140, 1981.
24. Reid MM, Craft AW, Walker W: Poor prognosis of T-cell leukemia in children. (letter) Lancet 2(8047):1074–1075, 1977.
25. Sallon SE, Ritz J, Pesando J, Gelber R, O'Brien C, Hitchcock S, Caral F, Schlossman S: Cell surface antigens: Prognostic implications in childhood acute lymphoblastic leukemia.

Blood 55:395–402, 1980.
26. Dow LW, Borlla L, Sen L, Aur RJ, George SL, Mauer AM, Simone JV: Initial prognostic factors and lymphoblast-erythrocyte rosette formation in 109 children with acute lymphoblastic leukemia. Blood 50:671–682, 1977.
27. Roper M, Crist W, Ragab A, Pullen J, Humphrey GB, Boyett J, Metzgar R, van Eys J, Nix W, Cooper M: Pre-B cell leukemia differs in its response to therapy. Blood 58(5):150A, 1981.
28. Jaffe S, Berard CW: Lymphoblastic lymphoma; A term rekindled with new precision. Ann Inter Med 89(3):415–417, 1978.
29. Nathwani BN, Kim H, Rappaport H: Malignant lymphoma, lymphoblastic. Cancer 38:964–983, 1976.
30. Nadler LM, Reinherz EL, Weinstein HJ, D'Orsi CJ, Schlossman SF: Heterogeneity of T-cell lymphoblastic malignancies. Blood 55(5):806–810, 1980.
31. Miller RW: Delayed radiation effects in atomic-bomb survivors. Science. 166:569–574, 1969.
32. Polley JR, Borges W, Yamazaki T: Incidence of leukemia in survivors of the atomic bomb in Hiroshima and Nagasaki, Japan. Am J Med 13:311, 1952.
33. Potolsky A, Creger WP: Radiation and drug therapies, and leukemia. Annu Rev Med 24:75–82, 1973.
34. Lange RD, Moloney WC, Yamazaki T: Leukemia in atomic bomb survivors. Blood 9:574, 1954.
35. Moloney WC, Kastenbaum MA: Leukemogenic effects of ionizing radiation on atomic bomb survivors in Hiroshima City. Science 121:308, 1955.
36. March HC: Leukemia in radiologists in a 20 year period. AM J M Sc 220:282, 1950.
37. Ulrich H: The incidence of leukemia in radiologists. New Engl J Med 234:45, 1946.
38. Schwartz AD, Lee H, Baum ES: Leukemia in children with Wilms' tumor. J Pediatr 87:374–376, 1975.
39. Aksoy M: Benzene and leukemia. Lancet I:441, 1978.
40. Vigliana EC, Forni A: Benzene and leukemia. Environ Res 11:122–127, 1976.
41. Manning MD, Carroll BE: Some epidemiological aspects of leukemia in children. JNCI 19(6):1087–1094, 1957.
42. Miller RW: Neoplasia and Down's syndrome. Ann NY Acad Sci 171:637–644, 1970.
43. German J, Bloom D, Passarge E: Bloom's syndrome. Surveillance for cancer in affected families. Clin Genet 12(3):162–168, 1977.
44. O'Gorman Hughes DW: Aplastic anaemia in childhood. III. Constitutional aplastic anaemia and related cytopenias. Med J Aust 1:519–526, 1974.
45. Hecht F, McCaw BK, Koler RD: Ataxia-telangiectasia-clonal growth of translocation lymphocytes. N Engl J Med 289:286–291, 1973.
46. Lilly F, Pincus T: Genetic control of murine viral leukemogenesis. Adv Can Res 17:231–277, 1973.
47. Meruelo D, Lieberman M, Ginzton N, Deak B, McDevitt HO: Genetic control of radiation leukemia virus-induced tumorigenesis. I. Role of the major murine histocompatibility complex, H-2. J Exp Med 146:1079–1087, 1977.
48. Meruelo D: A role for elevated H-2 antigen expression in resistance to neoplasia caused by radiation-induced leukemia virus. J Exp Med 149:898–909, 1979.
49. Sanderson AR, Mahour GH, Jaffe N and Das L: Incidence of HLA antigens in acute lymphocytic leukemia. Transplantation 16:672–673, 1973.
50. Rogentine GN, Trapani RJ, Yankee RA and Henderson ES: HL-A antigens and acute lymphocytic leukemia: The nature of the HL-A2 association. Tissue Antigens 3:470–476, 1973.

51. Albert ED, Nisperos B, Thomas ED: HLA antigens and haplotypes in acute leukemia. Leukemia Research 1:261–269, 1977.
52. Grumet FC: HLA and disease associations. Transplant Proc 9:1839–1844, 1977.
53. Lawler SD, Klouda PT, Smith PG, Till MM and Hardesty RM: Survival and the HLA system in acute lymphoblastic leukemia. Brit Med J 1:547–548, 1974.
54. Klouda PT, Lawler SD, Till MM, Hardesty RM: Acute lymphoblastic leukemia and HLA: a prospective study. Tissue Antigens 4:262–265, 1974.
55. Davey FR, Lachant NA, Dock NL, Hubbell C, Stockman JA and Henry JB: HLA antigens and childhood acute lymphocytic leukemia. Brit J Haematology 47(2):211–220, 1981.
56. DeBruyére M, Cornu G, Heremans-Bracke T, Malchaire J, Sokal G: HLA haplotypes and long survival in childhood acute lymphoblastic leukemia treated with transfer factor. Brit J Haematology 44(2):243–251, 1980.
57. Michel K, Hubbel C, Dock NL, Davey FR: Correlation of HLA- Drw3 with childhood acute lymphocytic leukemia. Arch Pathol Lab Med 105:560, 1981.
58. Révész T, Bencz'r M, Gyódi E, Petrányi GG, Schuler D: The association of HLA-DR5 antigen with longer survival in childhood leukemia. Brit J Haematol 48:508–509, 1981.
59. Budowle B, Acton RT, Barger BO, Blackstock R, Crist W, Go RCP, Humphrey GB, Ragab A, Roper M, Vietti T, Dearth J: Properdin factor B and acute lymphocytic leukemia (ALL) Cancer 50:2369–2371, 1982.
60. Pike MC, Smith PG: Clustering of Cases of Hodgkin's Disease and Leukemia. Cancer 34:1390–1394, 1974.
61. Smith PG, Pike MC, Till MM, Hardisty RM: Epidemiology of Childhood Leukemia in Greater London: A search for evidence of Transmission assuming a possibly long latent period. Br J Cancer 33:1–8, 1975.
62. Till MM, Hardisty RM, Pike MC, Doll R: Childhood Leukemia in Greater London: A search for evidence of clustering. Brit Med J 3:755–758, 1967.
63. Lock SP, Merrington M: Leukemia in Lewisham (1957-63). Brit Med J 3:759–760, 1967.
64. Knox G: Epidemiology of childhood leukemia in Northumberland and Durham. Brit J Prev Soc Med 18:17–24, 1964.
65. Mainwaring D: Epidemiology of acute leukemia of childhood in the Liverpool area. Brit J Prev Soc Med 20:189–194, 1966.
66. Meighan SS, Knox G: Leukemia in childhood: epidemiology in Oregon. Cancer 18:811–814, 1965.
67. Heath CW, Hasterlik RJ: Leukemia among children in a suburban community. Amer. J Med 34:796–812, 1963.
68. Pike MC, Smith PG: A case-control approach to examine diseases for evidence of contagion, including diseases with long latent periods. Biometrics 30:263–279, 1974.
69. Theilen GH: Public health aspects of animal tumor viruses. Theirogenology 6:331–342, 1976.
70. Cotter SM: Feline leukemia virus induced disorders in the cat. Vet Clin N Amer 6:367–378, 1976.
71. Hardy WD Jr, Old LJ, Hess PW, Essex M, Cotter S: Horizontal transmission of feline leukaemia virus. Nature 244:266–269, 1973.
72. Jarrett W, Jarrett O, Mackey L et al.: Horizontal transmission of leukemia virus and leukemia in the cat. JNCI 51:833–841, 1973.
73. Piper CE, Abt DA, Ferrer JF et al.: Seroepidemiological evidence of horizontal transmission of bovine C-type virus. Cancer Res 35(10):2714–2716, 1975.
74. Dutcher RM, Larkin EP, Marshak RR: Virus-like particles in cow's milk from a herd with high incidence of lymphosarcoma. JNCI 33:1055–1064, 1975.

75. Kettman R, Portetelle D, Mammerick M, Cleuter Y, DeKegel D, Galou M, Chysdael J, Burney A, Chantrenne H: Bovine leukemia virus: An exogenous RNA oncogenic virus. Proc Natl Acad Sci 73:1014–1018, 1976.
76. Ferrer JF, Abt DA, Bhatt DM, Marshak RR: Studies on the relationship between infection with bovine C-type virus, leukemia and persistent lymphocytosis in cattle. Cancer Res 34:893–900, 1974.
77. Kawakami TG, Huff SD, Buckley PM, Dungworth DL, Snyder SP, Gilden RV: C-type virus associated with gibbon lymphosarcoma. Nature 225:170–171, 1972.
78. Ioachim HL: Prevention of gross virus-induced leukemia in progeny of immunized female rats. Cancer Res 30:2661–2664, 1970.
79. Jarrett WFH, Crawford E, Martin WB, Davie F: A Virus-like Particle associated with Leukemia (Lymphosarcoma). Nature 202:567–569, 1964.
80. Allen DW, Cole P: Viruses and human cancer. N Engl J Med 286:70–82, 1972.
81. Francis DP, Essex M: Leukemia and lymphoma: Infrequent manifestations of common viral infections? A review. J Infect Dis 138(6):916–923, 1978.
82. Baxt W et al.: Human leukemic cells containing reverse transcriptase associated with a high molecular weight virus-related RNA. Nature 240:72, 1972.
83. Holland JF: The acute leukemias: In: Cecil Text of Med. 5th Ed. Vol. II, p. 1813, (eds., Beeson PB, McDermott W, Wyngaarden JB). WB Saunders Co., Philadelphia, 1979.
84. Gallo RC, Yong DS, Ting RC: RNA-dependent DNA polymerase of human acute leukemic cells. Nature 228:927, 1970.
85. Ioachim HL, Sabbath M, Andersson B, Keller S: Viral and chemical leukemia in the rat: Comparative study. JNCI 47(1):161–168, 1971.
86. Kalyanaraman VS, Sarngadharan MG, Nakao Y, Ito Y, Aoki T, Gallo RC: Natural antibodies to the structural core protein (p24) of the human T-cell leukemia (lymphoma) retrovirus found in the sera of leukemia patients in Japan, Proc Natl Acad Sci USA 79:1653–1657, 1982.
87. Catovsky D, Rose M, Goolden AWG, White JM, Bourikas G et al.: Adult T-cell lymphoma—Leukaemia in Blacks from the West Indies. Lancet 8273:643, 1982.
88. Hinuma Y, Nagata K, Hanaoka M, et al.: Adult T-cell leukemia: Antigen in an ATL cell line and detection of antibodies to the antigen in human sera. Proc Natl Acad Sci USA 78:6476–6480, 1981.
89. Gallo RC, Blattner WA, Reitz MS Jr, Ito Y: HTLV: The Virus of adult T-cell leukaemia in Japan and Elsewhere. Lancet 8273:683, 1982.
90. Mier JW, Gallo RC: Purification and some characteristics of human T-cell growth factor from phytohemagglutinin-stimulated lymphocyte-conditioned media. Proc Natl Acad Sci USA 77:6134–6138, 1980.
91. Essex M: Adult T-cell leukemia-lymphoma: Role of a human retrovirus. JNCI 69(4):981–985, 1982.
92. Gallo RC, Wong-Staal F: Retroviruses as etiologic agents of some animal and human leukemias and lymphomas and as tools for elucidating the molecular mechanism of leukemogenesis. Blood 60(3):545–557, 1982.
93. Donham KJ, Berg JW, Sawin RS: Epidemiologic relationship of bovine population and human leukemia in Iowa. Amer J Epidemiol 112(1):80–92, 1980.
94. Gupta P, Ferrer JF: Expression of Bovine Leukemia Virus Genome Is Blocked by a Non-immunoglobulin Protein in Plasma from infected cattle. Science 215:405–407, 1982.
95. Ferrer JF, Kenyon SJ, Gupta P: Milk of Dairy Cows Frequently contains a Leukemogenic Virus. Science 213:1014–1016, 1981.
96. Reif JS: Pet associated zoonoses. In: Current Vet Therapy VI (eds. Kirk RW et al.), p. 1433, WB Saunders Co., Philadelphia, 1977.

97. Levy SB: Cat leukemia: A threat to man? N Engl J Med 290(9):513–14, 1974.
98. Gilmore CE, Holzworth J: Naturally occurring feline leukemia: Clinical, pathologic, and differential diagnostic features. JAVMA 158:1013–1025, 1971.
99. Jarrett O, Laird HM, Hay D, Jarrett WFH: Feline leukemia. J Small Anim Pract 10:599–603, 1969.
100. Benveniste RE, Todaro GJ: Evolution of type C viral genes: Origin of feline leukemia virus. Science 190:886–888, 1975.
101. Hardy WD Jr., Hess PW, MacEwen EG, McClelland AJ, Zuckerman EE, Essex M, Cotter SM, Jarrett O: Biology of Feline leukemia virus in the natural environment. Cancer Res 36:582–588, 1976.
102. Hardy WD Jr: Immunopathology of Lymphoreticular Neoplasms (eds. Twomey JJ and Good RA), 129–180. Plenum, New York, 1978.
103. Cotter SM: Update on Feline Leukemia. In: Proceedings: American Animal Hospital Association 46th Annual Meeting, 119–121, 1979.
104. Francis DP, Essex M, Hardy WD, Jr.: Excretion of feline leukaemia virus by naturally infected pet cats. Nature 269:252–254, 1977.
105. Gardner MB, Rongey RW, Johnson EY, DeJournett R, Huebner JR: C-type tumor virus particles in salivary tissue of domestic cats. JNCI 47:561–565, 1971.
106. Hardy WD, Jr., Geering G, Old LJ, deHarven E, Brodey RS, McDonough S: Feline leukemia virus: occurrence of viral antigens in the tissues of cats with lymphosarcoma and other diseases. Science 166:1019–1021, 1969.
107. Hoover EA, Olsen RG, Mathes L et al.: Relationship between feline leukemia virus antigen expression and viral infectivity in blood, bone marrow and saliva of cats. Cancer Res 37:3707–3710, 1977.
108. Ladiges WC, DiGiacomo RF, Wardrop KJ, Hardy WD, Jr.: Prevalence and sequelae of feline leukemia virus infection in laboratory cats. JAVMA 179(11): 1206–1207, 1981.
109. Hardy WD, Jr: The Virology, Immunology and Epidemiology of the Feline Leukemia Virus. In: Feline Leukemia Virus, (eds. Hardy WD, Jr, Essex M, McClellan AJ), 33–78. Elsevier North Holland, Inc. 1980.
110. Holzworth J: Leukemia and related neoplasms of the cat. I. Lymphoid neoplasms. JAVMA 136:47–69, 1960.
111. Neilsen SW: Neoplastic diseases: In: Catcott: Feline Medicine and Surgery, American Veterinary Publication, Wheaton, 1964.
112. Laird HM, Jarrett O, Crighton GW and Jarrett WFH: An electron microscopic study of virus particles in spontaneous leukemia in the cat. JNCI 41:867–878, 1968.
113. Jarrett O, Laird HM, Hay D: Growth of feline leukemia virus in human cells. Nature 224:1208–1209, 1969.
114. Hardy WD, Jr., Suckerman EE, MacEwen EG, et al.: A feline leukemia and sarcoma virus induced tumor specific antigen. Nature 270:249–251, 1977.
115. Essex M, Cotter SM, Carpenter JL: Feline virus-induced tumors and the immune response: Recent developments. Am J Vet Res 34:809–812, 1973.
116. Hoover EA, Olsen RG, Hardy WD, Jr., Schaller JP, Mathes LE: Feline leukemia virus infection: Age-related variation in response of cats to experimental infection. JNCI 57:365–369, 1976.
117. Essex M, Cotter SM, Carpenter JL, Hardy WD, Jr., Hess P, Jarrett W, Schaller JP, Yohn DS: Feline oncornavirus-associated cell membrane antigen II. Antibody titers in healthy cats from household and laboratory colony environments. JNCI. 54:631, 1975.
118. Jarrett O: Growth of feline leukemia virus in human, canine, and porcine cells. Proc. 4th Int Symp on Comparative Leukemia Research, Cherry Hill, NJ, 1969.
119. Azocar J, Essex M: Susceptibility of human cell lines to feline leukemia virus and feline

sarcoma virus. JNCI 63:1179–1184, 1979.
120. Olsen RG, Mathes LE, Yohn DS: In Comparative Leukemia Research 1973, (eds. Ito Y, Dutcher RM), Krager/Basel, 419–429, 1975.
121. Caldwell GC, Baumgartener L, Carter C, Cotter S, Currier R, Essex M, Hardy W, Olson C, Olsen R: In: Comparative Leukemia Research 1975, (eds. Clemmesen J, Yohn DS), Karger/Basel, 238–241, 1976.
122. Sordillo PP, Markovich RP, Hardy WD Jr: Search for evidence of feline leukemia virus infection in Humans with leukemias, lymphomas, or soft tissue sarcomas. JNCI 69(2):333–337, 1982.
123. Francis DP, Essex M, Cotter SM, Gutensohn N, Jakowski R, Hardy WD Jr: Epidemiologic association between virus-negative feline leukemia and the horizontally transmitted feline leukemia virus. Cancer Lett 12:37–42, 1981.
124. Hardy WD Jr, McClelland AJ, Zuckerman EE, et al.: Development of virus non-producer lymphosarcomas in pet cats exposed to FeLV. Nature 288:90–92, 1980.
125. Sliski AH, Essex M, Meyer C, Todaro GJ: Feline oncornavirus associated cell membrane antigen (FOCMA): Expression on feline sarcoma virus-transformed nonproducer mink cells. Science 196:1336–1339, 1977.
126. Bross ID, Gibson R: Cats and childhood leukemia. J Med (BASEL) 1:180–187, 1970.
127. Penrose M: Cat Leukaemia. Brit Med J 1:755, 1970.
128. Bross ID, Bertell R, Gibson R: Pets and adult leukemia. AJPH 62(11):1520–31, 1972.
129. Fasal E, Jackson EW, Klauber MR: Mortality in California Veterinarians. J Chron Dis 19:293–306, 1966.
130. Botts RP, Edlavitch S, Payne G: Mortality of Missouri Veterinarians. JAVMA 149(5):499–504, 1966.
131. Schnurrenberger PR, Martin RJ, Walker JF: Mortality in Illinois Veterinarians. JAVMA, 170(10):1071–1075, 1977.
132. Blair A, Hayes HM Jr: Cancer and other causes of death among US veterinarians, 1966-1977. Int J Cancer 25:181–185, 1980.
133. Guthensohn N, Francis DP, Hardy WD, Jr., Essex M: In: Viruses in Naturally Occurring Cancer (eds. Essex M, Todaro G, ZurHausen H), Cold Spring Harbor Lab, New York, 1980.
134. Schneider R: The natural history of malignant lymphoma and sarcoma in cats and their associations with cancer in man and dog. JAVMA 157(11):1753–1758, 1970.
135. Hanes B, Gardner MB, Loosli CG, Heidbreder G, Kogan B, Marylander H, Huebner RJ: Pet association with selected human cancers: A household questionnaire survey. JNCI 45(6):1155–1162, 1970.
136. Safety Standards for Research Involving Oncogenic Viruses, Department of Health, Education and Welfare publication (NIH) 75-790, National Cancer Institute, 1974.
137. Essex M, Hardy WD Jr., Cotter SM, et al.: Naturally occurring resistant feline oncornavirus infections in the absence of disease. Infection and Immunity 11:470–475, 1975.
138. Hardy WD Jr: Immunodiffusion studies of feline leukemia and sarcoma. JAVMA 158:1060, 1971.
139. Maruyama K, Dmochowski L, Richard CG: A search for antural antibody against feline and murine leukemia antigen by mixed hemadsorption test. JAVMA 158:1076, 1971.

4. Inhibitors of Microtubule Formation

HIMAN STERNLICHT

A number of diverse chemical agents have been identified which perturb microtubule assembly and disassembly by interacting specifically with microtubule protein. Microtubules are found in all eukaryotic cells and are a major component of the mitotic spindle. Drugs that perturb microtubule polymerization and depolymerization in many cases are potent antimitotic agents with potential in cancer chemotherapy. In this chapter we review the pharmacology of a number of antimicrotubule drugs with emphasis on the mechanisms by which they alter microtubule function. To keep the review tractable, as the list of antimicrotubule agents is large, we confined ourselves primarily to the following drugs: colchicine and its derivatives; podophyllotoxins and nocodazole (competitive inhibitors of colchicine); the vinca alkaloids (*e.g.* vinblastine and vincristine); the macrolides (*e.g.*, maytansine); taxol; and griseofulvin. These drugs were chosen, in part, because they illustrate different mechanisms of assembly inhibition. Furthermore, most of these drugs have been found to be effective in cancer chemotherapy and many are in clinical use. Our review benefited from a number of excellent earlier reviews (see references [1–4]).

The inhibition of microtubule assembly has been studied by a variety of physical and biochemical methods, and our understanding of inhibition processes is constantly evolving. We confined our review mainly to studies done since 1975. Constraints of time and space caused us to focus on a select number of studies, and we found it necessary to omit many meritorious studies. Nevertheless we hope that this review, despite deficiencies, will help clarify the issues and will be of value to both the novice and practitioner in the field.

G. Bennett Humphrey et al. (eds), Adrenal and Endocrine Tumors in Children.

1. MICROTUBULES AND THEIR ASSEMBLY

1.1. Tubulin

Microtubules are polymeric structures which *in vivo* are observed to be several microns in length. They appear in electron micrographs as cylinder-like, hollow core structures of ~25 nm outer diamter and ~15 nm inner diameter (Figure 1), and display long-range order [5–7] which may be related to microtubule function. Microtubules assembled *in vitro* typically have walls that are made up of 14 protofilaments, while microtubules assembled *in vivo* typically have walls made up of 13 protofilaments [4, 8]. Tubulin, the major subunit protein of the microtubule, was originally identified by Taylor [9] in eukaryotic cells as a soluble protein which complexed colchicine tightly. One dimensional SDS gel electrophoresis of microtubule protein obtained from a variety of cell lines, as well as from brain – an organ rich in microtubules and commonly used as a source of microtubule protein, indicated that tubulin is the major component (~80–90%) of the microtubule [10–12] and suggested that tubulin is a heterodimer composed of two *ca* 55,000 molecular weight polypeptides, α and β. Cross-linking experiments done on tubulin in solution and also optical diffraction studies of electron micrographs of microtubules confirmed that tubulin exists predominantly as the heterodimer, $\alpha\beta$ [13, 14]. Structural studies further suggest that the microtubule is a polar structure with α and β subunits alternating along the longitudinal axis of the microtubule [14, 15]. This polarity appears to play an important role in the *in vivo* functions of the microtubule [16–18]. The *ca* 10–20% non-tubulin protein typically present in microtubule protein preparations are collectively referred to as microtubule associated proteins (MAPs), and at least several of these proteins appear to be conserved [18–21]. The biological functions of these minor proteins remain to be established. However, a number of the MAPs facilitate microtubule assembly and reduce the critical, *i.e.*, minimum tubulin concentrations required for assembly *in vitro* [22–24].

A comparison of the amino acid sequences of the NH_2-terminal region of tubulins derived from widely separated species [25] indicated that α and β are highly conserved proteins, changing only very slowly with evolution. Furthermore, α and β have very similar amino acid compositions [26, 27] suggesting that they may have evolved from a common precursor. In addition, α and β both have an unusual clustering of acidic residues, glutamic and aspartic acids, at thir carboxyl terminii which may play a role in assembly [28, 29]. Despite these similarities, peptide mapping studies [30], immunological studies of the cross-reactivities of antibodies to α and β [31], and hybridization studies using specific cloned tubulin cDNA [32] suggest that overall α and β chains have very different sequences and conformations. A

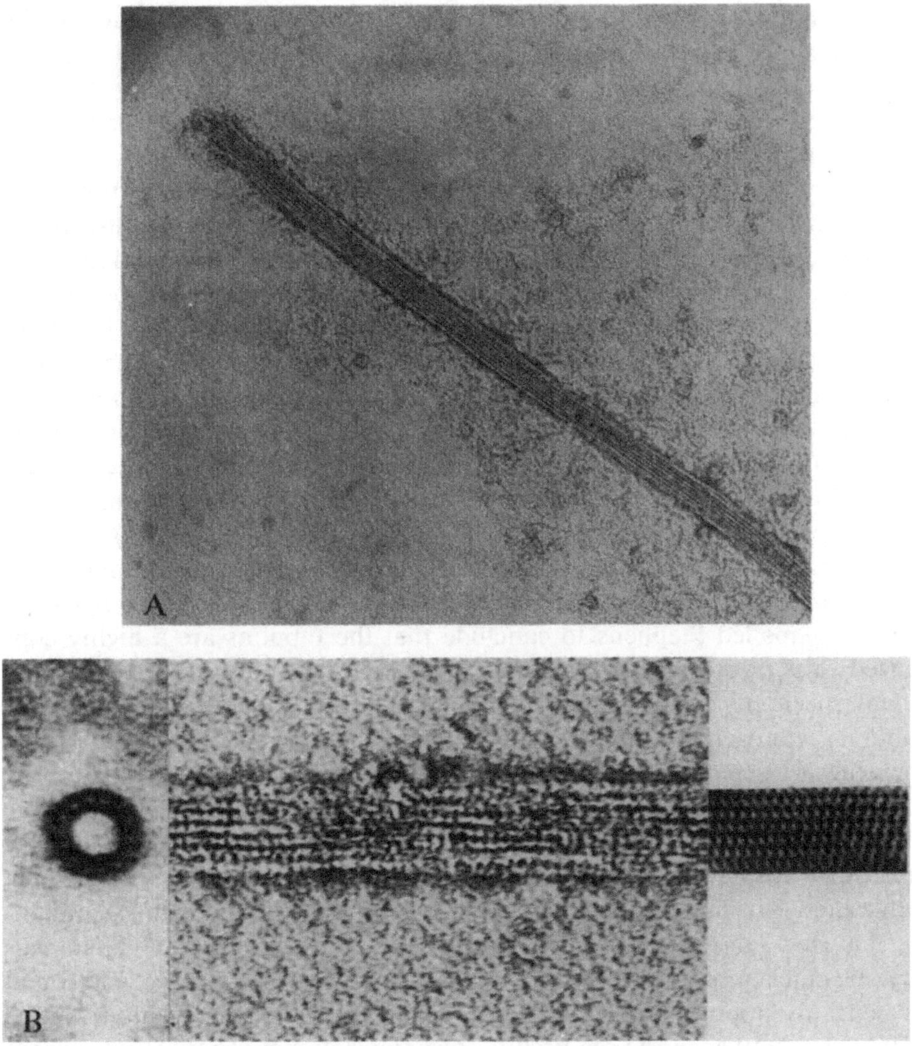

Figure 1. Electron micrography studies of reassembled dog fish microtubule protein (Courtesy Dr. George Langford). (*A*) A negatively stained microtubule. The microtubule is flattened against its carbon grid support, and in this flattened state measures 34–36 nm across. Six to seven axially aligned but slightly tilted filaments (the protofilaments) can be counted across the microtubule width. (*B*) (Left) A tannic acid stained thin section of a microtubule pellet showing the 14 protofilaments that typically make up the wall of reassembled microtubules. (Middle) An enlargement of a negatively stained microtubule showing alternating regions where protofilaments appear distinct then indistinct as one proceeds along the longitudinal axis. This banding, which shows a 96 nm axial repeat, arises from constructive and destructive interferences between negatively stained protofilaments on the front and backsides of the microtubule (183). (Right) An optical reconstruction of a negatively stained microtubule in which the contribution from the backside protofilaments was eliminated by optical filtering. The protofilaments from the front face appear distinct, and the quasiglobular nature of the tubulin subunits is also apparent.

determination of the amino acid sequences of the first 90 residues of the NH_2-terminal region of porcine brain tubulin [33] indicated that α and β have *ca* 45% homology, consistent with α and β being distinctly different proteins. Recently the complete amino acid sequences of α and β were deduced from the DNA sequences of α and β c-DNA [34].

There are two general classes of microtubules in cells: 'labile' cytoplasmic microtubules which can depolymerize and then repolymerize into the mitotic spindle during cell division; and 'stable' microtubules found in cilia, flagella, and in other specialized structures such as centrioles. Stable microtubule structures are generally resistant to such perturbations as low temperatures and drugs which depolymerize labile microtubules. Part of this stability arises from cross-bridging elements linking the microtubule components. Stephens [35] investigated the primary structural differences among tubulin subunits derived from 'stable' and 'labile' microtubule forms using tryptic peptide mapping. In all cases, irrespective of source, the tubulins were heterogeneous, usually consisting of several α and β populations. Major differences were observed between cytoplasmic tubulin and tubulin derived from cilia and flagella. However, the overall similarity in peptide maps led Stephens to conclude that the tubulins are a highly conserved class of proteins having local regions of variability to provide functional specificity. In a related study, Gozes and collaborators examined tubulin heterogeneity in rat brain during maturation. Using isoelectric focusing as a separative technique [36] and monoclonal antibodies as probes of tubulin structure [37], they identified 7 to 9 distinct isotubulins during maturation. These isotubulins were presumed to have different structures since they displayed different antigenic responses toward the monoclonal antibodies. Kirschner and colleagues [32] prepared bacterial clones containing inserted DNA specific for α and β tubulin, using mRNA from embryonic chicken brain and sea urchin egg as the initial templates, and found evidence for approximately 4 α and 4 β genes in the chicken genome, and a still larger number in the sea urchin. Post-translational modification further contributes to tubulin heterogeneity. Tubulins can undergo phosphorylation [38, 39], glycosylation [2, 40] and tryrosylation [41, 42]. *Thus it appears that the cell may have several kinds of tubulin dimer which it uses to assemble various kinds of microtubule structures.* How a cell sorts out these various kinds of tubulins for specific microtubule formation and function is presently unclear.

The X-ray structure of tubulin has not been determined. Insights into tubulin conformation has been derived from EM and low angle X-ray studies of microtubules, from spectroscopic studies, from secondary structure predictions based on sequence information, and from protein modification studies. Electron microscopy studies of microtubules, for example, indicate that tubulin is composed of two quasiglobular polypeptide chains [14, 15, 43]. Ventilla *et al.* [44] concluded from their circular dichroism studies that tubulin dimer consists of ~50% random coil conformation and varying amounts of α-helix and β-pleated sheet dependent on temperature. At 4 °C they observed *ca* 22% α-helix and *ca* 30% β-pleated sheet. At 25 °C, a temperature sufficiently high for tubulin to spontaneously assemble into microtubules, the percentage of α-helix in the dimer fell to zero while that of the β-pleated sheet increased to *ca* 50%. Similar results were obtained by Lee *et al.* [45] for calf brain tubulin. Ringel and Sternlicht [46] concluded from a carbon magnetic resonance study of microtubule protein prepared from bovine brain that tubulin dimer is a highly flexible protein with significant amounts of random coil conformation. The degree of random coil appeared to be independent of temperature. They speculated that the large degree of random coil conformation may be related to the ability of microtubules to bind and accommodate large numbers of diverse proteins. Ponstingl and his collaborators predict on the basis of their sequence data for the first 90 amino acid residues at the NH_2-terminal [33] and the first 200 amino acid residues at the COOH-terminal end [29, 47] that the NH_2-terminal region of α-tubulin is in an irregular conformation with no major hydrophobic region, and that the COOH-terminal region, with the exception of the highly acidic terminal 40 residues, is also in an irregular conformation with no major hydrophobic region.

Protein modification studies have been useful for identifying potential residues involved in the assembly process [2], and also for identifying residues that may be affected by antimitotic drugs (see Figure 1). Modification of 3 critical histidine residues will block assembly [48]. The sharp optimum for both assembly and colchicine binding at pH 6.7–6.8 which is close to the pK_a of the imidizole group may be related to these histidyl residues. Oxidation of 1 or 2 sulfhydryl groups out of approximately 7 sulfhydryls per monomer also blocks assembly [49, 50]. The efficacy of arsenical derivatives as antimitotic agents, discovered more than 50 years ago, is presumably related to the ability of these derivatives to react specifically with sulfhydryl groups on tubulin. Sternlicht *et al.* [51], reductively methylated the amino groups of tubulin with formaldehyde and sodium cyanoborohydride and found that the specific methylation of one highly reactive amino group on the α-chain prevents assembly. Furthermore, a comparison of the reductive methylation pattern of α and β tubulin suggests that the β-chain may be in a more random coil state than the α-chain. The earlier observation that formaldehyde is a potent antimitotic agent at concentrations order of magnitudes lower than that required for fixation of cells [52] is presumably related to the specific effects that formaldehyde has on tubulin.

Tubulin binds a large number of ligands. These include antimitotic drugs, nucleotides, and metal ions. There are high affinity sites for a number of metal ions such as Mg^{2+}, Ca^{2+} and Zn^{2+} [53, 54]. Mg^{2+} [55] facilitates assembly whereas Ca^{2+} inhibits assembly and will cause microtubules to depolymerize under appropriate conditions [56, 57]. Certain of the metal ions (*e.g.*, Zn^{2+}) induce the assembly of polymorphic forms such as tubulin sheets [58]. Tubulin has two tight binding sites for GTP [59, 60], one of which is exchangeable (the E-site), and several weak binding sites [61]. E-site GTP undergoes hydrolysis to GDP during assembly [62, 63]. The biological significance of GTP hydrolysis during polymerization has been the source of considerable speculation. Hydrolysis to GDP apparently is not essential for assembly as non-hydrolyzable analogs of GTP also induce assembly suggesting that nucleotides such as GTP may function, in part, as allosteric affectors of assembly. A detailed discussion of nucleotide and metal ion effects on assembly is beyond the scope of this review. The interested reader is referred elsewhere [2, 4, 64].

1.2. The Assembly Process

Microtubule assembly *in vitro* can be monitored by a variety of techniques such as turbidity changes [65] or viscosity changes [66] during polymerization, sedimentation analysis [65], dark-field microscopy [67] and electron microscopy [68]. The turbidity assay is a convenient and popular method as the degree of turbidity developed during assembly accurately reflects the total microtubule mass formed [69]. Microtubules can be isolated in large quantities from brain extracts by repeated cycles of assembly and disassembly using organic-type buffers (pH 6.6–6.9) supplemented with EGTA, Mg^{2+} and GTP [65]. Brain tubulin in turn can be used as carrier protein to isolate tubulin from other cellular sources. Assembly is carried out at elevated temperatures (~37 °C), and disassembly is accomplished by homogenizing the microtubules in the cold (~4 °C). After 2 or 3 cycles the assembly-disassembly procedure yields tubulin and small amounts of non-tubulin proteins, or MAPs that will copurify in essentially constant stoichiometry with tubulin during subsequent cycles of assembly and disassembly. The precise biological function of the MAPs is presently unclear. Two major classes have been identified [11, 23] – the high molecular weight (HMW) proteins ($\gtrsim$270,000 M.W.) and the tau proteins (~50,000–70,000 M.W.). Both classes facilitate microtubule assembly, presumably through their ability to stabilize both oligomer precursors and specific interactions between tubulin subunits in the microtubule [4]. HMW MAPs are major constituents of the filamentous projections or arms extending from the microtubules, often observed in electron micrographs of microtubules [6], while the tau protein are believed to be distributed on the surface of the microtubule with no projections apparent in electron micrographs [70]. Recent studies by Ludueña *et al.* [71] suggest that tau proteins stabilize longitudinal interactions between tubulins and facilitate assembly by catalyzing the formation of protofilaments whereas the HMW MAPs may stabilize lateral interactions and facilitate assembly by catalyzing association between protofilaments.

Microtubule formation *in vitro* occurs as a nucleated polymerization in which the nucleation step is thermodynamically less favorable than the elongation step [72, 73]. One consequence of the fact that nucleation is thermodynamically less favorable than elongation is that polymerization begins abruptly at a critical tubulin concentration, and has the appearance of a highly cooperative event. The critical concentration, *i.e.*, the minimum tubulin concentration required for assembly, is interpreted in this model of assembly as being equal to the apparent dissociation constant for tubulin bound at the microtubule ends. The smaller the critical tubulin concentration the greater is the affinity of the microtubule ends for tubulin. MAPs facilitate microtubule formation by reducing the critical tubulin concentration required for assembly [4]. Low concentrations of certain drugs, such as colchicine [74] and nocodazole [75], when bound to tubulin increase the critical tubulin concentrations required for assembly, *i.e.*, reduce the affinity of the microtubule ends for tubulin, whereas certain other drugs, such as taxol [76], decrease the critical tubulin concentration.

Considerable effort has been expended to identify the oligomer precursor(s) for the initiation of microtubule assembly *in vitro*. Sedimentation analysis studies [77, 78] done on cold (4 °C) non-assemblying microtubule protein preparations at conditions of pH and ionic strength which favor assembly at elevated temperature indicated that microtubule protein preparations at 4 °C were a mixture of tubulin dimer and double-ring oligomeric structures (M.W. $\sim 3 \times 10^6$, 30S-36S Svedberg constant). Since tubulin dimer would not readily assemble into microtubules once the oligomers were removed, it was thought that these ring structures were the nucleation centers in the microtubule polymerization reaction. Subsequent studies showed that this was a simplification [79–81]. The actual intermediates leading to microtubule formation still remain to be established. Kirschner and Williams carried out a time-course study of assembly with the aid of a rapid-spray technique which froze intermediate forms for electron microscopy examination [68, 82]. They reported a transitory buildup of spiral and twisted ribbon forms during the nucleation phase. The concentration of the ring species during assembly monotonically decreased from initial values suggesting that the ring species was a precursor to these other forms. Spiral and twisted ribbons disappeared as microtubules accumulated during the elongation phase. Little is known about drug effects on oligomeric intermediates in microtubule assembly. Both colchicine tubulin [83] and nocoda-zole tubulin [75] appear to associate with tubulin and MAPs into normal oligomeric structures. However, the early studies by Kirschner and Williams [82] suggested that colchicine may have perturbing effects on oligomers as it is capable of inducing aborted spiral and ribbon forms at high concentrations.

In vivo and *in vitro* assembly of microtubules differ in significant ways. *In vitro* assembly is characterized by the spontaneous formation of nucleation centers and the subsequent elongation of these centers into microtubules. As a consequence *in vitro* assembled microtubules are randomly distributed and randomly oriented in solution, and their lengths show a significant spread. *In vivo* assembly, on the other hand, appears to involve specialized structures such as centrioles and the precentriolar material, kinetochores, and basal bodies which function as nucleation centers. These structures are collectively referred to as microtubule organizing centers (MTOC) and control the spatial distribution and orientation of assembled microtubules [84]. Thus, cytoplasmic microtubules are not randomly distributed throughout the cell, often have very narrow ranges of length, and most are anchored at specific sites.

Immunofluorescence techniques using tubulin antibody as the primary antibody have been applied to a variety of cell lines [85–87] and have resulted in excellent fluorescent images of assemblying microtubules. In the case of interphase fibroblasts, such as 3T3 cells, microtubules can be seen radiating outward from the perinuclear region. If the cells are treated with antimicrotubule drug, cytoplasmic microtubules depolymerize while the resistant MTOC remain essentially intact. Upon recovery following removal of drug, microtubules are observed to elongate from the MTOC within the cell [88]. Various techniques have also been developed to decorate microtubules *in situ* [17, 89] so as to display their polarity. Microtubule assembly by MTOC occurs as a highly polar process with the so called 'minus' ends of the microtubules anchored on an organizing center, and the so called 'plus' ends free. Kirschner [18] proposed an interesting mechanism to explain how cells manage to suppress spontaneous assembly of microtubules, and preferentially assemble microtubules in a polar fashion on MTOC. He suggested that the GTP hydrolysis at the E-site is linked to assembly, and causes a disparity in the critical tubulin concentrations at the two ends, such that the 'minus' end of the microtubule has the higher critical concentration. *In vivo* this disparity would cause free, or unanchored microtubules, to be unstable relative to microtubules anchored by their 'minus' ends onto MTOC. *In vitro,* where both ends of the microtubule are free, this disparity in critical tubulin concentrations would manifest itself at steady-state as net disassembly of tubulin subunits from the 'minus' ends and net assembly at the 'plus' ends, *i.e.*, as a steady-state flux of tubulin subunits through the microtubule [90, 91].

Many factors appear to be involved in regulating microtubule assembly in cells. In addition to GTP [64], MAPs [19–24], and posttranslational modifications of tubulin [38–42] affecting assembly, there is evidence that cyclic AMP [39, 92, 93], pH [94] and Ca^{2+} [57] play roles in assembly regulation. Recently mitotic apparatii have been isolated by gentle procedures which avoid detergents [95]. In these studies numerous small vesicles with Ca^{2+} release and sequestering activity were found in association with the spindle fibers. Harris *et al.* studied the distribution of microtubules in sea urchin eggs through first cleavage using indirect immunofluorescence [96] and observed 'waves' of cytoplasmic microtubule breakdown followed by reorganization of the depolymerized microtubules into mitotic spindles. These 'waves' displayed spatial and temporal coherences, often overlapping within the same egg, and were attributed to waves of Ca^{2+} release and resequestering into vesicles. How antimitotic drugs affect these complex assembly processes within the cell remain to be determined.

2. ANTIMICROTUBULE DRUGS

Several classes of antimicrotubule drugs have been studied in some detail: *e.g.*, (i) colchicine and its competitive inhibitors, podophyllotoxin and nocodazole; (ii) the vinca alkaloids; (iii) maytansine; (iv) taxol and (v) griseofulvin (Figure 2). With the exception of griseofulvin, these drugs bind specifically to tubulin. Griseofulvin, on the other hand, binds specifically to a MAP protein [97]. New kinds of antimicrotubule drugs have recently been identified. Some have structural features very similar to previously studied drugs and presumably inhibit in similar manners, while others have structures very different from those in Figure 2 (*e.g.*, the marine cytotoxic agents [98, 99] whose modes of action remain to be established).

2.1. Colchicine and its competitive inhibitors

Colchicine (Figure 2) is one of the most extensively studied antimitotic drugs. Despite its potency and proven antineoplastic activity against tumors, it is not much used in cancer chemotherapy, presumably because of its toxicity. Colchicine is a potent antimicrotubule drug that affects microtubule assembly at substoichiometric concentrations relative to tubulin [100]. The molecular basis for the inhibition remains to be established, although several mechanisms have been proposed (see Figure 3). Tubulin is believed to have only one tight binding site for colchicine [59, 60], and appears to have one or more weak binding sites [46, 101, 102]. Furthermore, the tight binding complex (TC) is believed to be the direct inhibitor of assembly, while the weak bind sites are presently thought not to play a

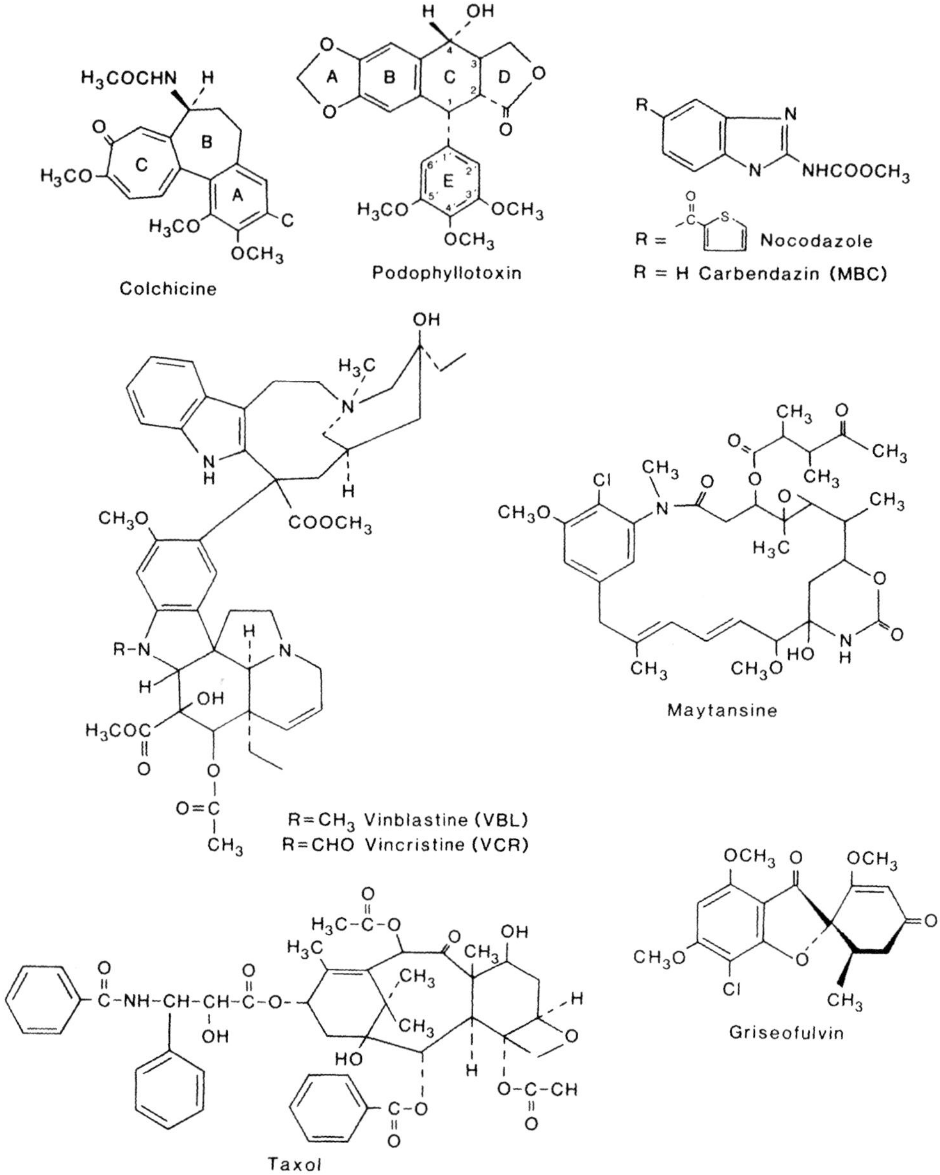

Figure 2. Structural formulas of colchicine, podophyllotoxin, nocodazole, MBC, vinblastine, vincristine, maytansine, taxol and griseofulvin.

role in inhibition. However, studies which convincingly demonstrate that these weak binding sites are indeed irrelevant remain to be done. The pH optimum for binding at the high affinity site is 6.7 [103], while kinetic measurements of the association and dissociation rate constants indicate a value of ~0.05 to 0.1 μM at 37 °C for its dissociation constant [104].

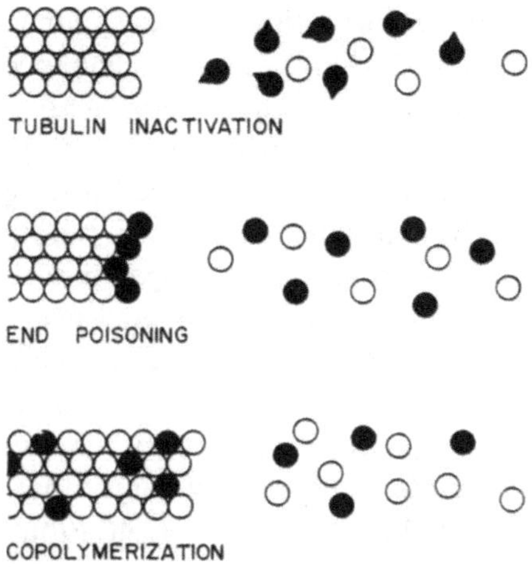

Figure 3. A pictorial representation of various mechanisms which have been proposed to explain colchicine inhibition of microtubule assembly.

Colchicine interacts anomalously with the tight binding site. The rate of equilibration is slow, and the binding is nearly irreversible. It has been suggested that binding to the tight site does not occur as a bimolecular reaction, but rather as a multistep process in which colchicine induces a conformational change in tubulin [105, 106]. Barnes *et al.* [101] have further proposed that the so called tight binding site may actually consist of two interacting sites, where the second site develops as a result of a conformational change induced in tubulin by colchicine bound at the first site. Ventilla *et al.* [44] proposed that tubulin exists in two conformations in equilibrium with each other, and that colchicine preferentially binds to and stabilizes one of the conformations. Circular dichroism [44] and nuclear magnetic resonance [46] studies have failed to detect significant conformational changes in tubulin upon colchicine binding, altough these spectroscopic results do not exclude the possibility that the conformational changes are subtle and are confined to localized region(s). Chemical modification studies support the hypothesis that colchicine induces a conformational change upon binding. Ludueña *et al.* [107] have reported that colchicine suppresses by more than 50% the reactivity of both α- and β-chain toward alkylation by iodoacetamide. Furthermore, competitive studies of TC and tubulin binding to tubulin-antibody [108] indicate a diminished ability of TC to bind to antibody, consistent with a conformation difference between TC and tubulin. Whether these putative protein conformation changes account for the anolamous colchicine binding behavior is unclear. Certain colchicine derivatives, such as colcemid (desacetyl-N-methyl colchicine), which inhibit assembly and mitosis as well as colchicine and presumably should induce similar kinds of protein conformation changes, bind rapidly and reversibly [109]. Colchicine undergoes a significant enhancement in its fluorescence upon binding to tubulin which may be indicative of a conformational change in colchincine itself [110]. This interpretation is supported by the recent study by Dietrich *et al.* which indicated a significant change in the circular dichroism spectrum of colchicine upon binding to tubulin [111].

The putative protein conformational changes induced by colchicine may be responsible for altered assembly in the presence of the drug. Purified tubulin exhibits a small intrinsic GTPase activity. David-Pfeuty *et al.* [112] found that microtubules assembled from purified tubulin display a markedly enhanced GTPase activity during assembly which appeared to be confined to the microtubule ends. They further found that colchicine is capable of activating the intrinsic GTPase activity of the tubulin dimer. The significance of this intriguing finding which suggests a link between colchicine and GTP function remains to be elucidated further. Sternlicht *et al.* [113] showed that one mode of assembly inhibition involved the copolymerization of tubulin and TC. They proposed that the altered protein conformation in TC may, in turn, cause small changes in tubulin-tubulin contacts which results in an increase in the free energy of assembly [74].

The colchicine site appears to be distinct from the polymerization site in tubulin. The two sites, for example, display markedly different sensitivities toward thermal denaturation [114, 115] and chemical modifications [48, 107]. Schmitt and Atlas [116] carried out affinity labelling of tubulin using bromocolchicine, an alkylating agent which is also a competitive inhibitor of colchicine, and concluded from their labelling patterns that colchicine binds tightly to the α-chain, and weakly at other sites in both α- and β-chains. The weak binding sites were presumed to be responsible for the anomalous labelling patterns observed in the presence and absence of colchicine. In a subsequent study Schmitt and Kram [117] showed that the bromocolchicine alkylated a cysteinyl residue. Whether this residue was one of the sulfhydryl groups identified by Kuriyama [49] and Nishida and Kobayashi [18] as essential for assembly was not established. Recently Sheir-Neiss *et al.* [119] identified a β-chain mutant in Aspergillus nidulans which was resistant to inhibition by nocodazole, a competitive inhibitor of colchicine. This could be interpreted as indicating that the colchicine site is on the β-chain, or at the α–β interface. However, Cabral *et al.* [120] have found single-step β-chain mutants in Chinese Hamster Ovary (CHO) cells that were simultaneously resistant to colchicine, colcemid, vinblastine and griseofulvin. Vinblastine binds at a different site than colchicine, while griseofulvin is presumed to bind to MAPs. The finding that the β-chain mutants were cross-reactive to all four drugs argues caution with respect to assigning the colchicine site to the β-chain. Simultaneous cross-reactivity might indicate that it is not the drug-binding sites which were altered in the β-mutants, but rather a critical interaction between β-tubulin and some other component in microtubule assembly.

Colchicine is a tropolone derivative with three rings: one aromatic ring (A) with three methoxy groups; one twisted seven carbon ring (B) with a substituted amino group; and one seven-carbon tropolone ring (C) with one oxy and one methoxy group (Figure 2). Derivatives were synthesized in an effort to elucidate the relationship between colchicine structure and activity [1, 121, 122]. Binding *per se* did not render a derivative active. Certain minimum structural features needed to be present in order for the derivatives to be inhibitors. The structure-activity studies indicated the following: The trimethoxy groups on the phenyl ring *A* are essential for activity as their removal renders the drug inactive. (The trimethoxy phenyl moeity present in podophyllotoxin [Figure 2] presumably serve a similar purpose.) The position of the oxy and methoxy groups on ring *C* is also important, as *iso-colchicine* which has their positions interchanged, is several order of magnitude less potent than colchicine. *Colchiceine* which has a hydroxyl rather than a methoxy group on ring *C* is inactive. The polycyclic nature of the drug appears to be essential for activity. For example, 2-methoxy tropone is inactive, although it binds well to tubulin [122]. Similarly, 1,2,3-trimethoxybenzene is inactive. However, the bicyclic compound obtained by linking rings *A* and *C, i.e.,* 2-methoxy-5(2′,3′,4′-trimethoxyphenyl) tropone is fully active despite its lack of a *B* ring. Curiously, despite the finding that the *B* ring is not essential for activity, a derivative of colchicine in which one fluorine replaces a hydrogen on the N-acetyl group on ring *B,* is several order of magnitude more potent as a mitotic poison than colchicine [123]. On the other hand, *desacetamidocolchicine,* a derivative in which the acetamido group on the *B* ring is replaced by a proton, is as active as colchicine [122].

Podophyllotoxin (Figure 2), an alkaloid extracted from the root of the MAY apple, is an effective inhibitor of microtubule assembly. However, toxic side effects have severely limited its use as an antineoplastic agent. Less toxic derivatives have been synthesized, and two derivatives, VP-16-213 and VM-26, have been very effective in the treatment of leukemias and solid tumors [124]. However, these two derivatives do not inhibit tubulin assembly [125], and function by degrading DNA [126]. Podophyllotoxin is a competitive inhibitor of colchicine binding [127], and like colchicine inhibits assembly at substoichiometric concentrations [128]. It has one tight-binding site per tubulin dimer, and binds optimally at the same pH as does colchicine. Furthermore, the tight-binding site decays at a similar rate as that for colchicine, and can be stabilized by the same ligands, sucrose, and vinblastine, which stabilize the colchicine site [127]. Both podophyllotoxin and colchicine markedly suppress the reactivity of α- and β-chains of tubulin towards alkylation by iodoacetamide [107]. Podophyllotoxin binding differs from colchicine in being relatively rapid, and also reversible [129]. In addition, podophyllotoxin binding does not enhance the intrinsic GTPase activity of tubulin upon binding, although it inhibits the polymerization-linked GTPase activity displayed by microtubule ends [112]. Podophyllotoxin also binds to tubulin at several low affinity sites [102]. The significance of these other sites is not known.

Structure-activity studies indicate that colchicine and podophyllotoxin most probably share a common trimethoxyphenyl binding region on tubulin with other portions of the two drugs binding to different residues in the tight binding site [127], and also indicate that the bicyclic AB ring of podophyllotoxin by itself is incapable of inhibiting assembly [125]. Derivatives which lack the D ring, as well as those which lack a closed C ring also do not inhibit microtubule assembly [125]. Kelleher concluded from a competitive inhibition study of colchicine binding in the presence of podophyllotoxin derivatives that the conformation about the lactone ring (D) may be of importance in determining tubulin binding activity [130]. Loike *et al.* [125] and Brewer *et al.* [131] examined this possibility further and concluded from a stereochemical study using magnetic resonance that the podophyllotoxin binding site on tubulin has strict steric requirements in the region where position 12 of ring D interacts with tubulin. The magnetic resonance results further indicated that one of the preferred rotamer conformations for the ethylidene glucoside moiety of VP-16-213 is over the H-11 proton of ring *D*, and suggested that VP-16-213 and VM-26 do not inhibit microtubule assembly, possibly because the bulky glucoside moiety sterically interferes with the ability of the *D* ring to bind. Loike and Horwitz [126] correlated the ability of VP-16-213 and VM-26 to degrade intracellular DNA with the presence of a 4′-hydroxyl group on ring *E* and predicted that other apropriately designed 4′-hydroxyl derivatives could be exceptionally potent antitumor agents capable of arresting cells in metaphase as well as degrading DNA.

Nocodazole (Figure 2), a benzimidazole derivative first synthesized for use as a fungicide, is a potent inhibitor of microtubule assembly and mitosis. Its efficacy as an antitumor agent appears to be partly due to its direct antimitotic effects, and partly due to its perturbing effects on subcellular organization in nondividing cells [132]. De Brabander *et al.* [133] reported that *in vivo* microtubules of malignant cells are more susceptible to the action of nocodazole than are nonmalignant cells, and further suggested that this rather high degree of specificity *in vivo* for malignant cells may explain the very low bone marrow and neuronal toxicity of this drug. Hoebeke *et al.* [134] and Brodie *et al.* [135] have suggested that nocodazole competitively inhibits colchicine binding even though there is no apparent structural similarity between the two compounds. Davidse and Flach [136] reported that nocodazole and colchicine are both competitive inhibitors of a nocodazole analog, carbendazim, (MBC), while podophyllotoxin does not inhibit MBC binding to tubulin. This could suggest that the benzimidazole derivatives bind to that portion of the colchicine site which is not shared by podophyllotoxin. Nocodazole binds rapidly and reversibly to tubulin with a dissociation half-life at 37 °C that is apparently less than 1 minute [134]. Nocodazole, like colchicine, inhibits assembly at substoichiometric concentrations of drug. Lee *et al.* [75], carried out a variety of spectroscopic studies of nocodazole inhibition of calf brain tubulin, and found that low to moderate concentrations of drug inhibited microtubule assembly by a process that did not appear to directly involve MAPs. Furthermore, the critical tubulin concentrations required for assembly in the presence of nocodazole increased with increasing nocodazole concentrations suggesting that the affinity of the microtubule ends for tubulin were a decreasing function of the nocodazole concentration. Similar findings were reported in earlier studies of colchicine inhibition [74, 113] where inhibition was attributed to the effects of a copolymerization reaction between tubulin and tubulin-colchicine complex. Lee *et al.* further concluded that the formation of a nocodazole-tubulin complex apparently induces conformational changes in tubulin which increases the exposure of sulfhydryl and tyrosine residue.

2.2. Vinca alkaloids

The vinca alkaloids (Figure 2) are extensively used in cancer chemotherapy where they inhibit at low concentrations. These drugs are bifunctional indole derivatives formed from catharantine and vindoline moiety which separately have little or no activity. Vincristine (VCR) and vinblastine (VBL), the two alkaloid forms most commonly used in chemotherapy, differ at one carbon position (Figure 2). Both appear to be equally effective at blocking microtubule assembly, and at perturbing preformed microtubules [137]. However, they differ significantly with respect to their chemotherapeutic effectiveness and toxicities [138, 139]. Those differences could indicate drug-dependent differences in transport, absorption and metabolism in different tissue types, but may also reflect differential effects on biological processes other than microtubule assembly and disassembly [140].

The vinca-alkaloids are potent inhibitors of microtubule assembly. They bind at sites different from colchicine, and are non-competitive inhibitors of assembly. Unlike colchicine, vinca binding is rapid and reversible [141, 129]. However, like colchicine the vincas inhibit assembly at concentrations substoichiometric to tubulin. Himes *et al.* [137], for example, found in studies of bovine brain tubulin that ~1 mole of alkaloid per

7 moles of tubulin caused essentially complete inhibition of assembly, while Wilson *et al.* [142] found in a study of chick embryo brain tubulin that very much smaller ratios of vinca to tubulin had significant effects on the rates of assembly. Vincas also induce tubulin to aggregate into forms other than microtubules. *In vivo,* VBL induces paracrystal formation within the cell [143]. Paracrystals are composed of hexagonally packed macrotubules that have diameters of ~32 nm and walls made up of two spiralling protofilaments [144]. *In vitro,* tetrameter aggregates [145], rings [146] and spirals [147] have been observed. Donoso *et al.* [148] found that MAPs stabilize the spiral structure obtained with VCR *in vitro*, possibly by functioning as polycations [149], and suggested that MAPs are also necessary for vinca-induced paracrystal formation. At present, it is thought that vinca-alkaloids inhibit microtubule assembly by a mechanism different from that involved in the induction of aggregated forms.

Lee *et al.* [145] and Wilson *et al.* [150] reported that tubulin has two high-affinity vinblastine binding sites per dimer. In addition, several low-affinity sites have been detected [129]. The high affinity sites are unstable and decay, binding progressively more weakly with time [150]. However, ligands such as colchicine and sucrose can stabilize the high-affinity sites [150, 151]. Values of *ca* $2 \times 10^4\ M^{-1}$ to $6 \times 10^6\ M^{-1}$ have been reported for the high-affinity binding constant at 37 °C. The reason for this wide variation is not known, but may reflect species-dependent differences in binding, or possibly decay of the high-affinity sites prior to the binding measurements. Bhattacharyya and Wolff reported one high-affinity and one low-affinity site for rat brain tubulin [151]. The low-affinity site did not appear to be a decay product of a high-affinity site. They suggested that the high-affinity site was involved in microtubule inhibition, while the low-affinity site was involved in tubulin aggregation and paracrystal formation. This interpretation, which ascribes inhibition and aggregation as the effects of VBL binding to two different sites, is supported by a recent comparative study by Ludueña *et al.* [152] of the effects of VBL and maytansine on microtubule assembly and tubulin aggregation.

The vincas, like colchicine, also induce conformation changes in tubulin. VBL, for example, stabilizes GTP [153] and colchicine binding [103], perturbs the UV spectrum and intrinsic fluorescence of tubulin [152], and suppresses the reactivity of tubulin toward alkylation by iodoacetamide [108]. Unlike colchicine and podophyllotoxin which suppress alkylation of α and β-chains about equally, VBL preferentially suppresses alkylation of the α-chain. In addition, the low-affinity binding site appears to alter certain residues at the tubulin surface [152]. David-Pfeuty *et al.* [112] found that the vincas, like colchicine, inhibit the large spontaneous GTPase activity that develops at the microtubule ends during assembly but, unlike colchicine, they do not enhance the intrinsic GTPase activity of tubulin. Furthermore, the vincas also inhibit the colchicine-induced GTPase activity of tubulin. David-Pfeuty *et al.* interpreted the differences in the response of tubulin to colchicine and vincas as indicating that these drugs induce differential conformational changes in tubulin which have differential effects on the longitudinal and lateral bonds formed between tubulins in the microtubule polymer.

2.3. Maytansine

Maytansine (Figure 2), an ansa macrolide of considerable antitumor potency [154], is obtained from plants of the genera Maytenus and Putterlickia. Maytansine binds rapidly and reversibly to tubulin [141], and is a competitive inhibitor of vinca alkaloid binding [141, 155]. Colchicine has no effect on maytansine binding. Maytansine and the vinca alkaloids have comparable binding constants, share a common binding site, although an additional site or attachment position specific for maytansine appears to be present [141]. Maytansine may inhibit tubulin polymerization by interfering with certain critical-SH groups necessary for assembly [156]. Like the vincas, it inhibits assembly substroichiometric. Unlike the vincas, as well as colchicine and podophyllotoxin, maytansine appears capable of inducing rapid microtubule disassembly *in vitro* when added to microtubules at end state [157]. Furthermore, maytansine enhances alkylation by iodoacetamide [157], an effect opposite to that obtained with VBL, suggesting that maytansine may have different conformation effects on tubulin.

A number of maytansine analogs have been synthesized and used to probe structure-activity relationships [154, 158, 159]. The stoichoimetry of maytansine binding appears to be two per tubulin molecule. Bhattacharyya and Wolff [155] reported that maytansine competes with VBL for both the high and low affinity sites. Mandelbaum-Shavit *et al.* [141] found that maytansine was capable of completely displacing bound VCR. If maytansine indeed binds to the low-affinity site which is presumed to be responsible for vinca-induced aggregation of tubulin [151], its effects on tubulin must somehow be different as maytansine does not induce aggregation. In this connection, Ludueña *et al.* [152] found differing effects on the intrinsic fluorescence of tubulin. While maytansine competitively inhibited the VBL-induced quenching associated with VBL binding at the high-affinity site, it did not alter the VBL-induced fluorescence shift associated with VBL binding at the low-affinity site. These results suggested that either maytansine does not bind at the low-affinity site, or it produces a different conformational effect upon binding at that site.

2.4. Taxol

Taxol (Figure 2), a drug isolated from the western Yew [160], has significant antineoplastic activity toward leukemias [161]. Its mechanism of action appears to be very different from most antimitotic drugs in that taxol *stabilizes* microtubules and *promotes* microtubule assembly [76]. This increase in microtubule stability affects the ability of cells to assemble and disassemble microtubules in a controlled manner [162]. *In vitro* studies suggest that maximal stabilization occurs at stoichiometric concentrations of taxol relative to tubulin, and that the dissociation rate constant for tubulin bound to microtubule is significantly reduced relative to the association rate constant [3, 76]. *In vitro* studies further indicate that taxol significantly decreases the critical tubulin concentration required for assembly, and the extent of the decrease suggests that the apparent free energy of assembly in the presence of drug is reduced by several kilocalories [3].

Taxol induces both MAP-free and GTP-depleted preparations to assemble into microtubules. The microtubules are generally small, and often ribbon-like structures are observed during the initial stages of assembly. Microtubules assembled in the presence of taxol differ from normally assembled microtubules in that they are completely resistant to depolymerization by cold (4 °C) and by 4 mM $CaCl_2$ [3, 76]. These effects are observed both in the presence and absence of GTP. Taxol effects on assembly are similar to the effects produced by Guanyl-5′-methylenediphosphonate (GMP(CH_2)pp), a GTP analog incapable of being hydrolyzed at the α–β phosphate linkage [163]. The significance of this similarity is presently unclear. However, taxol does not affect GTP binding to tubulin, and both GTP and GDP will hydrolyze in its presence during assembly. The molecular mechanism by which taxol achieves its unusual effects thus remains to be established.

2.5. Griseofulvin

Griseofulvin (Figure 2), an antibiotic first isolated from Penicillum griseofulvum, is a potent antifungal agent. It inhibits microtubule assembly at relatively high concentrations (20–200 μM), and arrests mitosis in metaphase. Griseofulvin differs from other antimicrotubule drugs in that its inhibitory action can be explained by a specific binding to MAPs [97]. While some investigators [164, 165] have reported that the drug also binds to tubulin, these sites may represent nonspecific binding [97]. How griseofulvin interacts with MAPs, and with which class of MAPs, to inhibit assembly is not known.

2.6. Endogenous inhibitors

Various investigators have speculated on the biological significance of the drug-binding sites, and have suggested that there might be endogenous inhibitors which bind to these sites, and which play a role in microtubule assembly. Sherline *et al.* [166] reported finding endogenous, competitive inhibitors of colchicine binding in rat brain. These inhibitors appeared to be particulate, protein in nature, and confined primarily to the microsomal fraction. Some inhibitory activity was detected in the cytosol, and ascribed to a ~250,000 M.W. protein. Whether the cytosolic protein represented a unique protein, or one that leaked out of the microsomes, was not established. Sherline *et al.* suggested that these inhibitors function in the cell by binding and sequestering non-polymerized tubulin, and thereby controlling the concentration of cytosolic tubulin available for microtubule assembly. Lockwood [167], using a different isolation procedure, reported finding several endogenous inhibitors in cytosol extracts of calf brain. One was a *ca* 15,000 M.W. protein, and the other a small heat stable peptide <5,000 M.W. At present, the significance of these various findings remain speculative. Whether there are endogenous inhibitors which bind at the vinca sites is not known.

3. MECHANISMS OF INHIBITION

The mechanisms by which drugs inhibit microtubule assembly and disassembly are complex and only poorly understood. In the previous section we alluded to the perturbing effects that antimicrotubule drugs have on tubulin conformation [106, 152, 75], -SH groups [118], GTPase activity [112], MAP availability [168] and tubulin dissociation rate constants [3]. The antimitotic activity of these drugs are presumably related to their *in vitro* mechanisms of action, but other factors undoubtedly also contribute to their antimicrotubule action *in vivo* (*c.f.* [96, 169]). A critical review of all the various mechanisms that have been proposed to explain antimicrotubule drug action is beyond the scope of this brief article. Instead, we focus on colchicine and the vinca alkaloids, two of the most intensely studied drug families, and review the various models that have been proposed to explain their *in vitro* effects on microtubule assembly and disassembly. Curious puzzles have emerged from studies of the mechanisms of action of colchicine. The elucidation of these puzzles is currently a very active area of research which should contribute significantly to our understanding of microtubule function.

3.1. Colchicine

Various models have been proposed to explain colchicine effects on microtubule assembly (Figure 3). Initially (Figure 3 top panel), it was thought [170] that colchicine inhibited microtubule assembly by depleting the pool of available subunit protein. This was presumed to occur by complexing with tubulin to form the assembly-incompetent species, TC. According to this simple model, half-maximal inhibition of assembly should occur when ~50% of the tubulin was complexed with colchicine. However, in 1973 Olmsted and Borisy reported that inhibition occured substoichiometrically, *i.e.,* that only a small fraction of the theoretical number of colchicine binding sites need to be complexed in order for *in vitro* assembly to be completely inhibited by colchicine [100]. This observation was confirmed by Wilson *et al.* [171] who also observed that substoichiometric amounts of podophyllotoxin and vinblastine inhibited microtubule assembly [171]. In an earlier study which preceded the Olmsted and Borisy investigations, Borisy *et al.* [172] reported that if high concentrations of colchicine ($\gtrsim 100$ μM) are added to polymerizing mixtures of microtubule protein, microtubule assembly is abruptly arrested but microtubules which formed prior to the addition of colchicine do not disassemble. Larger apparent steady-state levels were observed the later the colchicine addition. Margolis and Wilson [173] suggested on the basis of these results (and the finding that colchicine did not bind to tubulin subunits within the microtubule) that microtubule ends were being perturbed. They proposed that TC, the tight-binding 1:1 complex of tubulin and colchicine, was the direct inhibitor of assembly, and suggested that once a microtubule assembly end acquires a sufficiently small number of TCs, a 'cap' or kinetic block is established at the microtubule end which inhibits further tubulin addition or dissociation (Figure 3, middle panel). Margolis *et al.* generalized the model and applied it to mitosis [174]. In a later study using bovine brain tubulin and ^{3}H-GTP to probe the rates of association and dissociation at steady-state, Margolis *et al.* [175] proposed that ~1 TC complex bound per microtubule assembly end at steady-state was capable of significantly reducing the normal equilibrium rates of tubulin association and dissociation from the microtubule end. In 1979 Sternlicht and Ringel [113] reported the results of a kinetic study of *de novo* microtubule assembly in the presence of low to moderate rate concentrations of TC (<10 μM) under conditions where spontaneous nucleation was suppressed by the addition of polyanion (heparin). Polymerization was induced by adding microtubule fragments (MTF), and assembly proceeded almost exclusively by dimeric protein addition to the MTFs which elongated into microtubules. The number of microtubules remained constant during the elongation reaction and equalled the number of MTFs added, a property which significantly simplified interpretation of assembly-kinetics [80]. Sternlicht and Ringel showed that as assembly proceeded in the presence of TC, the number of *assembly-competent* microtubule ends remain *constant* and essentially equal to the number of MTFs initially added to induce assembly. They interpreted their data as indicating that TC substoichiometrically inhibits elongation reactions by a mechanism other than end-poisoning, and proposed the *copolymerization* mechanism for inhibition (Figure 3, bottom panel). A similar conclusion was reached when they extended their studies to spontaneously assemblying tubulin in the presence of TC (no heparin) [74].

Sternlicht and Ringel proposed that: TC substoichiometric inhibits *de novo* microtubule assembly by copolymerizing with tubulin to form random copolymers; the copolymers formed in the presence of TC have assembly-competent ends but display altered assembly kinetics which correlate with the TC mole fraction in the copolymers; the apparent association rate constant for tubulin addition to microtubule ends is more sensitive to the TC content than the apparent dissociation rate constant for tubulin, and decreases with increasing TC mole fraction values in the copolymer; and the critical tubulin concentrations required for assembly increases with increasing TC mole fractions in the copolymer and increasing TC in the reaction mixture. The critical tubulin concentrations were taken as a measure of the apparent dissociation constant for tubulin bound to copolymer ends. In subsequent studies Sternlicht *et al.* [74] showed that a good first approximation inhibition at low to moderate TC concentration ($\lesssim 10\ \mu$M) does not directly involve MAPs, and proposed a predictive theory for modelling the copolymerization of tubulin and TC [176, 177]. Their theory related copolymer composition to the composition of the reaction mixture and to the affinity of the microtubule end for tubulin and TC. Assembly inhibition could be understood as resulting from the interplay of two effects: one where tubulin facilitates the incorporation of TC into the microtubule, and the second where TC inhibits the assembly of tubulin into microtubules. The molecular basis for the inhibition was not established. Sternlicht *et al.* [74] proposed that altered protein conformation in TC may increase the free energy of assembly by inducing small changes in tubulin-tubulin contacts when TCs are incorporated into copolymer or into oligomer intermediates. Whether structural perturbations (*e.g.*, altered microtubule lattice) or biochemical perturbations (*e.g.*, an altered polymerization dependent GTPase activity) or both underline the apparent increase in the free energy of assembly in the presence of TC remains to be established.

Podophyllotoxin appears to inhibit *de novo* assembly by a copolymerization mechanism [102]. Lee *et al.* [75] have reported that nocodazole, a competitive inhibitor of colchicine, also inhibits *de novo* assembly by increasing the critical tubulin concentration, and does so by a process which appears to be independent of or only weakly linked to MAP concentrations. These similarities between nocodazole and colchicine inhibitioin of *de novo* assembly most likely indicate that nocodazole and tubulin form a nocodazole-tubulin complex which also inhibits *de novo* assembly by a copolymerization mechanism. Farell and Wilson [178] carried out a study at steady-state of the effects of TC on reassembled microtubules from sea urchin sperm tail outer doublet tubulin, and obtained results compatible with the copolymerization model. Thus, there are currently two major models for colchicine inhibition of microtubule assembly. In the 'capping' or kinetic block model, microtubule ends are presumed to bind TC quasi-irreversibly with an affinity constant larger than that for tubulin. In addition, TCs at the microtubule end are presumed to cause a significant reduction in the normal steady-state rates of association and dissociation of tubulin dimer. Furthermore, end states reached in the presence of TC are not believed to be equilibrium end-states. For example, high concentrations of colchicine (TC) are observed to abruptly arrest assembly, and higher microtubule yields are obtained the later the colchicine (TC) addition. In the copolymerization model, TC complexes are presumed to reversibly bind to microtubule ends. The affinity of the microtubule ends for TC was estimated to be at least 5 to 6 times less than the affinity of the ends for tubulin, while the TC dissociation rate constants were estimated to be greater than that for tubulin. Furthermore, TC and tubulin are presumed to coassemble and reach equilibrium end-states.

Such disparate perceptions strongly argue that the inhibition process is not understood, and important aspects have yet to be elucidated. The two models were derived under differing conditions. The 'capping' model was proposed to explain the results of steady-state experiments where often relatively high colchicine or TC to tubulin ratios were used, while the copolymerization model was proposed to explain the results of *de novo* microtubule formation studies where TC to tubulin ratios in the reaction mixture were relatively low. Sternlicht and Ringel [113] suggested that concentration differences may underlie the disparate perceptions of the two models. Zackroff *et al.* [179] noted that inhibition by high concentrations of colchicine was reminiscent of the blocking effects that high concentrations of GDP have on microtubule protein assembly [180]. They proposed that microtubule elongation involves *cooperative* interactions between oligomers (tubulin-MAP complexes) at the microtubule ends, and that GTP is capable of stabilizing an obligatory binding step involving oligomer and ends. High concentrations of GDP [180] and colchicine [172] presumably prevent this stabilization. Their proposal relating colchicine inhibition to GTP function in microtubule assembly is strengthened by David-Pfeuty *et al.*'s finding of an endogenous GTPase activity, intrinsic to tubulin and linked to polymerization, which may be involved in TC inhibition [112]. Farell and Wilson [178] proposed that the capping phenomenon may be related to the TC to tubulin ratio in the solution. They suggest that when this ratio exceeds a critical value, the recovery phase in their proposed cycles of poisoning and recovery does not occur, and the ends become assembly-incompetent in the presence of TC. Sternlicht speculated [181] that the disparate perceptions of how colchicine inhibits assembly may be the result of two binding sites on tubulin. At low to moderate colchicine concentrations, the tight-binding site, presumably on the α-subunit [116], is occupied to give TC_α. Copolymers assembled from tubulin and TC_α display reduced *association* rate constants for tubulin addition to microtubule ends, while tubulin dissociation rate constants remain largely unaffected. At higher colchicine concentrations, a weaker site is occupied, possibly on the β-chain, and the concentration of drug-free subunits is significantly reduced. Furthermore, when both binding sites are occupied, the association as well as the *dissociation* rate constants are markedly reduced, and a 'capping' mechanism of inhibition is operative. There is suggestive evidence in support of this model. Ringel and Sternlicht [46, 102] were able to show from nuclear magnetic resonance studies of C-13 enriched colchicine, that there is at least one weak and rapidly exchanging site on tubulin ($K_{Diss} \gtrsim 200\ \mu M$). Barnes *et al.* [101] have proposed that there is a second colchicine binding site on tubulin, and suggested that the second site develops as a result of a conformational change induced in tubulin by colchicine bound at the first site. Oakley and Morris [182] have isolated β-tubulin heat sensitive mutants of *Aspergillus nidulans* which give rise to *hyperstable* microtubules in which disassembly is inhibited. Taxol perturbs microtubule function by generating hyperstable microtubules [3, 76]. The maximum stabilization occurs at stoichiometric (1:1) ratios of taxol and tubulin. Whether taxol binds to the β-chain is not known.

3.2. Vinca alkaloids

Vinca alkaloids inhibit microtubule assembly substoichiometrically [137, 171]. However, other processes, different from those proposed for colchicine [113, 173], may play important roles in vinca inhibition of *de novo* assembly. Himes *et al.* [137] reported that assembly is totally inhibited at 37 °C when microtubule protein preparations contain 1 VCR to ~7 tubulins. Ultracentrifuge studies of these mixtures indicated large changes in the sizes of the sedimentation species. The amount of 6 S (*i.e.*, tubulin dimer) and 30S forms decreased dramatically, and a new species with a sedimentation constant >45S appeared. Furthermore, short spiral forms extending over several tenths of a micron were observed when stoichiometric concentrations of VCR were added to microtubule protein preparations at 0 °C. The vincas, therefore, inhibit *de novo* assembly, at least in part, by inducing tubulin to aggregate into oligomeric forms incapable of participating in microtubule assembly. A similar mechanism does not appear to be operative in the case of colchicine as colchicine apparently does not significantly affect the distribution and types of oligomeric forms present in solution [83]. Nevertheless, Zackroff *et al.*, in their cooperative model of microtubule assembly [179], proposed that colchicine interferes with an obligatory binding step involving *catalytic* concentrations of oligomer intermediates.

Warfield *et al.* [147] found that the vincas had also a significant effect on *preformed* microtubules in that these drugs were capable of inducing a microtubule to macrotubule transition at 37 °C. Denoso *et al.* [148] examined further the effects that vincas have on preformed microtubules assembled either in the presence or absence of MAPs. When the VCR to protein ratios were much less than 1, they observed short, curly filamentous extensions at the microtubule ends. However, as they increased the vinca concentrations, they observed the complete depolymerization of MAP-free microtubules into amorphous globular material while MAP-containing microtubules gave rise to spiral-like structures (Figure 4) which appeared to be intermediate between microtubules and paracrystal forms. Spirals were seen to emerge from different parts of the microtubule, although the majority originated at the microtubules ends (Figure 4). In most cases these structures were extensions of single protofilaments but spirals containing 2 protofilaments were also observed. Maximum production of the spiral protofilaments occurred at a VCR to protein ratio of ~1, suggestive that perhaps

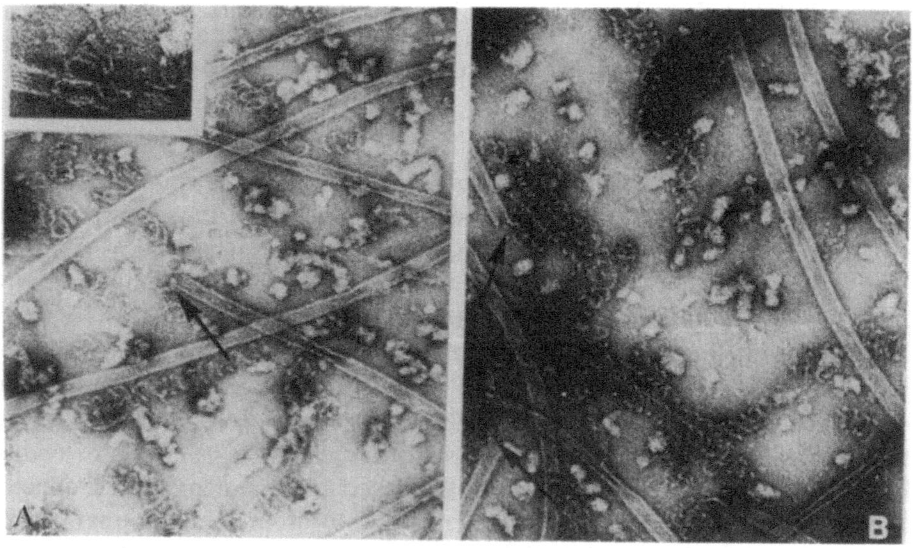

Figure 4. Electron micrograph of MAP containing microtubules treated with VCR (Courtesy of Dr. Richard Himes). (*A*) 15 minutes after the addition of VCR. *Inset*, spirals formed from one protofilament originating from the middle of a microtubule. (*B*) 15 minutes after a second addition of VCR. Each addition of VCR introduced 9 μM of VCR. Arrows in (*A*) and (*B*) point to spirals which are continuous with protofilaments of microtubules.

only the high-affinity vinca binding site was involved. Denoso *et al.* further showed that spirals will directly form from microtubules at 37 °C as well as spontaneously form at 0 °C in the presence of vincas, and suggested that vincas destabilize lateral interactions between tubulin subunits causing single protofilaments to unravel from the microtubule ends. MAPs apparently stabilize the single protofilament forms, presumably by interacting with two or more tubulin dimers within the protofilament, and prevent the protofilaments from depolymerizing. (See section on antimicrotubule drugs and reference [2] for related studies.)

Vincas appear to interact in a more complicated way with tubulin and microtubule than does colchicine, although there may be similarities in their modes of inhibition. David-Pfeuty *et al.* [112], for example, proposed that TC may function by destabilizing lateral interactions between protofilaments, while Zackroff *et al.* [179] proposed that there may be a complex relationship between colchicine inhibition and oligomeric forms. Polymorphic forms are readily seen when vincas are added to microtubules or microtubule protein preparations. The copolymerization [113] and end-poisoning [173] models derived from studies of colchicine inhibition do not appear to be immediately applicable to vinca inhibition. Whether these theories can be appropriately modified to accommodate the polymorphic effects of the vincas remains to be seen.

4. SUMMARY AND PROSPECTUS

Tubulin is a complex protein able to interact with a variety of drugs. The mechanisms by which drugs interact with tubulin and inhibit microtubules assembly and dissambly are not understood although considerable progress has been made these several years toward identifying the molecular bases for inhibition. Binding experiments have indicated that there are several drug binding sites. However, amino-sequence determinations by Ponstingl *et al.* have not revealed sequences suggestive of major hydrophobic pockets which could be involved in drug binding, while spectroscopic studies have indicated that tubulin has a high percentage of random coil structure, and a high degree of internal flexibility. The significance of these curious findings in terms of how tubulin functions and binds to drugs and MAPs remains to be established. Recently, Valenzuela *et al.* [34] have determined the essentially complete amino acid sequences of α- and β-polypeptide chains of chicken embryo brain tubulin. This sequence information should significantly facilitate further studies. Undoubtedly, new kinds of antimicrotubule and antimitotic drugs will also be uncovered in the next few years. Most probably, some of these will contribute toward a deeper understanding of microtubule function, and facilitate the design of new and highly potent antineoplastic agents.

ACKNOWLEDGEMENTS

This work was supported in part by an American Cancer Society Grant CH-99B to Himan Sternlicht. The author wishes to thank Drs. George Langford and Richard Himes for the use of several electron micrographs.

REFERENCES

1. Dustin P: Microtubule Poisons. In: Microtubules, Springer-Verlag Publishers, 1978, p 166–225.
2. Ludueña RF: Biochemistry of tubulin. In: Microtubules, Roberts K, Hyams J (eds), Academic Press, 1979, p 66–116.
3. Schiff P, Horwitz S: Tubulin, a target for chemotherapeutic agents. In: Molecular action and targets for cancer chemotherapeutic agents, Academic Press, 1980, p 483–505.
4. Kirschner M: Microtubule assembly and nucleation. In: International Review of Cytology, Vol. 54, Bourne G, Danielli J (eds), 1978, p 1-71.
5. Amos L: Arrangement of high molecular weight associated proteins on purified mammalian brain microtubules. J Cell Biol 72:642–654, 1977.
6. Kim H, Binder L, Rosenbaum J: The periodic association of MAP_2 with brain microtubules *in vivo*. J Cell Biol 80:266–276, 1979.
7. Mendelkow E, Thomas J, Cohen H: Microtubule structure at low resolution by X-ray diffraction. Proc Natl Acad Sci USA 74:3370–3374, 1977.
8. Pierson G, Burton P, Himes R: Alterations in number of protofilaments in microtubules assembled *in vitro*. J Cell Biol 76:223–228, 1978.
9. Taylor E: The mechanism of colchicine inhibition of mitosis. I. Kinetics of inhibition and the binding of H^3-colchicine. J Cell Biol 25:145–160, 1965.
10. Murphy D, Borisy G: Association of high-molecular-weight proteins with microtubules and their role in microtubule assembly. Proc Natl Acad Sci USA 72:2696–2700, 1975.
11. Sloboda R, Dentler W, Rosenbaum J: Microtubule-associated proteins and the stimulation of tubulin assembly *in vitro*. Biochemistry 15:4497–4505, 1976.
12. Bryan J, Wilson L: Are cytoplasmic microtubules heteropolymers? Proc Natl Acad Sci USA 8:1762–1766, 1971.
13. Ludueña R, Shooter E, Wilson L: Structure of the tubulin dimer. J Biol Chem 252:7006–7014, 1977.
14. Erickson H: Microbutule surface lattice and subunit structure and observations on reassembly. J Cell Biol 60:153–167, 1974.
15. Amos L, Baker T: The three-dimensional structure of tubulin protofilaments. Nature 279:607–612, 1979.
16. Bergen L, Kuriyama R, Borisy G: Polarity of microtubules nucleated by centrosomes and chromosomes of chinese hamster ovary cells *in vitro*. J Cell Biol 84:151–159, 1980.
17. Heidemann S, McIntosh J: Visualization of the structural polarity of microtubules. Nature 286:517–519, 1980.

18. Kirschner M: Implications of treadmilling for the stability and polarity of actin and tubulin polymers *in vivo.* J Cell Biol 86:330–334, 1980.
19. Nagle B, Doenges K, Bryan J: Assembly of tubulin from cultured cells and comparison with the neurotubulin model. Cell 12:573–586, 1977.
20. Sherline P, Schiavona K: Immunofluorescence localization of proteins of high molecular weight along intracellular microtubules. Science 198:1038–1040, 1977.
21. Cleveland D, Spiegelman M, Kirschner M: Conservation of microtubule associated proteins. J Biol Chem 254:12670–12678, 1979.
22. Lee J, Tweedy N, Tinasheff S: *In vitro* reconstitution of calf brain microtubules: effects of macromolecules. Biochemistry 17:2783–2790, 1978.
23. Cleveland D, Hwo S, Kirschner M: Purification of tau, a microtubule-associated protein that induces assembly of microtubules from purified tubulin. J Mol Biol 116:207–225, 1977.
24. Murphy D, Johnson K, Borisy G: Role of tubulin-associated proteins in microtubule nucleation and elongation. J Mol Biol 117:33–52, 1977.
25. Ludueña R, Woodward O: α- and β-tubulin separation and partial sequence Ann NY Acad Sci 253:272–283, 1975.
26. Ludueña R, Woodward D: Isolation and partial characterization of α- and β-tubulin from outer doublets of sea urchin sperm and microtubules of chick-embryo brain. Proc Natl Acad Sci USA 70:3594–3598, 1973.
27. Lu R, Elzinga M: Chromatographic resolution of the subunits of calf brain tubulin. Anal Biochem 77:243–250, 1977.
28. Lu R, Elzinga M: The primary structure of tubulin sequences of the carboxyl terminus and seven other cyanogen bromide peptides from the α-chain. Biochim Biophys Acta 537:320–328, 1978.
29. Ponstingl H, Little M, Krauhs E, Kempf T: Carboxy-terminal amino acid sequence of α-tubulin from porcine brain. Nature 282:423–424, 1979.
30. Cleveland D, Fischer S, Kirschner M, Laemmli U: Peptide by limited proteolysis in sodium dodecyl sulfate and analysis by gel electrophoresis. J Biol Chem 252:1102–1106, 1977.
31. Piperno G, Luck D: Microtubular proteins of Chlamydomonas reinhardtii. J Biol Chem 252:383–391, 1977.
32. Cleveland D, Lopata M, MacDonald K, Cowan N, Rutter W, Kirschner M: Number and evolutionary conservation of α- and β-tubulin and cytoplasmic β- and α-actin genes using specific cloned cDNA probes. Cell 20:95–105, 1980.
33. Krauhs E, Little M, Ade W, Kempf T, Hoter Warbinek R, Ponstingl H: 45% homology in the N-terminal 90 amino acid residues of α- and β-tubulin from porcine brain. In: Programme abstracts, 2nd international symposium on microtubules and microtubule inhibitors, Beerse (Belgium), p 63, 1980.
34. Valenzuela P, Quiroga M, Zaldivar J, Rutter W, Kirschner M, Cleveland D: Nucleotide and corresponding amino acid sequences encoded by α- and β-tubulin mRNAs. Nature 289:650–656, 1981.
35. Stephens R: Primary structural differences among tubulin subunits from flagella, cilia and the cytoplasm. Biochemistry 17:2882–2891, 1978.
36. Gozes R, Littauer U: Tubulin microheterogeneity increases with rat brain maturation. Nature 276:411–413, 1978.
37. Barnstable C, Gozes I: Monoclonal antibodies that recognize discrete forms of tubulin. J Cell Biol 87:251a, 1980.
38. Eipper B: Rat brain microtubule protein: purification and determination of covalently bound phosphate and carbohydrate. Proc Natl Acad Sci USA 69:2283–2287, 1972.

39. Lockwood A: Cyclic nucleotide dependent protein kinase as molecular regulators of cell morphology. In: Microtubules and microtubule inhibitors, De Brabander M, De Mey J (eds), Elsevier press, 1980, p 71–83.
40. Margolis RK, Margolis RU, Shelanski M: The carbohydrate composition of brain microtubule protein. Biochem Biophys Res Commun 47:432–437, 1972.
41. Raybin K, Flavin M: An enzyme tyrosylating α-tubulin and its role in microtubule assembly. Biochem Biophys Res Commun 65:1088–1095, 1975.
42. Thompson W, Deanin G, Gordon M: Intact microtubules are required for rapid turnover of carboxyl-terminal tyrosine of α-tubulin in cell culture. Proc Natl Acad Sci USA 76:1318–1322, 1979.
43. Crepeau R, McEwen B, Edelstein J: Differences in α and β polypeptide chains of tubulin resolved by electron microscopy with image reconstruction. Proc Natl Acad Sci USA 75:5006–5010, 1978.
44. Ventilla M, Cantor C, Shelanski M: A circular dichroism study of microtubule protein. Biochemistry 11:1554–1561, 1972.
45. Lee J, Frigon R, Tinasheff S: Structural stability of calf brain microtubule protein. Ann NY Acad Sci 253:284–291, 1975.
46. Ringel I, Sternlicht H: A study of tubulin flexibility and conformation. Fed Proc (in press), June 1981.
47. Ponstingl H, Little M, Krauhs E, Kempf T: Microheterogeneity in the amino acid sequence of the C-terminal 200 positions in α-tubulin from porcine brain. In: Programme abstracts, 2nd international symposium on microtubules and microtubule inhibitors, Beerse (Belgium), p 29, 1980.
48. Lee Y, Houston L, Himes R: Inhibition of the self-assembly of tubulin by diethylpyrocarbonate and photooxidation. Biochem Biophys Res Commun 70:50–57, 1976.
49. Kuriyama R: Further studies on tubulin polymerization *in vitro*. J Biochem (Tokyo) 77:23–31, 1975.
50. Nishidi E, Kobagashi T: Relationship between tubulin SH groups and bound guanine nucleotide. J Biochem (Tokyo) 81:343–347, 1977.
51. Sternlicht H, Ringel I, Szasz J, Burns R, Sherman G: Evidence for an essential lysine in microtubule assembly. J Cell Biol 87:251a, 1980.
52. Sentein P: Action of gluteraldehyde and formaldehyde on segmentation mitosis. Exp Cell Res 95:223–246, 1975.
53. Olmsted J, Borisy G: Ionic and nucleotide requirements for microtubule polymerization *in vitro*. Biochemistry 14:2996–3005, 1975.
54. Solomon F: Binding sites for calcium on tubulin. Biochemistry 16:358–36, 1977.
55. Gaskin F: *In vitro* microtubule assembly regulation by divalent cations and nucleotides. Biochemistry 20:1318–1322, 1981.
56. Weisenberg R: Microtubule formation *in vitro* in solutions containing low calcium concentrations. Science 177:1104–1105, 1972.
57. Welsh M, Dedman J, Brinkley B, Means R: Calcium-dependent regulator protein: localization in mitotic apparatus of eukaryiotic cells. Proc Natl Acad Sci USA 75:1867–1871, 1978.
58. Gaskin F, Kress Y: Zinc ion-induced assembly of tubulin. J Biol Chem 252:6918–6924, 1977.
59. Weisenberg R, Borisy G, Taylor E: The colchicine-binding protein of mammalian brain and its relation to microtubules. Biochemistry 7:4466–4479, 1968.
60. Bryan J: Definition of three classes of binding sites in isolated microtubule crystals. Biochemistry 11:2611–2616, 1972.
61. Jameson L, Caplow M: Effect of guanosine diphosphate on microtubule assembly and

stability. J Biol Chem 255:2284–2292, 1980.
62. Weisenberg R, Deery W, Dickinson P: Tubulin-nucleotide interactions during the polymerization and depolymerization of microtubules. Biochemistry 15:4248–4254, 1976.
63. Carlier M, Pantaloni D: Kinetic analysis of the correlation between tubulin assembly and GTP hydrolysis. In: Programme abstracts, 2nd international symposium on microtubule inhibitors, Beerse (Belgium), p 38, 1980.
64. Jacobs M: Tubulin and nucleotides. In: Microtubules, Roberts K, Hyams J (eds), Academic Press, 1979, p 255–277.
65. Gaskin F, Cantor R, Shelanski M: Turbidimetric studies of the *in vitro* assembly and disassembly of porcine neurotubules. J Mol Biol 89:737–758, 1974.
66. Kuriyama R, Sakai H: Viscometric demonstration of tubulin polymerization. J Biochem (Tokyo) 75:463–471, 1974.
67. Miki-Noumura T, Kamiya R: Shape of microtubules in solution. Exp Cell Res 97:451–453, 1976.
68. Kirschner M, Honig L, Williams R: Quantitative electron microscopy of microtubule assembly *in vitro*. J Mol Biol 99:263–276, 1975.
69. Berne B: Interpretation of the light scattering from long rods. J Mol Biol 89:755–758, 1974.
70. Zingsheim H, Herzog W, Weber K: Differences in surface morphology of microtubules reconstituted from pure brain tubulin using two different microtubule-associated probes: the high molecular weight MAP 2 proteins and tau proteins. Eur J of Cell Biol 19:175–183, 1979.
71. Ludueña R, Fellous A, Francon J, Nunez J, McManus L: A hypothesis on the role of tau and high molecular weight protein (MAP 2) in microtubule assembly. J Cell Biol 87:244a, 1980.
72. Oosawa F, Kasai M: Theory of linear and helical aggregations of macromolecules. J Mol Biol 4:10–21, 1962.
73. Johnson K, Borisy G: The equilibrium assembly *in vitro*. In: Molecules and cell movement, Inoué S, Stephens R (eds), Raven Press, 1975, p 119–139.
74. Sternlicht H, Ringel I, Szasz J: The copolymerization of tubulin and tubulin.cochicine complex in the absence and presence of associated proteins. J Biol Chem 255:9138–9148, 1980.
75. Lee J, Field D, Lee L: Effects of nocodazole on structures of calf brain tubulin. Biochemistry 19:6209–6215, 1980.
76. Schiff P, Fant J, Horwitz S: Promotion of microtubule assembly *in vitro* by taxol. Nature 277:665–667, 1979.
77. Olmsted J, Marcum J, Johnson K, Allen A, Borisy G: Microtubule assembly: some possible regulatory mechanisms. J Supramol Struct 2:429–450, 1974.
78. Kirschner M, Williams R, Weingarten M, Gerhart J: Microtubules from mammalian brain: some properties of their depolymerization products and a proposed mechanism for assembly and disassembly. Proc Natl Acad Sci USA 71:1159–1163, 1974.
79. Lee J, Timasheff S: The reconstitution of microtubules from purified calf brain tubulin. Biochemistry 14:5183–5187, 1975.
80. Bryan J: A quantitative analysis of microtubule elongation. J Cell Biol 71:749–767, 1976.
81. Scheele R, Borisy G: *In vitro* assembly of microtubules. In: Microtubules, Roberts K, Hyams J (eds), Academic Press, 1979, p 176-254.
82. Kirschner M, Williams R: The mechanism of microtubule assembly *in vitro*. J Supramol Struct 2:412–424, 1974.
83. Penningroth S: Colchicine binding to an oligomer of tubulin. Biochem Biophys Res Com-

mun 92:183–190, 1980.
84. Solomon F: Organizing microtubules in the cytoplasm. Cell 22:331–332, 1980.
85. Osborn M, Weber K: The display of microtubules in transformed cells. Cell 12:561–571, 1977.
86. Spiegelman B, Lopata M, Kirschner M: Multiple sites for the initiation of microtubule assembly in mammalian cells. Cell 16:239–252, 1979.
87. Brinkley B, Fuller G, Highfield D: Studies of microtubules in dividing and non-dividing mammalian cells using antibody to 6S bovine brain tubulin. In: Microtubules and microtubule inhibitors, Borger SM, de Branbander M (eds), North Holland Publishers, 1975, p 297–312.
88. Osborn M, Weber K: Cytoplasmic microtubules in tissue culture cells appear to grow from an organizing structure towards the plasma membrane. Proc Natl Acad Sci USA 73:867–871, 1976.
89. Haimo L, Telzer B, Rosenbaum J: Dynein bind to and crossbridges cytoplasmic microtubules. Proc Natl Acad Sci USA 76:5759–5763, 1979.
90. Margolis R, Wilson L: Opposite end assembly and disassembly of microtubules at steady state *in vitro.* Cell 13:1–8, 1978.
91. Bergen L, Borisy G: Head-to-tail polymerization of microtubules *in vitro.* Electron microscope analysis of seeded assembly. J Cell Biol 84:141–150, 1980.
92. Brinkley B, Fuller G, Highfield D: Cytoplasmic microtubules in normal and transformed cells in culture. Analysis by tubulin antibody immunofluorescence. Proc Natl Acad Sci USA 72:4981–4985, 1975.
93. Porter K, Puck T, Hsie W, Kelley D: An electron microscope study of the effects of dibutyryl cyclic AMP on chinese hamster ovary cells. Cell 2: 145–162, 1974.
94. Berlin R, Regula C, Pfeiffer J: Microtubule assembly and disassembly at alkaline pH. In: Microtubules and microtubule inhibitors, de Branbander M, De Mey J (eds), Elsevier Press, 1980, p 145–160.
95. Silver R, Cole D: Isolation of mitotic apparatus containing vesicles with calcium sequestering activity. Cell 19:505–516, 1980.
96. Harris P, Osborn M, Weber K: Distribution of tubulin-containing structures in the egg of the sea urchin from fertilization through first cleavage. J Cell Biol 84:668–679, 1980.
97. Roobol A, Gull K, Pogson C: Evidence that griseofulvin binds to a microtubule associated protein. FEBS Lett 75:149–153, 1977.
98. Gerwick W, Fenical W, Engen D, Clardy J: Isolation and structure of spatol, a potent inhibitor of cell replication from the brown seaweed spatoglossum schmittii. J Am Chem Soc 102:7991–7993, 1980.
99. Jacobs R, White S, Wilson L: Selective compounds derived from marine organisms: effects on cell division in fertilized sea urchin eggs. Fed Proc 40:26–29, 1981.
100. Olmsted J, Borisy G: Characterization of microtubule assembly in porcine brain extracts by viscometry. Biochemistry 12:4282–4289, 1973.
101. Barnes L, Roberson G, Williams R: Binding of colchicine and colchicine analogs to tubulin. Model evidence for two binding sites. Fed Proc 39:2162a, 1980.
102. Ringel I, Sternlicht H: Unpublished work.
103. Wilson L: Properties of colchicine binding protein from chick embryo brain. Interactions with vinca alkaloids and podophyllotoxin. Biochemistry 9:4999–5007, 1970.
104. McClure W, Paulson J: The interaction of colchicine and some related alkaloids with rat brain tubulin. Mol Pharmacol 13:560–575, 1977.
105. Wilson L, Friedkin M: The biochemical events of mitosis. II. The *in vivo* and *in vitro* binding of colchicine in grasshopper embryos and its possible relation to inhibition of mitosis. Biochemistry 6:3126–2135, 1967.

106. Garland D: Kinetics and mechanism of colchicine binding to tubulin: evidence for ligand-induced conformational change. Biochemistry 17:4266–4272, 1978.
107. Ludueña R, Roach M, Garrison P: Effect of drugs on the alkylation of tubulin. J Cell Biol 75:272a, 1977.
108. Morgan J, Ludueña R, Spooner B: Tubulin conformation changes induced by anti-mitotic drug binding. J Cell Biol 79:292a, 1978.
109. Banerjee A, Bhattacharyya B: Colcemid and colchicine binding to tubulin. FEBS Lett 99:333–336, 1979.
110. Bhattacharyya B, Wolff J: Promotion of fluorescence upon binding of colchicine to tubulin. Proc Natl Acad Sci USA 71:2627–2631, 1974.
111. Dietrich H, Williams R, Wilson L, Puett D: Changes in the circular dichroic spectrum of colchicine associated with tubulin binding. In: Programme abstracts, 2nd international symposium of microtubules and microtubule inhibitors, Beerse (Belgium), p 45, 1980.
112. David-Pfeuty T, Simon C, Panataloni D: Effect of antimitotic drugs on tubulin GTPase activity and self-assembly. J Biol Chem 254:11696–11702, 1979.
113. Sternlicht H, Ringel I: Colchicine inhibition of microtubule assembly via copolymer formation. J Biol Chem 254:10540–10550, 1979.
114. Barton J: Polymerization and colchicine binding: Two independent properties of tubulin. Biochim Biophys Acta 532:155–160, 1978.
115. Wiche G, Honig L, Cole R: Polymerizing ability of C_6 glial cell microtubule protein decays much faster than its colchicine binding activity. Nature 269:435–436, 1977.
116. Schmitt H, Atlas D: Specific affinity labelling of tubulin with bromocolchicine. J Mol Biol 102:743–758, 1976.
117. Schmitt H, Kram R: Binding of antimitotic drugs around cysteine residues of tubulin. Exp Cell Res 115:408–411, 1978.
118. Nishida E, Kobayashi T: Relationship between tubulin SH groups and bound nucleotides. J Biochem (Tokyo) 81:343–347, 1977.
119. Sheir-Neiss G, Lai M, Morris N: Indentification of a gene for β-tubulin in Aspergillus nidulans. Cell 15:639–647, 1978.
120. Cabral F, Sobel M, Gottesman M: CHO mutants resistant to griseofulvin have an altered β-tubulin. Cell 20:29–36, 1980.
121. Zweig M, Chignell C: Interaction of some colchicine analogs, vinblastine and podophyllotoxin with rat brain microtubule protein. Biochem Pharmacol 22:2141–2150, 1973.
122. Fitzgerald T: Molecular features of colchicine associated with antimitotic activity and inhibition of tubulin polymerization. Biochem Pharmacol 25:1383–1387, 1976.
123. Lettre H, Dönges K, Barthold H, Fitzgerald T: Synthese neuer colchicin-derivate mit hoher antimitotischer Wirksamkeit. Liebigs Ann 758:185–189, 1972.
124. Marthe G, Schwarzenberg L, Pouillart P. Oldham R, Weiner R, Jasmin C, Rosenfeld C, Hayat M, Misset J, Musset M, Schneider M, Amiel J, De Vassal F: Two epipodophyllotoxin derivatives, VP 16213 and VM 26 in the treatment of leukemias, hematosarcomas, and lymphomas. Cancer 34:985–992, 1974.
125. Loike J, Brewer C, Sternlicht H, Gensler W, Horwitz S: Structure-activity study of the inhibition of microtubule assembly *in vitro* by podophyllotoxin and its congeners. Cancer Res 38:2688–2693, 1978.
126. Loike J, Horwitz S: Effects of VP-16-213 on the intracellular degradation of DNA in Hela Cells. Biochemistry 15:5443–5448, 1976.
127. Cortese F, Bhattacharyya B, Wolff J: Podophyllotoxin as a probe for the colchicine binding site of tubulin. J Biol Chem 252:1134–1140, 1977.
128. Wilson L, Anderson K, Grisham L, Chin D: Biochemical mechanisms of action of microtubule inhibitors. In: Microtubules and microtubule inhibitors, Borgers M, de Branbander

M (eds), North Holland Publishers, 1975, p 103–113.
129. Wilson L: Microtubules as drug receptors: pharmacological properties of microtubule protein. Ann NY Acad Sci 253:213–231, 1975.
130. Kelleher J: Tubulin binding affinities of podophyllotoxin and colchicine analogues. Mol Pharmacol 13:232–241, 1977.
131. Brewer C, Loike J, Horwitz S, Sternlicht H, Gensler W: Coformational analysis of podophyllotoxin and its congeners. Structure-activity relationship in microtubule assembly. J Med Chem 22:215–221, 1979.
132. de Branbander M, Geuens G, Van de Veire R, Thoné F, Aerts F, Desplenter L, DeCree J, Borgers M: The effects of R17934 (NSC 238159), a new antimicrotubular substance on the ultrastructure of neoplastic cells *in vivo*. Eur J Cancer 13:511–528, 1977.
133. de Branbander M, Van de Veire R, Aerts F, Borgers M, Janssen P: The effects of methyl [5-(2-thienyl carbonyl)-1H-benzimidazol-2-yl carbamate, (R17934; NSC 238159], a new synthetic antitumoral drug interfering with microtubules on mammalian cells cultures *in vivo*. Cancer Res 36:905–916, 1976.
134. Hoebeke J, Van Nigen G, de Branbander M: Interaction of oncodazole (R 17934), a new antitumoral drug, with rat brain tubulin. Biochem Biophys Res Comm 69:319–324, 1976.
135. Brodie A, Potter J, Reed D: Effects of vinblastine, oncodazole, procarbazine, chlorambucil and bleomycin *in vivo* on colchicine binding activity of tubulin. Life Sci 24:1547–1554, 1979.
136. Davidse L, Flach W: Differential binding of methyl benzimidazol-2-yl carbamate to fungal tubulin as a mechanism of resistance to this antimitotic agent in mutant strains of Aspergillus nidulans. J Cell Biol 72:174–193, 1977.
137. Himes R, Kersey R, Heller-Bettinger I, Samson F: Action of the Vinca alkaloids vincristine, vinblastine, and desacetyl vinblastine amide on microtubules *in vitro*. Cancer Res 36:3798–3802, 1976.
138. Sweeney M, Cullinan G, Poore G, Gerzon K: Experimental antitumor activity of vinblastine amides. Proc Am Assoc Cancer Res 15:37, 1974.
139. Johnson I, Armstrong J, Gorman M, Burnet J: The Vinca alkaloids: a new class of oncolytic agents. Cancer Res 23:1390–1427, 1963.
140. Creasey W: Modifications in biochemical pathways produced by the vinca alkaloids. Cancer Chemother Rep 52:501–507, 1968.
141. Mandelbaum-Shavit F, Wolpert-Defillepes M, Johns D: Binding of Maytansine to rat brain tubulin. Biochem Biophys Res Commun 72:47–54, 1976.
142. Wilson L, Anderson K, Creswell K: On the mechanism of action of vinblastine. J Cell Biol 63:373a, 1974.
143. Bensch K, Malawista S: Microtubular crystals in mammalian cells. J Cell Biol 40:95–105, 1969.
144. Fujiwara K, Tilney L: Substructural analysis of the microtubule and its polymorphic forms. Ann NY Acad Sci 253:27–50, 1975.
145. Lee J, Harrison D, Timasheff S: Interaction of vinblastine with calf brain microtubule protein. J Biol Chem 250:9276–9282, 1975.
146. Erickson H: Negatively stained vinblastine aggregates. Ann NY Acad Sci 253:51, 1975.
147. Warfield R, Bouck G: Microtubule-macrotubule transitions: Intermediates after exposure to the mitotic inhibitor vinblastine. Science 186:1219–1220, 1974.
148. Donoso J, Haskins K, Himes R: Effect of microtubule-associated proteins on the interaction of vincristine with microtubules and tubulin. Cancer Res 39:1604–1610, 1979.
149. Haskins K, Donos J, Himes R: Spirals and paracrystals induced by vinca alkaloids: evidence that microtubule-associated proteins act as polycations. J Cell Sci 47:237–247,

1981.
150. Wilson L, Creswell K, Chin D: The mechanism of action of vinblastine. Binding of (acetyl-^{3}H) vinblastine to embryonic chick brain tubulin and tubulin from sea urchin sperm tail outer doublet microtubules. Biochemistry 14:5586–5592, 1975.
151. Bhattacharyya B, Wolff J: Tubulin aggregation and disaggregation: mediation by two distinct vinblastine-binding sites. Proc Natl Acad Sci USA 73:2375–2378, 1976.
152. Ludueña R, Ferrigini K, Roach M, Horowitz P: Contrasting effects of vinca alkaloids and ansa macrolides on the intrinsic fluorescence of tubulin. J Cell Biol 87:243a, 1980.
153. Tan L, Lagnado J: Effects of indole alkaloids and related compounds on the properties of brain microtubule protein. Biochem Soc Trans 3:121–124, 1975.
154. Kupchan S, Komoda Y, Court W, Thomas G, Smith R, Karim A, Gilmore C, Haltiwanger R, Bryan R: Maytansine, a novel antileukemic ansa macrolide from Maytenus ovatus. J Am Chem Soc 94:1354–1356, 1972.
155. Bhattacharyya B, Wolff J: Maytansine binding to the vinblastine sites of tubulin. FEBS Lett 75:159–162, 1977.
156. Remillard S, Rebhun L, Howie G, Kupchan S: Antimitotic activity of the potent tumor inhibitor Maytansine. Science 189:1002–1005, 1975.
157. Ludueña R, Roach M, McAda P: Correlation between the effects of drugs on microtubule assembly and on the alkylation of tubulin. J Cell Biol 79:289a, 1978.
158. Kupchan S, Sneden A, Branfman A, Howie G, Rebhun L, McIvor W, Wang R, Schnaitman T: Structural requirements for antileukemic activity among the naturally occurring and semisynthetic Maytansinoids. J Med Chem 21:31–37, 1978.
159. Higashide E, Asia M, Ootsu K, Tanida S, Kozai Y, Hasegawa T, Kishi T, Sugino Y, Yoneda M: Ansamitocin, a group of novel Maytansinoid antibiotics with antitumor properties from Nocardia. Nature 270:721–722, 1977.
160. Wani M, Taylor H, Wall M, Coggon P, McPhai A: Plant antitumor agents. VI. The isolation and structure of taxol, a novel antileukemic and antitumor agent from taxus brevifolia. J Am Chem Soc 93:2325–2327, 1971.
161. Wall M, Wani M: Antineoplastic agents from plants. Annu Rev Pharmacol Toxicol 17:117–132, 1977.
162. Schiff P, Horwitz S: Taxol stabilizes microtubules in mouse fibroblast cells. Proc Natl Acad Sci USA 77:1561–1565, 1980.
163. Sandoval I, McDonald E, Jameson J, Cuatrecasas P: Role of nucleotides in tubulin polymerization: effect of guanylyl 5′-methylene diphosphonate. Proc Natl Acad Sci USA 74:4881–4885, 1977.
164. Sloboda R, Malawista S, Van Blaricom, Creasey W, Rosenbaum J: Griseofulvin: *in vitro* microtubule assembly. J Cell Biol 70:290a, 1976.
165. Wehland J, Herzog W, Weber K: Interaction of griseofulvin with microtubules, microtubule protein and tubulin. J Mol Biol 111:329–342, 1977.
166. Sherline P, Schiavone K, Brocato S: Endogenous inhibitors of colchicine-tubulin binding in rat brain. Science 205:593–595, 1979.
167. Lockwood A: Molecules in mammalian brain that interact with the colchicine site on tubulin. Proc Natl Acad Sci USA 76:1184–1188, 1979.
168. Nunez J, Fellous A, Francon J, Lennon A: Competitive inhibition of colchicine binding to tubulin by microtubule-associated proteins. Proc Natl Acad Sci USA 76:86–90, 1979.
169. Salmon E, Begg D: Functional implications of cold-stable microtubules in kinetochore fibers of insect spermatocytes during anaphase. J Cell Biol 85:853–865, 1980.
170. Inoué S: The effect of colchicine on the microscopic and submicroscopic structure of the mitotic spindle. Exp Cell Res (Suppl) 2:305–314, 1952.
171. Wilson L, Anderson K, Grisham L, Chin D: Biochemical mechanisms of action of micro-

tubule inhibitors. In: Microtubules and microtubule inhibitors, Borgers M, de Brabander M (eds), North-Holland publishers, 1975, p 103–114.

172. Borisy G, Olmsted J, Klugman R: *In vitro* aggregation of cytoplasmic microtubule subunits. Proc Natl Acad Sci USA 69:2890–2894, 1972.

173. Margolis R, Wilson L: Addition of colchicine-tubulin complex to microtubule ends: the mechanism of substoichiometric colchicine poisoning. Proc Natl Acad Sci USA 74:3466–3470, 1977.

174. Margolis R, Wilson L, Kiefer B: Mitotic mechanism based on intrinsic microtubule behaviour. Nature 272:450–452, 1978.

175. Margolis R, Rauch C, Wilson L: Mechanism of colchicine-dimer addition to microtubule ends: implications for microtubule polymerization mechanism. Biochemistry 19:5550–5557, 1980.

176. Sternlicht H, Ringel I, Szasz J: A kinetic model for colchicine inhibition of microtubule assembly. Biophys Disc 32:445–448, 1980.

177. Sternlicht H, Ringel I, Szasz J: An analysis of the copolymerization of tubulin and tubulin.colchicine complex. Submitted for publication.

178. Farrell K, Wilson L: Proposed mechanism for colchicine poisoning of microtubules reassembled *in vitro* from Strongylocentrotus purpuratus sperm tail outer doublet tubulin. Biochemistry 19:3048–3054, 1980.

179. Zacroff R, Weisenber R, Deery W: Equilibrium and kinetic analysis of microtubule assembly in the presence of guanosine diphosphate. J Mol Biol 139:641–677, 1980.

180. Doery W, Zackroff R, Weisenberg R: Effects of microtubule associated proteins on assembly and stability of microtubule in colchicine and GDP. J Cell Biol 79:302a, 1978.

181. Sternlicht H: Unpublished work.

182. Oakley B, Morris R: β-tubulin mutants of Aspergillus nidulans defective for microtubule assembly and function. J Cell Biol 87:237a, 1980.

183. Langford G: Arrangement of subunits in microtubules with 14 protofilaments. J Cell Biol 87:521–525, 1980.

5. Biochemical Modulation as a Guide to Rational Combination Chemotherapy for the Treatment of Cancer

E.C. CADMAN, STEVEN GRANT and CHRIS C. BENZ

The treatment of cancer with drugs has led to significant improvement in response and survival of some patients with neoplastic disease. Unfortunately, the tumors which have benefited most from drug therapy account for a minority of the patients who have cancer. It is accepted from clinical trials that combinations of drugs generally lead to better results than that which follows treatment with only one drug. These drug combinations have often been chosen because of different proposed sites of drug action, different toxicity, or simply empirically without any logic. Seldom have drugs been combined in a sequential fashion dictated by the biochemical perturbations that result from the drugs to be used. A rational aproach to sequential drug therapy might allow for further improvement in the treatment of malignancy. If biochemical parameters could be identified which predict activation of a given drug or a given drug sequence, then perhaps characterization of cancer cells removed from the patient could be used to design the best possible therapy for that patient. Sequential use of certain drugs have been shown to be synergistic in their ability to inhibit animal tumors [1] and is not a new concept in the approach to improve cancer treatment. The interaction of drugs with either other drugs or natural metabolites has been an interest of many investigators [2–7].

This review will focus on the interaction of chemotherapeutic drugs on the de novo pyrimidine and purine synthetic pathways since many of the drugs available for cancer treatment are analogues of natural bases (for

Supported in part by the following sources: a Swebelius Award from the Yale Comprehensive Cancer Center, a National Cancer Institute Young Investigator Award, CA-24187; grants CA-09200 and CA-27130 from the National Cancer Institute and Grant CH-145 from the American Cancer Society. Dr. Grant is a fellow of the Leukemia Society of America and received support from the Cele Butwin foundation for Cancer Research and a Pharmaceutical Manufacturers Research Starter Grant. Dr. Cadman is a recipient of a Faculty Research Award from the American Cancer Society and is the person to whom reprint requests should be sent.

G. Bennett Humphrey et al. (eds), Adrenal and Endocrine Tumors in Children.

example, 5-fluorouracil) or nucleosides (for example, cytosine arabinoside).

1. 1-β-D ARABINOFURANOSYLCYTOSINE (Ara-C)

Ara-C is a deoxycytidine analogue with established anti-leukemic activity [8–11]. 5-Azadeoxycytidine (5-Aza-dCyd), also a deoxycytidine analogue, is the deoxy derivative of 5-Azacytidine, and also has been shown to have

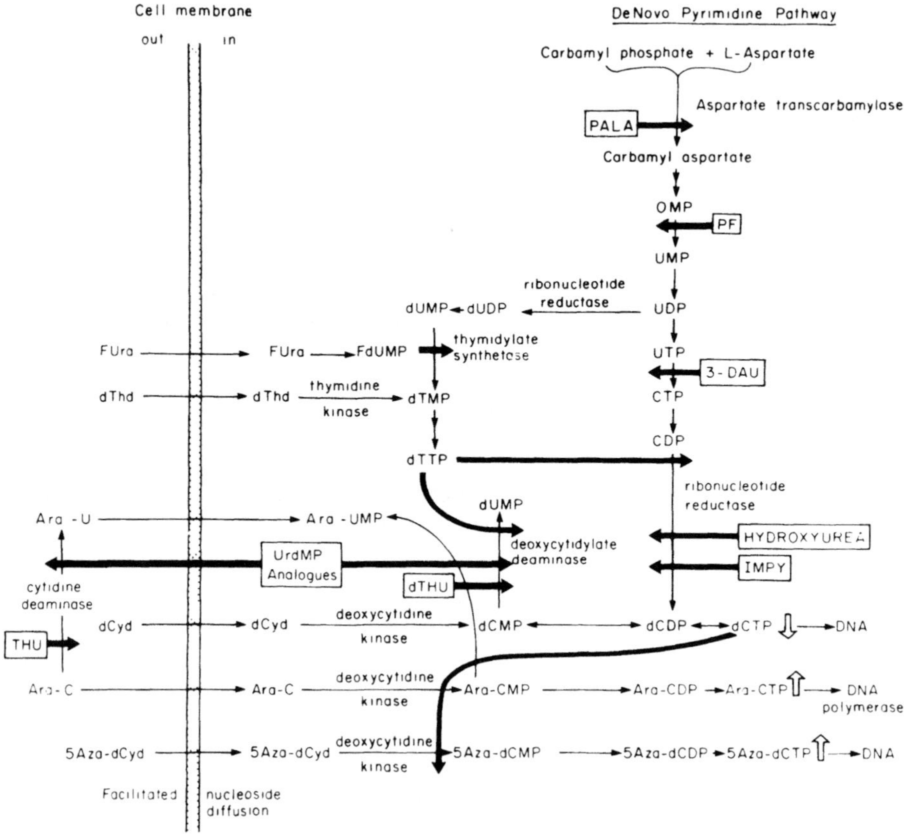

Figure 1. The modulation of cytosine arabinoside (Ara-C) and 5-Azadeoxycytidine (5Aza-dCyd) intracellular metabolism. The modulating drugs are in boxes with the dark arrows representing sites of inhibition. The open arrow at dCTP indicates a decrease while similar arrows pointing upward indicate an increase. Normally dCTP feedbacks on deoxycytidine kinase. A reduction in dCTP results in increased activity of this enzyme. PALA-[N-(Phosphonacetyl)-L-aspartate], PF – pyrazofurin, 3-DAU-3 deazauridine, IMPY – imidazopyrazole, FUra – 5-fluorouracil, dThd – thymidine, dCyd – deoxycytidine, THU – tetrahydrouridine, dTHU – deoxytetrahydrouridine.

anti-leukemic activity in murine leukemic cell lines [12–14]. Ara-C is thought to exert its cytotoxic effect through inhibition of DNA polymerase by the triphosphofylated metabolite, Ara-CTP [15, 16], although incorporation into DNA may also be an important contributor to the cytotoxicity [17]. The anti-tumor effects of 5-Aza-dCyd are presumably related to incorporation of the triphosphorylated metabolite into DNA [14–16, 18]. The rate-limiting step in the metabolism of both of these analogues is the conversion to the monophosphate nucleotide by the enzyme deoxycytidine kinase; resistance to both of these agents has been associated with decreased levels of this enzyme [19–21]. Since deoxycytidine kinase is under feedback constraint by deoxycytidine triphosphate (dCTP) [22], drugs capable of reducing intracellular levels of dCTP would be expected to enhance the metabolism of Ara-C and 5-Aza-dCyd (Figure 1).

1.1. Reduction of dCTP synthesis

The amount of dCTP present within a cell is the result of several factors which are, under usual circumstances, capable of maintaining this deoxynucleotide in the concentrations necessary for DNA synthesis (Figure 2). The synthesis of dCTP requires the reduction of the ribonucleotide, cytidine diphosphate (CDP) to deoxycytidine diphosphate (dCDP), which is subsequently phosphorylated to dCTP. If deoxycytidine (dCyd) is available in the culture media (or patient's blood), this nucleoside will enter the cell by facilitated diffusion. After entry into the cell, deoxycytidine kinase will phosphorylate dCyd to deoxycytidine monophosphate (dCMP) which can then be quickly converted to dCDP and finally to dCTP. There are two pathways by which dCTP can be reduced. Utilization of dCTP in the synthesis of DNA without simultaneous generation of dCTP will deplete intracellular dCTP. The deamination process which converts dCMP to deoxyu-

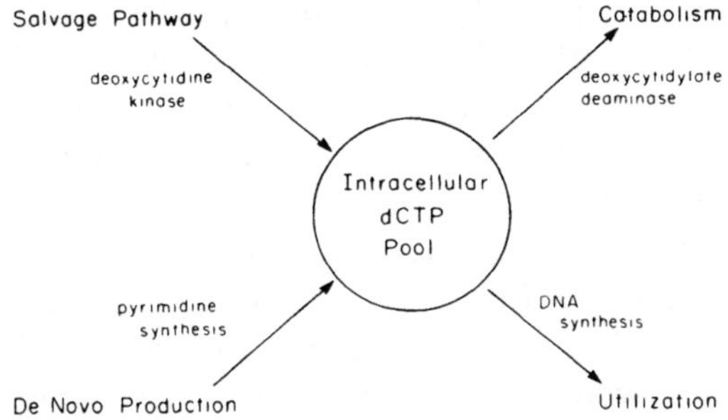

Figure 2. The conceptual modulation of intracellular dCTP. Because dCTP competes for DNA polymerase with Ara-CTP, the active derivative of Ara-C, and inhibits deoxycytidine kinase, the rate limiting enzyme responsible for phosphorylation of Ara-C, the concentration of this nucleotide is critical for Ara-C cytotoxicity.

ridine monophosphate (dUMP) resulting in the flow of dCTP to dCDP and then to dCMP can also be responsible for intracellular depletion of dCTP.

This knowledge of dCTP synthesis and utilization, when combined with the known inhibitory action of available drugs, leads to several theoretical drug combinations which are based on rational biochemical interactions. Many of the drug combinations which will be discussed are currently being investigated in clinical trials. It is important to realize that although these drug combinations may be scientifically reasonable, crucial investigations are needed to determine tissue selectivity (will the combination affect tumor cells to a greater extent than normal cells) and the dose and timing of drug administration.

Thymidine (dThd) is a nucleoside which is phosphorylated to thymidylate (dTMP) by thymidine kinase. The triphosphate derivative, dTTP, is capable of inhibiting ribonucleotide reductase, which results in a reduction of dCTP pools [23, 24]. This effect of dThd is associated with increased Ara-C accumulation into cells, increased Ara-CTP formation, and enhanced killing of cells treated with the sequence of dThd followed by Ara-C [25–28]. A similar observation with sequential dThd and 5-Aza-dCyd has also been reported [29].

Hydroxyurea is an inhibitor of ribonucleotide reductase [30] which produces reductions in intracellular concentrations of the deoxynucleotide triphosphates. The alterations in dCTP levels, however, have varied considerably [31, 32], which is probably related to the cell type studied and the dose and time of drug exposure. These variations from the anticipated dCTP reductions are a reminder that extrapolation of results directly from experimental tumor cells to the design of clinical protocols is not always appropriate. IMPY (imidazopyrazole) is a newer ribonucleotide reductase inhibitor which is currently being evaluated in the treatment of cancer patients [33]. Hydroxyurea [34, 35] and IMPY [35] increase the intracellular accumulation of Ara-C into L1210 cells and Novikoff Hepatoma cells respectively. As would be expected with a reduction in dCTP following these ribonucleotide reductase inhibitors, the active metabolite of Ara-C, Ara-CTP, was also increased which correlated with enhanced killing of the tumor cells [34]. This drug sequence has also been evaluated in the human promyelocytic leukemic cell line, HL-60. Similar reductions in dCTP levels, enhanced intracellular Ara-C accumulation and increased Ara-CTP formation occurred and were also correlated with synergistic cytotoxicity [36, 37].

These drugs could be antagonistic for cell kinetic reasons. Since cells can be prevented from synthesizing DNA by hydroxyurea, the subsequent administration of a drug which requires DNA synthesis to exert its cytotoxic effect would be theoretically less effective. Specifically, hydroxyurea followed by Ara-C could be an antagonistic drug combination. In one study, removing the hydroxyurea from the culture media before administering Ara-C resulted in a dramatic increase in cell death [37]. Presumably in this situation both the biochemical interaction and cell cycle kinetic effects of the drugs were optimized.

Pyrazofurin (PF) is a nucleoside analogue which as the monophosphorylated nucleotide is a tight binding inhibitor of orotodylate decarboxylase, the enzyme in the de novo pyrimidine synthetic pathway that converts orotidylate (OMP) to uridylate (UMP) [38, 39]. The result of this inhibition is a reduction in the ribonucleotide and deoxynucleotide pools. Consequently, a similar enhancement of Ara-C cytotoxicity could be expected when PF is given before Ara-C and, in fact, has been reported [35, 38].

PALA (N-[Phosphonacetyl]-L-Aspartate) is a transition state analogue inhibitor of L-aspartate transcarbamyolase, the enzyme catalyzing the second step in the de novo pyrimidine synthetic pathway [40]. This drug has been shown to be effective in the treatment of Lewis Lung carcinoma implanted in mice [41] and is currently being evaluated in patients with cancer [42]. The intracellular nucleotide and deoxynucleotide levels of several experimental tumors are reduced following exposure to PALA [43–45]. If these biochemical alterations also occur in human leukemic cells, then the sequential administration of PALA followed by Ara-C or 5-Aza-dCyd would have a rational biochemical basis also.

Deazauridine (DAU) is a uridine analogue which is cytotoxic to several experimental cell lines [46]. After entry into the cell, DAU is rapidly phosphorylated to the nucleoside triphosphate, which is an inhibitor of CTP synthetase [47, 48]. The consequence of the inhibition of this metabolic step which aminates UTP to CTP is a marked reduction in CTP concentration [49]. This results in less CDP, the substrate for ribonucleotide reductase, and therefore less dCDP and finally, less dCTP [50]. These interactions provide an explanation for the enhanced cytotoxicity observed when DAU precedes Ara-C [35, 50]. DAU has other effects which are also theoretical reasons for this sequential synergism. These will be presented in the section discussing the degradation of Ara-C.

1.2. Enhanced catabolism of dCTP

Deoxycytidylate deaminase converts dCMP to dUMP and is an important catabolic step in maintaining and increasing dUMP concentrations when the methylation of dUMP to dTMP is inhibited (Figure 3). Methotrexate prevents the regeneration of tetrahydrofolate (THF) from dihydrofolate (DHF) by inhibiting the enzyme dihydrofolate reductase (DHFR). The consequence of this reduction in tetrahydrofolate is a concomitant reduction

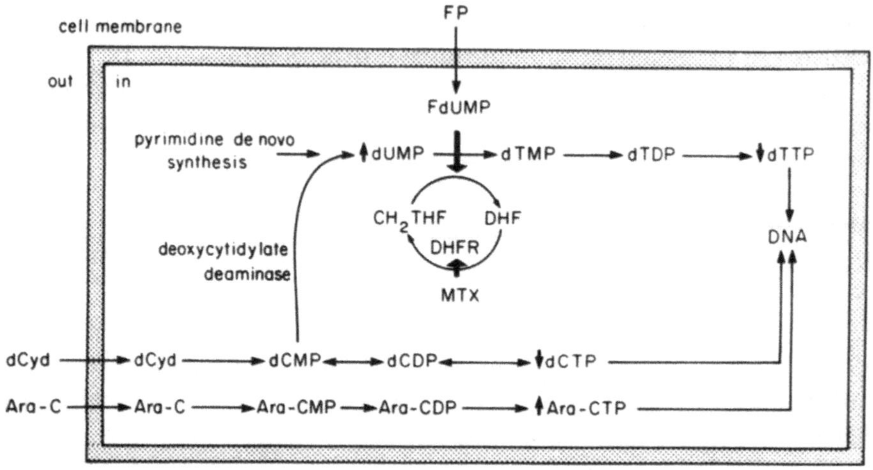

Figure 3. The modulation of Ara-C metabolism by either methotrexate (MTX) or Fluoropyrimidines (FP). The consequence of inhibiting thymidylate synthesis (dMTP) either directly by the FP derivative, FdUMP, or indirectly by MTX is an increase in dUMP primarily from the deamination of deoxycytidylate (dCMP). This results in a decrease in dCTP which allows an increase intracellular conversion of Ara-C to Ara-CMP and eventually greater quantities of Ara-CTP. CH_2THF — 5,10 methylenetetrahydrofolate, DHF — dihydrofolate, DHFR — dihydrofolate reductase.

of 5,10 methylenetetrahydrofolate (CH_2THF), the folate compound required by dTMP synthetase for the conversion of dUMP to dTMP. In cells affected by methotrexate, there is an increase in intracellular dUMP, which is primarily the result of the deamination of dCMP to dUMP [51]. Therefore cells exposed to methotrexate would be expected to have less intracellular dCTP which would allow greater intracellular phosphorylation of Ara-C to Ara-CTP. Many investigators have studied this drug combination. In some instances the cytotoxic results have been synergistic [52–54] and antagonistic [55–57].

A recent study did document that concentrations of methotrexate, which nearly totally inhibited dTMP formation in L1210 cells, did result in synergistic cytotoxicity [58]. The cytotoxicity was also associated with a reduction in dCTP levels and an increase in intracellular Ara-CTP. These effects of methotrexate on Ara-C metabolism and cytotoxicity were improved somewhat by also adding 2′-deoxyadenosine to cell cultures. The 2′-deoxyadenosine caused an increase in dATP levels which, through feedback inhibition of ribonucleotide reductase, resulted in a reduction in the synthesis of dCTP [59]. In this circumstance there was both an increased catabolism and a reduction in synthesis of dCTP.

The fact that in some instances this drug combination has been reported to be synergistic and antagonistic emphasizes again that different cells behave differently and that drug dose and drug scheduling are very important. Ideally, tumor cells from the patient to be treated should be evaluated to better define the parameters which are necessary for maximizing the desired effects.

The fluoropyrimidines (5-fluorouracil, 5-fluorouridine, and 5-fluoro-2′-deoxyuridine) inhibit dTMP synthetase when converted to 5-fluoro-2′-deoxyuridine monophosphate (FdUMP). Therefore these drugs should have a similar effect on Ara-C metabolism and cytotoxicity as did methotrexate. In fact, nearly identical results have been obtained [60]. Doses which completely inhibited dTMP formation were associated with the lowest dCTP concentrations, the greatest intracellular Ara-C accumulation, the highest Ara-CTP concentrations, and the greatest killing of cells. Because each of the three fluoropyrimidines requires different enzymes for the initial phosphorylation process, these drugs might allow for a greater selectivity between various normal and neoplastic tissues.

1.3. Reduced catabolism of Ara-C

The degradation of Ara-C occurs at the level of the nucleoside (Ara-C to Ara-U) and nucleotide (Ara-CMP to Ara-UMP) by cytidine and deoxycytidylate deaminases respectively [61]. The clinical importance of these enzymes has not been absolutely established, although some investigations have found that greater Ara-C deamination is associated with less cytotoxicity [62]. Other studies have not been so convincing [63]. It is logical, however, to attempt to prevent catabolism of Ara-C, or the nucleotide Ara-CMP, to an inactive derivative.

Tetrahydrouridine (THU) is a potent inhibitor of cytidine deaminase [64] and will inhibit the deamination of Ara-C [64–66]. This uridine analogue has also been found to increase Ara-CTP formation in human leukemic cells [67]. Because cytidine deaminase is present in the blood, it was not surprising to find that when THU was administered to patients just before a dose of Ara-C the resultant blood concentration of Ara-C was increased up to four-fold [68]. Likewise, it was not unexpected that this drug combination resulted in greater clinical toxicity [69].

Deoxytetrahydrouridine will inhibit dCMP deaminase [70] and would be expected to augment cytotoxicity of Ara-C in cells which have the capacity to phosphorylate Ara-C. Since dUMP has been reported to inhibit dCMP deaminase [71], other uridine analogues were recently evaluated as inhibitors of this deaminase reaction [72]. DAU monophosphate was found to be a competitive inhibitor of dCMP deaminase [72] and could help explain the synergistic interaction reported between DAU and Ara-C [35, 73]. FdUMP, the fluoropyrimidine derivative which inhibits dTMP synthetase, also inhibited dCMP deaminase [72]. Both drugs, DAU monophosphate and

FdUMP, were also capable of inhibiting cytidine deaminase. In both of these instances, each drug could have a double effect on Ara-C metabolism. One effect would lower dCTP pools, which would allow greater quantities of Ara-C to be phosphorylated by dCyd kinase. The other effect would be the reduction in the deamination of Ara-C and its intracellular phosphorylated derivatives.

Increased intracellular thymidine triphosphate will also inhibit the deamination of dCMP to dUMP [50, 74, 75]. Therefore dThd could also have a dual effect on Ara-C metabolism, depending on the extent of the influence of dTTP in the ribonucleotide reductase and deoxycytidylate deaminase activity. These effects obviously might be considerably different in different tissues where the target enzymes may have different initial rates for conversion of their respective substrates (Km) and different maximal rates for conversion which are determined to a large extent on the total amount of enzyme present (Vmax) within the cell.

2. 5-AZACYTIDINE

5-Azacytidine (5-Aza-Cyd) is a cytidine analogue in which the 5 carbon is replaced by a nitrogen [76]. This drug has been effective in the treatment of human acute myelogenous leukemia [77–79]. 5-Aza-Cyd is phosphorylated by uridine-cytidine kinase to the monophosphate derivative [80], which is the limiting step in the conversion of 5-Aza-Cyd to the active metabolite, 5-Aza-CTP.

Uridine-cytidine kinase is the enzyme responsible for converting uridine and cytidine to UMP and CMP. This enzyme is capable of salvaging these two nucleosides from the medium to maintain pyrimidine ribonucleotide pools [81–87]. Pyrazofurin (PF) treatment inhibits pyrimidine synthesis at the decarboxylation of OMP to UMP and results in a reduction of UTP and CTP, both feedback modulators of uridine-cytidine kinase [80]. Therefore when 5-Aza-Cyd is given after PF exposure, cells accumulate increased quantities of 5-Aza-Cyd which eventually leads to greater 5-Aza-CTP levels; the result is enhanced cell killing [88, 89].

Because the anti-tumor activity of 5-Aza-Cyd depends on the incorporation of 5-Aza-CTP into RNA [90–93], a reduction in CTP, which competes with this nucleotide analogue for entry into RNA, would enhance the incorporation of 5-Aza-CTP into newly forming RNA. DAU, which inhibits the synthesis of CTP does, in fact, result in an augmented incorporation of this fraudulant nucleotide into RNA. This effect is also associated with increased cytotoxicity when DAU precedes 5-Aza-Cyd [94].

PALA, as would be expected, also results in enhanced intracellular accumulation of 5-Aza-Cyd and is a synergistic cytotoxic drug combination [95]. Both PF and PALA would be expected to also enhance the intracellular metabolism and cytotoxicity of FUrd, the fluoropyrimidine analogue of uridine.

3. METHOTREXATE

Methotrexate (MTX) is a tight binding inhibitor of dihydrofolate reductase (DHFR). The cytotoxicity of this agent depends on several factors which include the binding characteristics of methotrexate to DHFR, the intracellular concentrations of methotrexate and DHFR and the intracellular concentration of the folate cofactors required for cellular metabolism. However, the predominant factor required of a cell for methotrexate cytotoxicity to occur is the synthesis of DNA. Thymidylate (dTMP) continues in the presence of methotrexate until the 5,10 methylenetetrahydrofolate pools are reduced (CH_2THF). Without the capacity to transfer the methyl group to dUMP, dTMP synthesis ceases and therefore DNA synthesis can not continue. In addition, the tetrahydrofolate pools are necessary for methylation at two enzymatic steps in de novo purine synthesis, and therefore the creation of purines is also affected by methotrexate. This methotrexate cytotoxicity can be prevented by supplying thymidine (dThd), a source of dTTP, and hypoxanthine, or inosine, a source of purine bases beyond the methy-

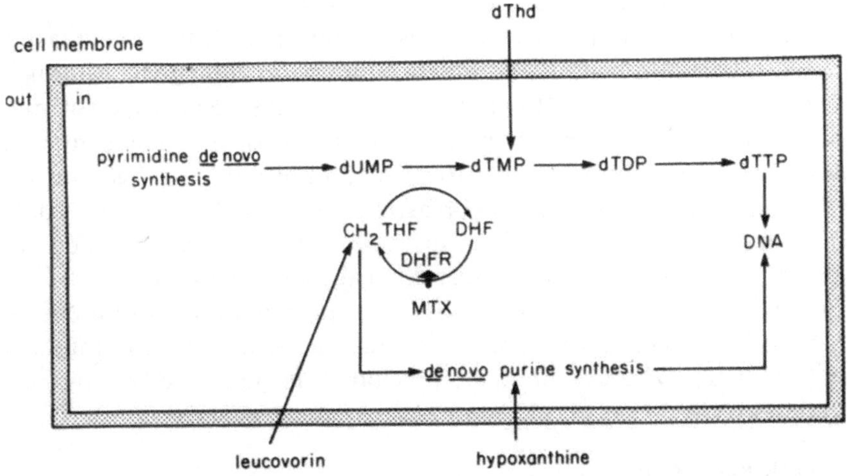

Figure 4. The methods of rescuing cells from the inhibitory effects of methotrexate (MTX). When the tetrahydrofolate pools are depleted both dTMP and purine synthesis are inhibited, and the reversal requires either replenishment of the tetrahydrofolate pools by leucovorin, or thymidine (dThd) and hypoxanthine which bypass the MTX induced blockade.

lation steps in the de novo purine synthetic pathway [96]. Leucovorin (5-formyltetrahydrofolate) can be converted to CH_2THF within the cell and therefore also rescue the cell from potential methotrexate cytotoxicity [96] (Figure 4).

Since the biochemical perturbations induced by methotrexate can easily be circumvented, the consideration that major differences between these described methotrexate effects on normal and neoplastic cells could be exploited by rescuing normal cells and not the cancer was a logical clinical approach. Leucovorin was first demonstrated to improve the therapeutic efficacy of methotrexate in mice bearing L1210 leukemia in 1966 [97]. The effectiveness of leucovorin rescue to improve methotrexate cytotoxicity is dependent on the tumor being treated. The best results have been observed in methotrexate resistant cell lines [98].

Leucovorin rescue has been used extensively in the treatment of human malignancy [99]. Unfortunately few clinical trials have been performed comparing the higher dose methotrexate and leucovorin rescue with doses of methotrexate which do not require rescue. Currently the use of high doses of methotrexate which require leucovorin to prevent toxicity can not be recommended as routine therapy.

Thymidine as a rescue agent in patients treated with methotrexate has recently been used by several investigators [100–102]. Prior to clinical use, animal studies confirmed the ability of dThd to prevent methotrexate toxicity [103]. The important observation was that several human cell lines were afforded protection by dThd while some cancer cell lines treated with methotrexate were unaffected by dThd [104–106].

The ability of dThd to selectively rescue normal cells from neoplastic cells exposed to methotrexate is the ideal chemotherapeutic goal. Although this selectivity is poorly understood, nor does it always occur, experimental evidence suggests that normal bone marrow and gastrointestinal mucosa, the major sites of methotrexate host toxicity, do not require exogenous purines to the same extent that some neoplastic cells do [101, 103, 107, 108]. The dose of dThd and duration of the infusion of this deoxynucleoside are also important determinants for protection against host toxicity.

Because dThd has a plasma ½ life of approximately 10 minutes, and is not absorbed when given orally, it must be given by continuous infusion [100, 102]. This requirement precludes the use of dThd rescue on a routine basis.

4. 5-FLUOROURACIL

5-Fluorouracil (FUra) is a drug which is an effective antitumor agent for the treatment of several human malignancies. The cytotoxicity is the result of two nucleotide derivatives; 5-fluorodeoxyuridylate (FdUMP) which inhibits thymidylate (dTMP) synthetase and 5-fluorouridine triphosphate (FUTP) which is incorporated into RNA. Complete protection of FUra cytotoxicity in several cell lines requires both dThd and uridine (Urd) to be present indicating that these two FUra derivatives act in concert to kill cells [109]. However, some cells can be protected from FUra by dThd alone, indicating the major lethal effect in this circumstance is from the inhibition of dTMP formation [110, 111].

FUra enters cells by facilitated diffusion and can then be converted to nucleotides by several possible enzymatic pathways (Figure 5). The predominant metabolitic pathway is the conversion of FUra to FUMP by orotate phosphoribosyltransferase which requires 5-phosphoribosyl-1-pyrophosphate (PRPP) [111, 112]. FUMP is then phosphorylated to the toxic metabolites FdUMP and FUTP. Therefore, if the rate-limiting metabolic step in FUra metabolism, FUMP formation, can be increased, then enhanced cytotoxicity should result. A review of these complex interactions has been published [113].

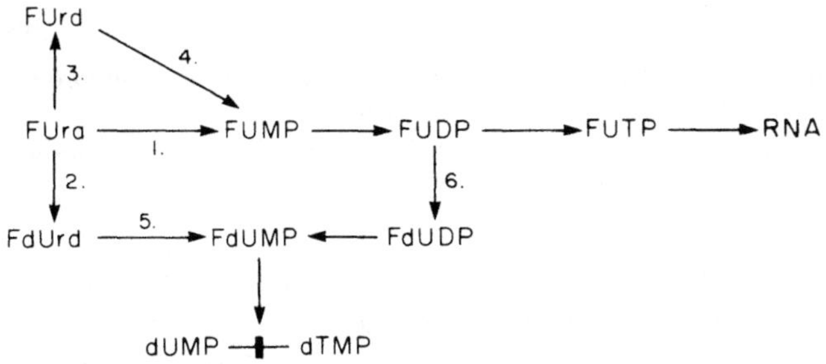

Figure 5. The metabolism of 5-fluorouracil (FUra). The enzymes are: 1. orotatephosphoribosyl transferase, 2. thymidine phosphorylase, 3. uridine phosphorylase, 4. uridine-cytidine kinase, 5. thymidine kinase, 6. ribonucleotide reductase. FdUMP inhibits thymidylate synthetase and FUTP is incorporated into RNA.

One mechanism by which this metabolic process can be increased is to provide greater quantities of the required cofactor, PRPP. The first committed step in de novo purine synthesis also requires PRPP for the amidophosphoribosyl transfer reaction which forms phosphoribosylamine. The end products of purine synthesis influence the rate of PRPP production and utilization. Therefore, inhibitors of de novo purine synthesis would be expected to result in increased intracellular PRPP concentrations which could now be used in the conversion of FUra to FUMP.

Methotrexate, as just described, will indirectly result in inhibition of de novo purine synthesis by the depletion of the folate cofactors necessary for continued purine synthesis. The consequence of this methotrexate inhibition is, as expected, an increased intracellular concentration of PRPP, which in turn is associated with increased intracellular nucleotide metabolism of FUra (Figure 6). Both toxic metabolites were also increased (FdUMP and

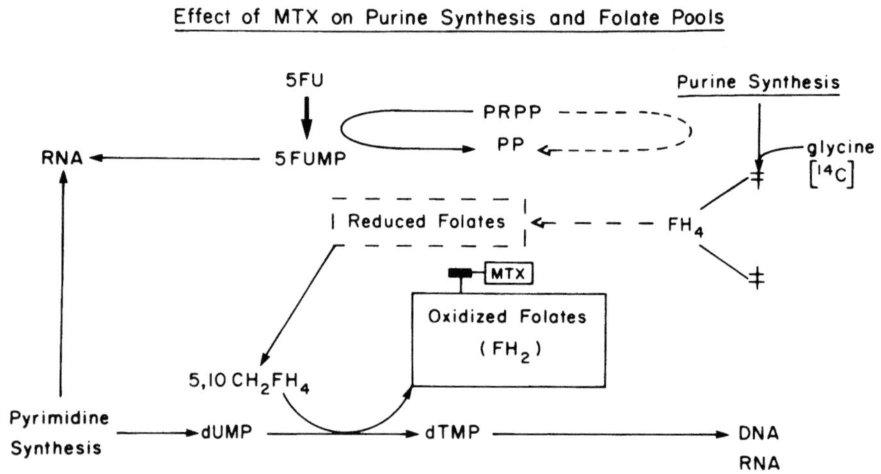

Figure 6. The effect of methotrexate (MTX) on purine synthesis and 5-fluorouracil metabolism (5FU). Because of the depleted reduced folates, purine synthesis ceases allowing the phosphoribosyl pyrophosphate (PRPP) which would have been utilized for de novo purine synthesis to be used for the conversion of 5FU to 5FUMP.

FUTP) which were correlated with a synergistic killing of L1210 cells [114, 115]. Similar observations have also been reported with the human breast cancer cell cultures, 47-DN, and human colon tumor cell cultures, HCT-8 [116, 117]. Because the antipurine effect of methotrexate depends on the depletion of the tetrahydrofolate pools which occurs during the synthesis of dTMP, the effect of methotrexate on FUra metabolism is only observed in cells which are synthesizing DNA [118]. Therefore, the modulation of methotrexate on FUra in a given cancer will depend on the fraction of the tumor synthesizing DNA during the exposure of methotrexate. For example, the 47-DN cells which have a doubling time of 30 hours, require a 24 hour methotrexate exposure to maximize the synergistic killing which follows the sequence of MTX before FUra. The optimal exposure period of methotrexate in L1210 cultures which have a doubling time of 12 hours is 6 hours.

Other agents which directly inhibit de novo purine synthesis have also been found to enhance FUra metabolism and cytotoxicity when given prior to FUra administration [119] (Figure 7). The drug, 6-methylmercaptopurine ribonucleoside (MeMPR) which inhibits amidophosphoribosyltransferase

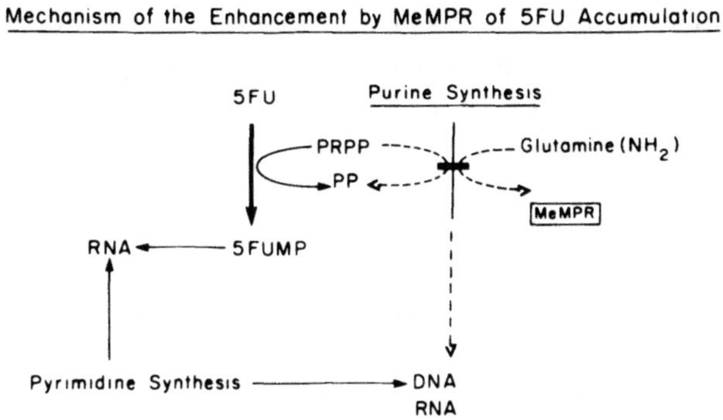

Figure 7. The effect of methylmercaptopurine ribonucleoside (MeMPR) on 5-fluorouracil (5FU) metabolism. As in figure 6, the inhibition of purine synthesis leads to increased PRPP concentrations which are used to increase the conversion of 5FU to 5 FUMP.

and increases PRPP also enhances FUra metabolism [119]. The other inhibitors of purine synthesis, 6-diazo-5-oxo-L-norleucine (DON), Azaserine (Aza), and L-alanosine (L-Ala) had similar effects on FUra. The inhibitor of PRPP synthetase, 7-deazadenosine, (tubercidin, Tbc) reduced PRPP concentrations and decreases FUra nucleotide formation. If tubercidin is given to cell cultures before the anti-purine drugs are added, the enhancing effect on FUra metabolism is prevented [119]. Therefore the cytotoxicity of the sequence of tubercidin before FUra would be expected to be antagonistic.

Preliminary clinical trials of methotrexate preceding FUra by 1 hour has resulted in tumor responses in women with advanced breast cancer that exceeds that which would have been expected [120]. Further clinical evaluation of this drug sequence is required to determine appropriate drug dosages and interval between methotrexate and FUra. In addition, determination of selectivity between tumor cells and neoplastic cells remains to be evaluated. For example, if enhanced FUra metabolism were to occur identically following these agents in normal and neoplastic cells, then nothing will have been achieved by the drug sequence. Therefore, these drug sequences should not be routinely administered to patients without concomitant investigations to evaluate tissue selectivity.

Agents which also require PRPP for nucleotide formation compete with FUra for this cofactor. Hypoxanthine, which is converted to inosine monophosphate (IMP) by hypoxanthineguanine phosphoribosyltransferase, will substantially reduce the enhanced FUra metabolic conversion and cytotoxicity [119, 121]. In a similar fashion, purine nucleosides which can be utilized but do not require PRPP, unlike the purine bases, will result in enhanced FUra cytotoxicity [122]. Although PRPP levels were not measured, the reduced need for PRPP for de novo purine synthesis could allow this cofactor to be available for conversion of FUra to FUMP.

The other mechanism which has been proposed for the enhancement in cytotoxicity which has been observed when nucleosides and (or) deoxynucleosides are given with FUra to cell cultures is that these nucleosides are acted on by the appropriate phosphorylase providing a ribose 1-phosphate or deoxyribose 1-phosphate respectively for the conversion of FUra to FUrd or FdUrd (Figure 5) [111, 122].

The other modulating effect on FUra metabolism involves the natural substrate for orotate phosphoribosyltransferase, orotate. PALA [N-(phosphonacetyl)-L-aspartate], which inhibits the first committed step in de novo pyrimidine synthesis, aspartate transcarbamoylase, results in a marked reduction in the synthesis of orotate [43–45]. Therefore, pretreatment of cell cultures with PALA will also result in an enhancement of FUra conversion to FUMP [119]. Pyrazofurin, which inhibits the decarboxylation of OMP to UMP, results in an elevation of orotate levels [38, 39]. Therefore, orotate will compete with FUra for PRPP at the same enzyme, orotate phosphoribosyltransferase. The kinetic properties of this enzyme favor the conversion of orotate to OMP rather than FUra to FUMP [112]. This explains the observation that pretreatment of cell cultures with pyrazofurin abrogates the FUra enhancing effect of MTX and the antipurine agents [119].

The concept that an inhibitor of purine synthesis which is associated with increased intracellular PRPP concentration could result in enhanced cytotoxicity when given before a second drug which requires PRPP for activation is not new. DON and azaserine when administered first in sequence had been previously shown to act synergistically with 6-mercaptopurine (6MP) and 6-thioguanine (6TG), the latter being purine base analogues which require the transfer of the ribose and phosphate from PRPP for metabolic activation [1, 123–126].

The incorporation of FUra into RNA can adversely affect the function of RNA and presumably therefore be a factor in the lethality of FUra [127–142]. Since the agents just discussed all influence the initial metabolic step in FUra metabolism, any increase in FUMP formation would also result in an increase in both the lethal derivatives of FUra, FdUMP and FUTP. Thymidine has been observed capable of increasing FUra incorporation into RNA which is associated with improved anti-tumor activity of FUra [133, 143]. The mechanism by which dThd enhances FUra activity has not been clearly elucidated, however, this sequential drug combination has been noted to result in enhanced interference with the processing of RNA [142]. Other possible ways in which dThd can influence FUra activity include the saturation of the degradative enzymatic system. The serum ½ life of FUra in patients who are receiving continuous infusions of dThd is prolonged, presumably from the saturation of these catabolic enzymes in the liver [144]. Although dThd infusion offered protection in patients given high doses of methotrexate, the dThd resulted in enhanced FUra toxicity [144], presumably the result of prolonged serum concentrations of FUra.

SUMMARY

The biochemical principles that contribute to the rational modulation of cytosine arabinoside, 5-Azacytidine, methotrexate and 5-Fluorouracil have been discussed. The influence of modulation agents on the cell cycle are important factors since the target drugs each are more susceptible in cells synthesizing DNA [145]. Although this review has only addressed the biochemical rationale of these drug combinations, the best possible drug sequencing must consider both the biochemical and cytokinetic effects. Caution should be used in extrapolating these drug sequences for the treatment of human malignancy until appropriate studies are performed to determine the proper drug doses and sequencing intervals.

REFERENCES

1. Sartorelli AC: Approaches to the combination chemotherapy of transplantable neoplasms. Prog Exp Tumor Res 6:228–288, 1965.
2. Grindey GB, Nichol CA: Interaction of drugs inhibiting different steps in the synthesis of DNA. Cancer Res 32:527–531, 1972.
3. Goldin A: *In vivo* metabolite — antimetabolite relationships in antitumor therapy. Adv Enzyme Regul 16:65–77, 1978.
4. Barlogie B, Plunkett W, Raber M, Latreille J, Keating M, McCredie K: *In vivo* cellular and pharmacological studies of 1-β-D-Arabinofuranosylcytosine and 3-Deazauridine chemotherapy for relapsing acute leukemia. Cancer Res 41:1227–1235, 1981.
5. Jackson RC, Harrap Kr: Computer models of anticancer drug interaction. Pharmacol Ther 4:245–280, 1979.
6. Grindey GB, Cheng YC: Biochemical and kinetic approaches to inhibition of multiple pathways. Pharmacol Ther 4:307–327, 1979.
7. Block A: Metabolic conditioning and metabolic actuation: experimental approaches to cancer chemotherapy involving combinations of metabolites and antimetabolites. Cancer Chemother Rep 58:471–477, 1974.
8. Cozzarelli NR: The mechanism of action of inhibitors of DNA synthesis. Annu Rev Biochem 46:641–668, 1977.
9. Bodey GP, Freireich EJ, Monto RW, Hewlitt TS: Cytosine arabinoside therapy for acute leukemia in adults. Cancer Chemother Rep 53:59–66, 1969.
10. Clarkson BD, Dowling MD, Gee TS: Treatment of acute leukemia in adults. Cancer 36:775–795, 1975.
11. Eillison RR, Holland JF, Weill M et al.: Arabinosyl cytosine: a useful agent in the treatment of acute leukemia in adults. Blood 32:507–523, 1968.
12. Momparler RL, Goodman J: *In vitro* cytotoxic and biochemical effects of 5-Aza-2′deoxycytidine. Cancer Res 37:1636–1639, 1977.

13. Sorm F, Vesely J: Effect of 5-Aza-2'deoxycytidine against leukemic and hematopoietic tissues in AKR mice. Neoplasma 15:339–343, 1968.
14. Vesely J and Cihak A: Incorporation of a potent antileukemic agent, 5-Aza-2'deoxycitidine into DNA of cells form leukemic mice. Cancer Res 37:3684–3689, 1977.
15. Furth JJ and Cohen JS: Inhibition of mammalian DNA polymerase by the 5'-triphosphate of 1-β-D Arabinofuranosylcytosine and (5'-triphosphate of) arabino-furanosyladenine. Cancer Res 28:2061–2067, 1968.
16. Graham FL, Whitmore GF: Studies in mouse L-cells on the incorporation of 1-β-D Arabinofuranosylcytosine into DNA and on inhibition of DNA polymerase by 1-β-D Arabinofuranosylcytosine, 5'-triphosphate. Cancer Res 20:1046, 1979.
17. Kufe DW, Major PO, Egan EM, Beards GP: Correlation of cytotoxicity with incorporation of Ara-C into DNA. J Biol Chem 255 (19):8997–9000, 1980.
18. Cihak A: Transformation of 5-Aza-2'deoxycytidine-^{3}H and its incorporation in different systems of rapidly proliferating cells. Eur J Cancer 14:17–24, 1978.
19. Schrecker AW: Metabolism of 1-β-D Arabinofuranosylcytosine in leukemia L1210: Nucleoside and nucleotide kinases in cell free extracts. Cancer Res 30:632–634, 1970.
20. Tattersall MHN, Saneshaguru K, Hoffbrand AV: Mechanism of resistance of human acute leukemia cells to cytosine arabinoside. Br J Hem 27:39–46, 1974.
21. Vesely J, Cihak A, Sorm F: Characteristics of mouse leukemic cells resistant to 5-azacytidine and 5-Aza-2'deoxycytidine. Cancer Res 28:1995–2000, 1968.
22. Martin DS, Stolfi RL, Sawyer RC, Nyak R, Spegelman S, Young C, Woodcock T: An overview of Thymidine. Cancer 45(6):1117–1128, 1980.
23. Bjursell G Reichard P: Effects of thymidine on deoxyribonucleoside triphosphate pools and deoxyribonuclei acid synthesis in Chinese Hamster ovary cells. J Biol Chem 248:3904–3909, 1973.
24. Lowe JK, Grindey GB: Inhibition of growth rate and deoxyribonucleoside triphosphate concentrations in cultured leukemia L1210 cells. Mol Pharmacol 12:177–184, 1976.
25. Grant S, Lehman C, Cadman E: Augmentation of 1-β-D Arabinofuranosyl cytosine intracellular accumulation and increased cytotoxicity in L1210 cells following thymidine exposure. Cancer Res 40:1525–1531, 1980.
26. Harris AW, Reynolds EC, Finch LR: Effect of thymidine on the sensitivity of cultured mouse tumor cells to 1-β-D Arabinofuranosylcytosine. Cancer Res 39:538–541, 1979.
27. Danhauser LL, Rustum YM: Effect of thymidine on the toxicity, anti-tumor activity, and metabolism of 1-β-D Arabinofuranosylcytosine in rats bearing a chemically induced colon carcinoma. Cancer Res 40:1274–1280, 1980.
28. Kinahan JJ, Kowal EP and Grindey GB: Biochemical and antitumor effects of the combination of thymidine and 1-β-D Arabinofuranosylcytosine against leukemia L1210. Cancer Res 41:445–451, 1981.
29. Grant S, Rauscher F III, Jakubowski A, Cadman E: Enhancement of intracellular accumulation and anti-tumor effect of 5-Aza-2' deoxycytidine by thymidine in L1210 cells. Proc Am Soc Clin Oncol C 56:332, 1980.
30. Krakoff IH, Brown NC, Reichard P: Inhibition of ribonucleoside diphosphate reductase by hydroxyurea. Cancer Res 28:1559–1565, 1968.
31. Skoog L, Bjursell G: Nuclear and cytoplasmic pools of deoxyribonucleoside triphosphate in Chinese Hamster ovary cells. J Biol Chem 249:6434–6438, 1974.
32. Walters RA, Tokey RA, Ratcliff RL: Cell-cycle-dependent variations of deoxyribonucleoside triphosphate pools in Chinese Hamster ovary cells. Biochim Biophys Acta 319:336–347, 1973.
33. Yap BS, Murphy WK, Burgess MA et al.: Phase-I clinical evaluation of 2,3-dihydro-1H-imidazolo [1,2b] pyrazole. Cancer Treat Rep 63:1849–1851, 1979.

34. Walsh CT, Craig RW, Agarwal RP: Increased activation of 1-β-D arabinofuranosylcytosine by hydroxyurea in L1210 cells. Cancer Res 40:3286–3292, 1980.
35. Plagemann PGW, Marz R, Wohlheuter RM: Transport and metabolism of deoxycytidine and 1-β-D arabinofuranosylcytosine into cultured Novikoff rat hepatome cells, relationship to phosphorylation, and regulation of triphosphate synthesis. Cancer Res 38:978–989, 1978.
36. Rauscher FD III, Cadman E: Enhancement of cytosine arabinoside metabolites and antitumor effect by hydroxyurea in human promyelocytic leukemia HL-60. Submitted to Cancer Res.
37. Unpublished observations (Cadman and Grant).
38. Cadman EC, Dix DE, Handschumacher RE: Clinical, biological, and biochemical effects of purzofurin. Cancer Res 38:682–688, 1978.
39. Dix DE, Lehman CP, Jakubowski A, Moyer JD, Handschumacher RE: Pyrazofurin metabolism, enzyme inhibition and resistance in L5178Y cells. Cancer Res 39:4485–4490, 1979.
40. Swyrd EA, Seaver SS, Stark GR: N-(phosphonacetyl)-L-aspartate, a potent transition state inhibitor of aspartate transcarbomylase, blocks proliferation of mammalion cells in culture. J Biol Chem 249:6945–6950, 1974.
41. Jayarom HN, Cooney DA, Viotica DT et al.: Mechanism of sensitivity and resistance of murine tumors to N-(phosphonacetyl)-L-aspartate (PALA). Cancer Treatment Rep 63:8:1291–1301, 1979.
42. Hart RD, Ohnuma T, Holland JF: Initial clinical study with N-(Phosphonacetyl)-L-aspartic acid (PALA) in patients with advanced cancer. Cancer Treat Rep 64:617–624, 1980.
43. Moyer JD, Handschumacher RF: Selective inhibition of pyrimidine synthesis and depletion of nucleotide pools by N-(Phosphonacetyl)-L-aspartate. Cancer Res 39:3089-3094, 1979.
44. Moyer JD, Smith PA, Handschumacher RE: Effects of N-(Phosphonacetyl)-L-aspartate (PALA) on circulating pyrimidine nucleosides nucleotide pools and nucleic acid synthesis. Proc Am Assoc Cancer Res 21:443, 1980.
45. Momparler RL, Vesely J, Momparler LF, Revard GE: Synergistic action of 5-Aza-2′ deoxycytidine and 3-Deazauridine on L1210 leukemic cells and EMT_6 tumor cells. Cancer Res 39:3822–3827, 1979.
46. Wong MD, Bloch A: Studies on the mode of action of 3-deazapyrimidines 1. Metabolism of 3-deazauridine and 3-deazacytidine in microbial and tumor cells. Biochem Pharmacol 21:1063–1073, 1972.
47. Brockman RW, Shaddix SC, Williams M, Nelson JA, Rose LM, Schabel FM Jr: The mechanism of action of 3-deazauridine in tumor cells sensitive and resistant to arabinosylcytosine. Ann NY Acad Sci 255:501–521, 1975.
48. McPortland RP, Wong MC, Block A, Winfeld H: Cytidine-5-triphosphate synthetase as a target for inhibition by the antitumor agent 3-deazauridine. Cancer Res 34:3107–3111, 1974.
49. Grant S, Cadman E: Altered 5-azacytidine metabolism following 3-deazauridine treatment of L5178Y and human myeloblasts. Cancer Res 40:4000–4006, 1980.
50. Jackson RC: The regulation of thymidylate biosynthesis in Novikoff hepatoma cells and the effects of amethopterin, 5-Fluorodeoxyuridine, and 3-deazauridine. J Biol Chem 253(20):7440–7446, 1978.
51. Fridland A: Effect of methotrexate on deoxyribonucleotide pools and DNA synthesis in human lymphocytic cells. Cancer Res 34:1883–1888, 1974.
52. Hoovis ML, Chu MY: Enhancement of the antiproliferative action of 1-β-D arabinofuranosylcytosine by methotrexate in murine leukemic cells (L5178Y). Cancer Res 33:521–525,

1973.
53. Avery TL, Roberts D: Dose-related synergism of cytosine arabinoside and methotrexate against murine leukemia L1210. Eur J Cancer 10:425–429, 1974.
54. Edelstein M, Vietti T, Valeriote F: The enhanced cytotoxicity of combinations of 1-β-D arabinofuranosylcytosine and methotrexate. Cancer Res 35:1555–1558, 1975.
55. Tattersall MHN, Connors TA, Harrap KR: Interaction of methotrexate and cytosine arabinoside. Lancet II:1378–1379, 1972.
56. Tattersall MHN, Harrap KR: Combination chemotherapy the antagonism of methotrexate and cytosine arabinoside. Eur J Cancer 9:229–232, 1973.
57. Grindey GB and Nichol CA: Interaction of drugs inhibiting different steps in the synthesis of DNA. Cancer Res 32:527–531, 1972.
58. Cadman E, Eiferman F: Mechanism of synergistic cell killing when methotrexate precedes cytosine arabinoside. J Clin Invest 64:788–797, 1979.
59. Jackson RC, Harkrader RJ: Synergistic and antagonistic interactions of methotrexate and 1-β-D arabinofuranosylcytosine in hepatoma cells. Biochem Pharmacol 30:223–229, 1981.
60. Grant S, Cadman E: The influence of the fluoropyrimidines on 1-β-D arabinofuranosylcytosine metabolism and cytotoxicity. Submitted to Cancer Research.
61. Chabner BA, Myers CE, Coleman CN, Johns DG: The clinical pharmacology of antineoplastic agents (first of 2 parts). New Engl J Med 292 (21):1107–1113, 1979.
62. Stewart CD, Burke PJ: Cytidine deaminase and the development of resistance to arabinosyl cytosine. Nature New Biol 233:109–110, 1971.
63. Tattersall MHN, Ganeshaguru K, Hoffbrand AV: Mechanisms of resistance of human acute leukemia cells to cytosine arabinoside. Br J Haematol 27:39–46, 1974.
64. Camiener GE: Studies of the enzymatic deamination of aracytidine. V. Inhibition *in vitro* and *in vivo* by tetrahydrouridine and other reduced pyrimidine nucleosides. Biochem Pharmacol 17:1981–1991, 1968.
65. White VM, Mellett LB, El Dareer SM: The effect of tetrahydrouridine (H_4U) on the metabolism of arabinosylcytosine (Ara-C) in tumorbearing mice. Pharmacologist 17:202, 1975.
66. El Dareer SM, Mulligan LT Jr, White V et al.: Distribution of [^{3}H] cytosine arabinoside and its products in mice, dogs and monkeys and effect of tetrahydrouridine. Cancer Treat Rep 61:395–407, 1977.
67. Chou TC, Arlin Z, Clarkson BD et al.: Metabolism of 1-β-D arabinofuranosylcytosine in human leukemic cells. Cancer Res 37:3561–3570, 1977.
68. Kreis W, Woodcock TM, Gordon CS, et al.: Tetrahydrouridine: Physiologic disposition and effect upon deanimation of cytosine arabinoside in man. Cancer Treat Rep 61:1347–1353, 1977.
69. Wong PP, Currie VW, Mackey RW, Krakoff IH, Tan CTC, Burchenal JH, Young CW: Phase I evaluation of tetrahydrouridine combined with cytosine arabinoside. Cancer Treat Rep 63:1245–1249, 1979.
70. Maley F, Maley GF: Tetrahydrodeoxyuridylate: A potent inhibitor of deoxycytidylate deaminase. Arch Biochem Biophys 144:723–729, 1971.
71. Maley GF, Maley F: Nucleotide interconversions in embryonic and neoplastic tissues. I. The conversion of deoxycytidylic acid to deoxyuridylic acid and thymidylic acid. J Biol Chem 234(11):2975–2980, 1959.
72. Drake JC, Hande KR, Fuller RW, Chabner BA. Cytidine and deoxycytidylate deaminase inhibition by uridine analogs. Biochem Pharmacol 29:807–811, 1980.
73. Yamamoto CM, Lauzon GJ and Paterson ARP: Toxicity of combinations of arabinosylcytosine and 3-deazauridine toward neoplastic cells in culture. Biochem Pharmacol

27:181–186, 1978.
74. Maley F, Maley GF: On the nature of a sparing effect by thymidine on the utilization of deoxycytidine. Biochemistry 1:847–851, 1962.
75. Maley GF, Maley F: The purification and properties of deoxycytidylate deaminase from chick embryo extracts. J Biol Chem 239:1168–1176, 1964.
76. Piskala A, Sorm F: Nucleic acids components and their analogues. LI. Synthesis of 1-Glycosyl derivatives of 5-azauracil and 5-azacytidine. Coll Czech Chem Commun 29:1060–1076, 1964.
77. Karon M, Sieger L, Leimbrock S, Finkelstein JZ, Nesbit ME, Swaney JJ: 5-Azacytidine: A new active agent for the treatment of acute leukemia. Blood 42:359–365, 1973.
78. Lomen PL, Baker LH, Neil GL, Samson MK: Phase I study of 5-Azacytidine (NSC-102816) using 24-hour continuous infusion for 5 days. Cancer Chem Rep 59 (Part 1):1123–1126, 1975.
79. Wiernik PH: Advances in the management of acute nonlymphocytic leukemia. Arch Intern Med 136:1399–1403, 1976.
80. Lee T, Karon M, Momparler RL: Kinetic studies on phosphorylation of 5-azacytidine with the purified uridine-cytidine kinase from calf thymus. Cancer Res 34:2482–2488, 1974.
81. Canellakis ES: Pyrimidine metabolism. II. Enzymatic pathways of uracil anabolism. J Biol Chem 337:329–338, 1957.
82. Krystal G, Scholefield PG: The partial purification and properties of uridine kinase from Ehrlich ascites tumor cells. Can J Biochem 51:379–389, 1973.
83. Orengo A: Regulation of enzymic activity by metabolites, 1. Uridine cytidine kinase of Novikoff ascites rate tumor. J Biol Chem 224:2204–2209, 1969.
84. Reichard P, Skold O: Formation of uridine phosphates from uracil in extracts of Ehrlich ascites tumor. Acta Chem Scand 11:17–23, 1957.
85. Skold O: Uridine kinase from Ehrlich ascites tumor: purification and properties. J Biol Chem 235:3272–3279, 1960.
86. Vesely J, Cahik A, Sorm F: Characteristics of mouse leukemia cells resistant to 5-azacytidine and 5-Aza-2′-deoxycytidine. Cancer Res 28:1995–2000, 1968.
87. Vesely J, Cahik A, Sorm F: Association of decreased uridine and deoxycytidine kinase with enhanced RNA and DNA polymerase in mouse leukemic cells resistant to 5-azacytidine and 5-Aza-2′-deoxycytidine. Cancer Res 30:2180–2186, 1970.
88. Cadman E, Eiferman F, Heimer R, Davis L: Pyrazofurin enhancement of 5-azayctidine antitumor activity in L5178Y and human leukemia cells. Cancer Res 38:4610–4617, 1978.
89. Chiuten DF, Muggia FM, Johnson RK: Antitumor activity of pyrazofurin in combination with 5-azacytidine against murine P388 and L1210 leukemias and colon carcinoma 26. Cancer Treat Rep 63:1857–1862, 1979.
90. Cahik A, Broucek J: Dual effect of 5-azacytidine on the synthesis of liver ribonucleic acids. Biochem Pharmacol 24:2497–2507, 1972.
91. Cahik A, Tykva R, Sorm F: Incorporation of 5-azacytidine and cytidine into RNA of mouse Ehrlich ascites tumor cells. Coll Czech Chem Commun 31:3015–3019, 1966.
92. Jurovicik M, Raska K, Sormova Z, Sorm F: Anabolic transformation of a novel antimetabolite, 5-azayctidine, and evidence for its incorporation into ribonucleic acids. Coll Czech Chem Commun 30:3370–3377, 1965.
93. Li LH, Olin EJ, Buskirk HH, Reineke LM: Cytotoxicity and mode of action of 5-azacytidine on L1210 leukemia. Cancer Res 30:2760–2769, 1970.
94. Grant S, Cadman E: Altered 5-azacytidine metabolism following 3-deazauridine treatment of L5178Y and human myeloblasts. Cancer Res 40:4000–4006, 1980.
95. Grant S, Rauscher F III, Jakubowski A, Cadman E: Effect of N-(Phosphonacetyl)-L-

aspartate on 5-azacytidine metabolism in P388 and L1210 cells. Cancer Res 41:410–418, 1981.

96. Hakala MT, Taylor E: The ability of purine and thymidine derivatives and of glycine to support the growth of mammalian cells in culture. J Biol Chem 234:126–128, 1959.
97. Goldin A, Venditti JM, Kline I, Mantel N: Eradication of leukaemic cells (L1210) by methotrexate and methotrexate plus citrovorum factor. Nature 212:1548–1550, 1966.
98. Sirotnak FM, Moccio DM, Dorick DM: Optimization of high-dose methotrexate with leucovorin rescue therapy in the L1210 leukemia and sarcoma 180 murine tumor models. Cancer Res 38:345–353, 1978.
99. Bertino JR: 'Rescue' techniques in cancer chemotherapy: Use of leucovorin and other rescue agents after methotrexate treatment. Sem Oncol 4:203–216, 1977.
100. Howell SB, Ensminger WD, Krishan A, Frei E III: Thymidine rescue of high-dose methotrexate in humans. Cancer Res 38:325–330, 1978.
101. Semon JH, Grindey GB: Potentiation of the antitumor activity of methotrexate by concurrent infusion of thymidine. Cancer Res 38:2905–2911, 1978.
102. Ensminger WD, Frei E III: The prevention of methotrexate toxicity by thymidine infusions in humans. Cancer Res 37:1857–1863, 1977.
103. Grindey GB, Semon JH, Pavelic ZP: Modulation versus rescue of antimetabolite toxicity by salvage metabolites administered by continuous infusion. Antibiot Chemother 23:295–304, 1978.
104. Borsa J, Whitmore GF: Studies relating to the mode of action of methotrexate. II. Studies on sites of action in L-cells *in vitro.* Mol Pharmacol 5:303–317, 1969.
105. Roberts D, Warmath EV: Methotrexate inhibition of CCRF-CEM cultures of human lymphoblasts. Eur J Cancer 11:771–782, 1975.
106. Grindey GB, Moran RG, Werkheiser WC: Approaches to the rational combination of antimetabolites for cancer chemotherapy. In Drug Design (E.J. Ariens, ed), Academic Press, N.Y., Vol. 5 pp 169–249, 1975.
107. Howell SB, Mansfield SJ, Taetle R: Thymidine and hypoxanthine requirements of normal and malignant human cells for protection against methotrexate cytotoxicity. Cancer Res 41:945–950, 1981.
108. Nederbragt H, Uitendaal MP, Van der Grint L, Leyva A, Pinedo HM: Reversal of methotrexate inhibition of colony growth of L1210 leukemia cells in semoisolid medium. Cancer Res 41:1193–1198, 1981.
109. Madoc-Jones H, Bruce WR: On the mechanism of the lethal action of 5-fluorouracil on mouse L cells. Cancer Res 28:1976–1981, 1968.
110. Evans RM, Laskin JD, Hakala MT: Assessment of growth-limiting events caused by 5-fluorouracil in mouse cells and in human cells. Cancer Res 40:4113–4122, 1980.
111. Laskin JD, Evans RM, Slocum HK, Burke D, Hakala MT: Basis for natural variation in sensitivity to 5 fluorouracil in mouse and human cells in culture. Cancer Res 39:383–390, 1979.
112. Reyes P: The synthesis of 5-fluorouridine 5-phosphate by a pyrimidine phosphoribosyltransferase of mammalian origin. 1. Some properties of the enzyme form P-1534J mouse leukemia cells. Biochemistry 8:2057–2062, 1969.
113. Heidelberger C: Fluorinated pyrimidines and their nucleosides. Antineoplastic and immunosuppressive agents, Part 2, Handbook of Experimental Pharmacology, eds. Sartorelli AC and Johns DG. (Springer, New York). Vol 38, pp 193–241, 1974.
114. Cadman E, Heimer R, Davis L: Enhanced 5-fluorouracil nucleotide formation after methotrexate administration: explanation for drug synergism. Science 205:1135–1137, 1979.
115. Cadman E, Heimer R, Benz C: The influence of methotrexate pretreatment on 5-fluorour-

acil metabolism in L1210 cells. J Biol Chem 256 (4):1695–1704, 1981.
116. Benz C, Schoenberg M, Choti M, Cadman E: Schedule-dependent cytotoxicity of methotrexate and 5-fluorouracil in human colon and breast tumor cell lines. J Clin Invest 66:1162–1165, 1980.
117. Benz C, Cadman E: Modulation of 5-fluorouracil metabolism and cytotoxicity by antimetabolite pretreatment in human colorectal adenocarcinoma HCT-8. Cancer Res 41:994–999, 1981.
118. Benz C, Cadman E: Biochemical alterations during unperturbed suspension growth of L1210 cells. Cancer Res 41:157–163, 1981.
119. Cadman E, Benz C, Heimer R, O'Shaughnessy J: The effect of de novo purine synthesis inhibitors on 5-fluorouracil metabolism and cytotoxicity. Biochem Pharmacol, in press.
120. Gewirtz AM, Cadman EC: Preliminary report on the efficacy of sequential methotrexate, 5-fluorouracil in advanced breast cancer. Cancer (Accepted).
121. Yoshida M, Hoshi A, Kuretani K: Prevention of antitumor effect of 5-fluorouracil by hypoxanthine. Biochem Pharmacol 27 (24):2979–2982, 1978.
122. Santelli G, Valeriote F: *In vivo* potentiation of 5-fluorouracil cytotoxicity against AKR leukemia by purines, pyrimidines, and their nucleosides and deoxynucleosides. JNCI 64:69–72, 1980.
123. Nelson JA, Parks RE Jr: Biochemical mechanisms for the synergism between 6-thioguanine and 6-(methylmercapto) purine ribonucleoside in sarcoma 180 cells. Cancer Res 32:2034–2041, 1972.
124. Scholar EM, Brown PR, Parks RE Jr: Synergistic effect of 6-Mercaptopurine and 6-Methylmercaptopurine ribonucleoside on the levels of adenine nucleotides of sarcoma 180 cells. Cancer Res 32:259–269, 1972.
125. Paterson ARP, Wang MC: Mechanism of the growth inhibition pontentiation arising from combination of 6-mercaptopurine with 6-(methylmercapto) purine ribonucleoside. Cancer Res 30:2379–2387, 1970.
126. Paterson ARP, Moriwaki A: Combination chemotherapy: Synergistic inhibition of lymphoma L5178Y cells in culture and *in vivo* with 6-mercaptopurine and 6-(methylmercapto) purine ribonucleoside. Cancer Res 29:681–686, 1969.
127. Glazer RI, Peale AL: The effect of 5-fluorouracil on the synthesis of nuclear RNA in L1210 cells *in vitro*. Mol Pharmacol 16:270–277, 1979.
128. Kaplan AS, Ben-Porat T: The action of 5-fluorouracil on the nucleic acid metabolism of pseudorabies virus-infected and non-infected rabbit kidney cells. Virology 13:78–92, 1961.
129. Mandel HG: The incorporation of 5-fluorouracil into RNA and its molecular consequences. Progress in Molecular and Subcellular Biology, ed. Hahn FE (Springer, New York). Vol. 1, pp 82–135, 1969.
130. Wilkinson DS, Cihak A, Pitot HC: Inhibition of ribosomal ribonucleic acid maturation in rat liver by 5-fluoroorotic acid resulting in the selective labeling of cytoplasmic messenger ribonucleic acid. J Biol Chem 246 (21):6418–6427, 1971.
131. Wilkinson DS, Crumley J: The mechanism of 5-fluorouridine toxicity in Novikoff hepatoma cells. Cancer Res 36:4032–4038, 1976.
132. Wilkinson DS, Pitot HC: Inhibition of ribosomal ribonucleic acid maturation in Novikoff hepatoma cells by 5-fluorouracil and 5-fluorouridine. J Biol Chem 248 (1):63–68, 1973.
133. Wilkinson DS, Tisty TD, Hanas RJ: The inhibition of ribosomal RNA synthesis and maturation in Novikoff hepatoma cells by 5-fluorouridine. Cancer Res 35:3014–3020, 1975.
134. Willen R, Stenram U: RNA synthesis in the liver of rats treated with 5-fluorouracil. Arch Biochem Biophys 119:501–503, 1967.

135. Carrico CK, Glazer RI: Effect of 5-fluorouracil on the synthesis and translation of polyadenylic acid-containing RNA from regenerating rat liver. Cancer Res 39:3694–3701, 1979.
136. Ardalan B, Cooney DA, Jayaram HN, Carrico CK, Glazer RI, MacDonald J, Schein PS: Mechanisms of sensitivity and resistance of murine tumors to 5-fluorouracil. Cancer Res 40:1431–1437, 1980.
137. Glazer RI, Legraverend M: The effect of 5-fluorouridine 5′-triphosphate on RNA transcribed in isolated nuclei *in vitro.* Mol Pharmacol 17:279–282, 1980.
138. Glazer RI, Legraverend M: The effect of 5-fluorouridine 5′-triphosphate on RNA transcribed in isolated nuclei *in vitro.* Mol Pharmacol 17:279–282, 1980.
139. Glazer RI, Hartman KD: The effect of 5-fluorouracil on the synthesis and methylation of low molecular weight nuclear RNA in L1210 cells. Mol Pharmacol 17:245–249, 1980.
140. Glazer RI, Legraverend M: The effect of 5-fluorouridine 5′-triphosphate on RNA transcribed in isolated nuclei *in vitro.* Mol Pharmacol 17:279–282, 1980.
141. Cory JG, Breland JC, Carter GL: Effect of 5-fluorouracil on RNA metabolism in Novikoff hepatoma cells. Cancer Res 39:4905–4913, 1979.
142. Carrico CK, Glazer RI: Augmentation by thymidine of the incorporation and distribution of 5-fluorouracil in ribosomal RNA. Biochem Biophys Res Commun 87:664–670, 1979.
143. Spiegelman S, Sawyer R, Nayak R, Ritzi E, Stolfi R, Martin D: Improving the anti-tumor activity of 5-fluorouracil by increasing its incorporation into RNA via metabolic modulation. Proc Natl Acad Sci USA 77 (8):4966–4970, 1980.
144. Kirkwood JM, Ensminger W, Rosowsky A, Papathanasopoulos N, Frei E III: Comparison of pharmacokinetics of 5-fluorouracil and 5-fluorouracil with concurrent thymidine infusions in a Phase I trial. Cancer Res 40:107–113, 1980.
145. Hill BT: Cancer chemotherapy, the relevance of certain concepts of cel cycle kinetics. Biochim Biophys Acta 516:389–417, 1978.

6. Psychological Intervention for Pain in Pediatric Cancer Patients

SUSAN M. JAY and CHARLES H. ELLIOTT

1. INTRODUCTION AND OVERVIEW

Pain is a frequently encountered experience for the child with cancer. The diagnosis of malignancy is accompanied by a panoply of bloodtests, injections, vena punctures, and periodic bone marrow aspirations and lumbar punctures (spinal taps) which are administered at frequent intervals over a period of years. In addition, the disease process, particularly in the final stages, can cause severe pain for the pediatric cancer patient. The coping capacities of pediatric cancer patients are challenged and sometimes overtaxed by this arduous series of aversive events which must be mastered during the adjustment process if the child is to emerge from this life-threatening situation with emotional and physical well-being. Psychology, as a discipline, has much to offer pediatric oncology in the area of assessment and management of pain.

Unfortunately, the problem of pediatric pain has been sorely neglected both in the medical and psychological literature. A review of major pediatric and nursing texts reveals little concern with the problem of pain management in children, a bitter irony given that few medical conditions or situations do not involve some type of pain experience. The psychological literature since 1960 is replete with theory, research, and clinical application in the area of pain management with adults, yet the literature on assessment and management of pain in children is characterized almost exclusively by anecdotal reports and by the absence of systematic, controlled research.

This neglect of pediatric pain as an area of inquiry and intervention was illustrated by Eland and Anderson [1] who conducted a thorough search of the literature from 1970 through 1975. The search produced 1380 articles on pain, yet only 33 of these dealt with pediatric pain. Furthermore, the 33 articles were almost all related to differential diagnosis and contained little or no information on assessment of children's pain behavior or methods of

G. Bennett Humphrey et al. (eds), Adrenal and Endocrine Tumors in Children.

intervention. Such a lack of information on such a clinically-relevant topic is somewhat bewildering for the medical or psychological practitioner who routinely encounters pediatric cancer patients with needle phobias, severe conditioned anxiety about bone marrows, and/or uncontrollable behavior to such an extent that medical procedures are difficult to administer (not to mention the less intense forms of distress and anxiety related to the regimen of diagnostic and therapeutic procedures).

The intent of the authors in this chapter is to counter this trend by providing clinically-relevant, yet data-based information concerning the assessment and management of pain in pediatric cancer patients. The nature of pain is conceptualized by the authors as a trimodal behavioral construct consistent with Sander's [2] definition: Pain is conceptualized as an interaction of overt, covert, and physiological responses that are capable of being produced by tissue damage or irritation but may also be produced and maintained by other antecedent or consequent stimulus conditions. Overt pain responses refer to verbal and nonverbal behavioral responses such as complaining, grimacing, screaming, requesting pain medication. Covert pain responses refer to a person's subjective thoughts, attitudes, perceptions, and images during painful experiences. The physiological response mode is characterized by autonomic, pyramidal, extrapyramidal, and biochemical reactions to a stimulus. Although physiological pain responses are generally generated by tissue damage or insult, the importance of antecedent and consequential environmental and psychosocial factors in shaping and/or perpetuating certain pain responses will be addressed.

In this chapter, the authors will first address the distinction between acute and chronic pain in children. Methods of assessing overt, covert, and physiological pain responses will be outlined and the importance of factors such as parental expectations, individual coping styles, environmental contingencies, and cognitive-developmental variables will be discussed. Intervention techniques which are used in reducing acute and/or chronic pain in children with cancer will be reviewed and the use of medication in pain reduction will be briefly discussed. Intervention techniques which are used in reducing acute and/or chronic pain in children with cancer will be reviewed and the use of medication in pain reduction will be briefly discussed. A 'package' of behavior therapy techniques developed by the authors will be discussed in detail. Initial data on the use of these techniques has suggested effectiveness in reducing children's distress during bone marrow aspirations and lumbar punctures. Finally, issues of clinical application will be discussed and problems encountered in applying psychological intervention in a medical setting will be reviewed.

1.1. Acute versus chronic pain

The acute-chronic dimension is addressed almost solely in the adult literature wherein sharp differences in etiology, mechanisms, physiopathology, function, diagnosis and therapy of acute versus chronic pain are assumed [3]. The distinction is less clear in pediatric oncology although the authors will attempt to delineate differences in the following discussion since the distinction holds implications for assessment, treatment planning and treatment outcome.

Acute pain and its associated physiological, psychological, and behavioral responses are almost invariably caused by noxious or tissue-damaging stimulation in relation to bodily insult or disease and is rarely caused *primarily* by psychological factors [3]. Acute pain serves an adaptive function as a signal of organic pathology or insult and prompts medical attention and/or diagnosis. For example, the leukemic child may complain of acute onset of severe headaches and subsequent tests may indicate central nervous system relapse. Also, acute pain may be a response to noxious physical experiences involving needles such as vena punctures, bone marrow aspirations, and lumbar punctures in which the child perceives the needle puncture as a painful physical insult. In such cases the child's perceptions and fearful cognitions may greatly intensify the actual physiological pain experience and extreme conditioned anxiety may develop. Varni [4] makes the point that although acute and chronic pain may be differentiated in terms of neurophysiological etiology, it is the severe intensity of the acute pain experience and the fear component which most clearly differentiates acute pain from chronic pain. For example, one observes an acute pain response in the child who develops such severe conditioned anxiety about bone marrow aspirations that he/she has to be physically restrained for the procedure to be performed. In contrast, the child with terminal disease may experience much chronic pain, but the fear component of that pain is generally outweighed by factors such as lethargy, apathy, withdrawal, and irritability.

In the adult literature, the term 'chronic pain' denotes a specific syndrome which may not be directly applicable or as easily generalized to pediatric patients. Adult chronic pain, in its most pathological form, has no biological function and is a function of reinforcing psychological and environmental factors, even though it may have originally had an organic etiology. Chronic pain, in its less psychopathological form, may refer to long-standing intractable pain caused by severe insult or progressive disease. Chronic pain is characterized by certain affect and/or 'chronic pain behaviors' including depressed mood, sleep and appetite disturbances, inactivity and general physical disability. These responses are often reinforced and maintained by socioenvironmental factors and secondary gains (attention, lack of responsibility, insurance benefits, narcotic dependence).

Chronic pain in children is a less well-defined syndrome but may have similar characteristics to adult chronic pain. In this chapter, the authors will discuss chronic pain largely in the context of pain resulting from progressive malignant disease or in some cases from iatrogenic origin. Common examples of such chronic pain include headaches, bone pain, phantom limb pain, and mouth ulcers caused by chemotherapy. Acute pain will be defined as pain resulting from specific, time-limited noxious events resulting in physical insult (injections, vena punctures, bone marrow aspirations, lumbar punctures) and/or temporary physical impairment (surgical pain).

2. ASSESSMENT

2.1. Overt, behavioral pain responses

Various techniques have been used to assess behavioral indicators of pain. These techniques can be divided into three categories: (a) global rating scales; (b) indirect measures and (c) behavioral observational scales. Assessment of overt, behavioral indices of pain is generally conducted by someone other than the patient (medical staff, observers, parents). Rating scales of exhibited pain behaviors such as crying, screaming, verbal expressions of pain and protest have been used successfully by nurses observing pediatric cancer patients undergoing painful medical procedures such as bone marrow aspirations and lumbar punctures [5, 6]. In these studies, nurses were asked to rate children's behavioral distress on a one to seven point Likert type scale with one indicating 'no evidence of distress' and seven indicating 'extreme, uncontrollable distress'. These ratings correlated highly with more objective observational scores of distress.

Indirect measures of pain behavior may be assessed by documenting medication requests, or 'well' behaviors such as time spent walking, standing, playing, talking [7, 8]. Such measures may be problematic in assessing children's pain levels since many children are reluctant to ask for pain medication because the fear of needles and shots may be more aversive than the pain itself [1]. Also, children who are not in severe or acute distress will often engage in play activities despite experienced pain. However, Varni [9] demonstrated the success of self-regulation techniques in managing bleeding and arthritic pain in a 9-year-old hemophilic child by using assessment measures such as dosages of pain medication, physical therapy measures, school days missed, and hospitalizations. Measures such as these provide only an indirect assessment of pain *per se,* but have an intrinsic value of their own in assessing a child's overall functioning.

Behavioral observation scales are probably the most objective and reliable techniques in assessing behavioral indicators of pain. Observational methods involve the use of observers who observe the child in a particular situation for a specified time interval and document the occurrence of specified behaviors which suggest pain or distress. Two observation scales have been reported in the pediatric oncology literature, both of which were designed to measure acute distress behaviors of pediatric cancer patients undergoing bone marrow aspiration procedures and lumbar punctures. The first scale, the Procedure Behavior Rating Scale (PBRS), developed by Katz, Kellerman, and Siegel [6] consists of 25 operationally-defined behaviors indicative of distress (cry, scream, verbal expression of pain, etc.) which are coded by observers for occurrence during medical procedures. Katz *et al.* suggest that the word 'distress' be used to encompass both constructs of anxiety and pain since they are often difficult to distinguish in clinical situations.

Jay and Elliott developed the Observation Scale of Behavioral Distress (OSBD) which constituted a revised version of the PBRS. The OSBD consists of 13 operationally-defined behaviors indicative of distress in children. The OSBD was designed with the following features which were intended to further refine the Procedural Behavior Rating Scale: (a) behaviors are recorded in continuous 15-second intervals within each of the 4 phases of the procedure rather than recorded once for occurrence or nonoccurrence over an entire phase; (b) each behavioral category in the OSBD is weighted according to intensity since most observers would agree that screaming and flailing are more intense and salient indicators of distress than verbal expressions of anxiety and pain. The OSBD behavioral categories and their respective intensity weights are as follows: Cry (1.5), Scream (4.0), Physical Restraint (4.0), Verbal Resistance (2.5), Requests Emotional Support (2.0), Muscular Rigidity (2.5), Verbal Fear (2.5), Verbal Pain (2.5), Flail (4.0), Nervous Behavior (1.0) and Information Seeking (1.5).* Initial data has suggested that the OSBD constitutes a reliable and valid measure of children's pain/distress and may be particularly useful in time-limited acute clinical situations which involve pain/distress for children (injections, vena punctures, various diagnostic and treatment procedures). A study investigating the validity of the OSBD indicated that children's OSBD distress scores were significantly correlated with children's self-rated pain measures, nurses' ratings, and parent-rated measures of distress (Jay *et al*; 1983). Additional studies are being conducted to further substantiate the validity of the OSBD.

* The OSBD and information concerning development, scoring, reliability, and validity can be obtained from the first author: Susan Jay, Psychosocial Program, Hematology-Oncology, Children's Hospital of Los Angeles, 4650 Sunset Blvd., Los Angeles, California 90027.

2.2. Covert, self-report pain responses

Covert indices of pain or distress include the patient's self-reports of his/her experienced pain, thoughts, images, or feelings during pain-related situations. Numerical (0 to 100) and adjective ('slight' to 'agonizing' pain) rating scales have been used frequently with adults [2]. Visual analog scales are also popular in the adult literature and consists of a vertical or horizontal line with one end labeled 'no pain' and the other, 'pain as bad as it could be' [10]. Patients mark the point on the line which indicates their level of pain intensity.

Self-report measures of pain and fear were used by Katz, Kellerman and Siegel [11] in a study of pediatric cancer patients (four years and older) undergoing bone marrow aspirations. Pain was assessed by showing the child a visual representation of a 'pain thermometer' which was gradated on a o ('no hurt') to 100 ('the most hurt possible') point scale. The child was instructed to 'point to the place that shows how much you hurt'. Fear was assessed by the use of seven 'fear faces' with the number one face representing 'not being scared at all' (smile) and the number seven face representing 'the most scared possible' (frown). The child was instructed to 'choose the face that shows how scared you were during the bone marrow aspiration'. Katz *et al.* reported that self-report measures of fear were more highly correlated with observed behavior than self-report measures of pain. A more recent report [12] indicated that pain thermometer ratings were significantly correlated ($r = .67$, $p < .02$) with observed behavior in children ages 8 years and older. Thus, in young children, the assessment of self-reported pain is somewhat problematical and less reliable than for older children. It is unlikely that children younger than seven or eight can reliably discriminate and translate experienced pain into gradated visual representations such as on a 1 to 100 point thermometer or discriminate quantitative pain adjectives ('extremely', 'a little', 'agonizing', etc.) which have been useful in assessing pain levels in adults.

2.3. Physiological pain responses

Although physiological measures can be very useful in assessing pain experiences, many methodological problems remain to be resolved. Specific patterns and relationships between physiological responses and pain experiences have not been well-established due to variability of responses elicited by different pain stimuli and because of wide individual differences in pain responses [13]. One of the major problems in using physiological responses as measures of anxiety and pain is that responses in the covert (self-report), overt (behavioral) and physiological systems typically do not correlate highly and research has not determined which is the most valid measure [14]. Such discrepancies are likely due to the fact that the different response systems can be shaped differentially by environmental events [15]. Physiological measures which are suggested in the literature as being related to pain experience include increased respiration rate, increased muscular tension, elevated systolic and diastolic blood pressure, increased pulse rate, and skin resistance [13].

Very few studies have employed physiological measures of pain/distress in children. Melamed and Siegel [16] found the Palmar Sweat Index to be a useful measure of children's preoperative and postoperative anxiety. Peterson and Shigetomi [17] used pulse rate and temperature as measures of pre- and post-operative anxiety but found that these measures did not correlate with other measures of anxiety, nor did they discriminate between treatment groups. The current authors are investigating the relationship between pulse rate, observational measures of distress, nurse ratings of distress, and self-report ratings of pain in pediatric cancer patients undergoing bone marrow aspirations and lumbar punctures. Further research on the use of physiological responses in the assessment and intervention of pain experiences in children is definitely warranted.

2.4. Other relevant environmental and psychological factors

Pain behavior in children may be influenced and shaped by a number of psychosocial and environmental factors. Identification of antecedent, concurrent, and consequent stimuli may elucidate certain variables which serve to intensify and/or maintain a child's response to painful stimuli. Fordyce [7] described an explicit interview for identifying numerous relevant controlling factors such as: (a) what happens just before and just after pain behavior? (b) how do significant others react to the child's pain behavior? (c) what makes the pain better and what makes it worse?

Parental behavior is a particularly important variable to assess in the process of examining the intensity and duration of children's pain behaviors. Parental attitudes towards pain and parental expectations may mediate children's perceptions and reactions. Jay *et al.* [12] found a strong positive relationship between parental anxiety and children's distress during bone marrow aspirations. The author's clinical experiences suggest that, with a few exceptions, the children who cope most effectively with traumatic medical procedures are those whose parents are supportive yet expect their children to cope well and who do not reinforce pain behaviors with overwhelming amounts of sympathy, nurturance, or attention. Nor do these parents openly display their own personal anxiety and distress. Clinical observation further suggests that some children whose parents choose not to be present during painful medical procedures actually cope very effectively and seem to accept such procedures as a grim fact of life without catastrophizing about the pain and fear. Shaw and Routh [18] found that when receiving injections, children exhibited more negative behavior if their mothers were present than children whose mothers were asked to stay in the waiting room. However, further research is needed to clarify the dynamics between parental behavior and children's coping capacities. It is too early to make specific recommendations to practitioners concerning the absence or presence of parents during medical procedures.

Assessment of expectations and reactions of medical staff may also reveal similar contingencies operating in relation to children's pain behaviors. The response of physicians and nurses to children's distress (attention, anxiety, prescribing medication, calm reassurance) may differentially influence children's reactions to pain. The question has not been resolved concerning how much attention is optimal in giving a child needed support during stressful situations yet simultaneously conveying the message that he/she can manage and cope with stressful situations.

Pain experiences are mediated by age and developmental factors. Research has shown that distress levels of pediatric cancer patients undergoing bone marrow aspirations under the age of 7 years are 5–10 times higher than children older than 7 years [12]. Such heightened distress in preschool children is likely related to their immature cognitive processes and to the meaning that they attribute to the painful experience. Preschool children generally have a limited understanding of logical cause-and-effect relationships which often results in distorted conceptions and misattributions in relation to pain and illnes [19, 20]. For example, Sheridan [21] noted that many younger children believe that it is possible to bleed to death from blood tests. Furthermore, many young children perceive pain and illness as punishment for bad deeds and thoughts [22]. Certainly such fearful fantasies and misattributions intensify the distress in young children who have to undergo painful medical procedures on a routine basis. Conditioned anxiety responses may also develop which make intervention even more difficult [6].

The context of the child's pain effects pain tolerance in children [23]. Previous experiences may shape the child's expectations and coexisting physical status (fatigue, discomfort, anxiety and depression) can certainly influence pain tolerance. Often, children with cancer exhibit decreased pain tolerance in the terminal stages of the disease. The effect of previous experiences upon children's distress levels during bone marrow aspirations is unclear in the research literature. Katz *et al.* [6] reported that pediatric cancer patients did not 'habituate' or adjust to such procedures over time, while Jay *et al.* [12] did find that patients became less distressed over time and with experience. However, such habituation may take as long as 2 years for the preschool child. Jay *et al.* speculated that the discrepancy in results may have been related to differences in clinic population and in staff-patient ratio. In small clinics such as the one at Oklahoma Children's Memorial Hospital, intense personal relationships develop between the patients and the medical staff. Furthermore, it is the authors' subjective clinical impression that most children's anxiety and distress decrease as they begin to develop warm, trusting relationships with the medical personnel who administer the procedures.

Assessment of children's cognitive coping styles is important in planning intervention and in predicting treatment outcome. Cognitive styles include dimensions such as internal-external locus of control [24], repression-sensitization, minimization-vigilant focusing [25], and monitor-distractor [26]. Locus of control refers to a person's perception of whether life events are controlled and influenced by oneself (internal) or by external forces such as fate, luck, and chance. Neuhauser *et al.* [24] found that children who have high internal control perceive themselves as having more control over the healing process. Although Jay *et al.* [12] found no relationship between locus of control and children's distress levels during painful medical procedures, further research is needed to clarify how children's perceived control over illness and pain relate to coping processes.

The three cognitive styles described in the adult literature (repression-sensitization, minimization-vigilant focusing, and monitor-distractor) all describe a similar construct. Persons referred to as repressors, minimizers, or distractors are those who tend to use selective inattention, denial, avoidance of information and rationalization when dealing with a stressful event. On the other hand, persons referred to as sensitizers, vigilant focusers, and monitors are those who cope with stressful events by actively seeking information, focusing on details, and practicing coping skills. Although little or no research has investigated such dimensions in children, the authors' clinical experience confirms discrepant cognitive styles in children which differentially influence efficacy of intervention. For example, in a treatment outcome study designed to reduce distress in pediatric cancer patients undergoing bone marrow aspirations and lumbar punctures, the use of filmed modeling (showing a film of a child undergoing such procedures utilizing effective coping techniques) actually appeared to increase the distress levels in two children who began to cry as they watched the procedures in the film. Such children could be referred to as minimizers, repressors, or distractors in contrast to the majority of children who were able to utilize the information in the film to their benefit. Such observations point to the necessity of matching intervention techniques with individual cognitive styles for optimal intervention outcome.

3. PSYCHOLOGICAL INTERVENTION FOR ACUTE PAIN

3.1. Painful medical procedures

Pediatric cancer patients frequently protest vena punctures, bone marrow aspirations, and lumbar punctures. The anxiety and distress produced in anticipation of these procedures is sometimes so severe that children (and often parents) exhibit symptoms such as nausea, vomiting, insomnia, nightmares, and skin rashes prior to the procedures. Young children often exhibit their distress during procedures behaviorally (kicking, fighting, screaming) to such an extent that physical restraint is necessary and it is very difficult for the medical staff to conduct the procedures. Due to the traumatic nature of bone marrows and lumbar punctures, it may take as long as two-three years for children to 'adjust' to the procedures or to encounter them without extreme distress and trauma [12]. A similar problem which warrants psychological intervention is severe anticipatory nausea and vomiting prior to intravenous chemotherapy which often occurs in older children and adolescents.

Hypnosis has been the most frequently reported intervention for acute distress and pain in pediatric cancer patients. Unfortunately, to date, no systematic controlled studies of the effectiveness of hypnosis in pain/anxiety control with children have been reported in the literature. Two such studies are in progress however, and offer promising results [27, 28]. Hilgard and Morgan [29] reported that formal hypnotic procedures were not effective with children under the age of 6 years who were undergoing bone marrow aspirations and lumbar punctures. Hilgard and LeBaron [30] presented an interesting and informative discussion concerning the use of hypnosis with pediatric cancer patients undergoing bone marrow aspirations. The authors found that the efficacy of hypnosis in this situation depended, in part, on the level of measured hypnotizability of the child.

However, more favorable results have been reported with older children and with children undergoing less traumatic procedures. Olness [31] and LaBaw, Holton, Tewell, and Eccles [32] reported that self-hypnosis was effective in modifying nausea and vomiting associated with chemotherapy and/or radiation and in reducing pain and distress during medical procedures. More sophisticated, data-based studies on hypnosis and relaxation training with adult cancer patients strongly suggest the effectiveness of such intervention for anticipatory nausea and vomiting [33, 34] and for pain control [35].

Modification of such hypnotic techniques for use with pediatric cancer patients offers much potential in reducing distress, pain, and anxiety and the need for systematic investigation of such intervention cannot be overstated. Gardner and Olness' [23] book on hypnosis and hypnotherapy with children is the most comprehensive compilation of information concerning application of hypnosis to pediatric problems and is recommended for those practitioners interested in applying hypnotic techniques with children. Methods of teaching hypnoanalgesea or pain control to children are outlined and include the following examples: (a) direct suggestions – 'Just imagine painting numbing mediation on your back'; (b) distancing suggestions – 'Imagine yourself in the mountains'; (c) suggestions for feelings antithetical to pain – 'Think of the funniest thing you ever did'; (d) distraction techniques such as storytelling or games; and (e) directing attention to the pain itself.

Behavior therapy offers a promising intervention alternative for reduction of pain-related behaviors in children. Behavior therapy techniques were used successfully by Jay *et al.* [36] in reducing behavioral distress of young cancer patients (3–9 years) undergoing bone marrow aspirations and lumbar punctures. The behavior therapy 'package' included the following components: filmed modeling, breathing exercises, reinforcement, emotive imagery, and behavioral rehearsal. These intervention techniques will be discussed in detail in the last section of the chapter. Elliott and Olson [37] also found that a similar package of stress management techniques (attention-distraction, relaxation, emotive imagery, and reinforcement) was effective in reducing children's pain-related behavior during medical treatments for burn injury. LeBaron and Zeltzer [38] reported the effectiveness of behavioral techniques (distraction, encouragement, reinforcement of 'well' behavior, and relaxation) in reducing vomiting and disability associated with intensive regimens of chemotherapy.

3.2. Surgery

Children with solid tumors may undergo one or more surgical procedures for biopsies and removal of the tumor. Hospitalization and surgery are stressful, painful and anxiety-producing experiences that can lead to transient or long-term disturbance, particularly if the child is not adequately prepared [39]. Psychological intervention can be helpful in alleviating anticipatory anxiety, in helping the child cope with post-surgical pain, and in facilitating post-surgical recovery.

The experience of surgery presents a situation in which fear, anxiety, pain, and emotional distress are all elements in the child's reactions. The pain in such a situation is usually associated with medical procedures (vena punctures, shots, bloodtests) and with postoperative surgical pain. Both pharmacological agents and psychological intervention strategies have the potential for reducing the sensory, cognitive, and affective components of surgery-related pain.

Preoperative instruction constitutes the form of psychological intervention most frequently used, the purpose of which is to provide information to the child, encourage emotional expression, and to establish a relationship of trust between the child and the medical staff [40]. Many hospitals offer innovative programs to prepare parents and children for hospitalization and surgery prior to the child's admission [41]. Preadmission 'parties' for patients may include tours of the induction room, recovery room, hospital playroom, x-ray equipment, physical therapy, and hospital rooms. Children are introduced to the surgeon, anaesthesiologist, and to the nurses who will be caring for them in order to foster a friendly, trusting relationship. Johnson [42] describes a program in a children's hospital that combines a puppet show with a tour of the hospital followed by a discussion period. The topics of fear, pain, anaesthesia, and the recovery room are discussed by the puppets and slides are shown of such equipment as intravenous tubes and traction [42]. Puppet therapy [43] and play therapy [44] have also been used to prepare children for painful medical procedures and surgery during hospitalization. These techniques give the child the opportunity to act out and/or express fears and perceptions concerning procedures while simultaneously providing information through exposure to medical equipment.

The usefulness and importance of such preparation in helping children cope with surgical procedures and in reducing postoperative adjustment problems is clear. Unfortunately, research studies investigating the efficacy of preoperative preparation suffer from numerous methodological flaws including inadequate measurement techniques and uncontrolled variables. However, one exception is a well controlled study by Melamed and Siegel [16] who demonstrated the effectiveness of filmed modeling in reducing children's anxiety concerning surgery. Children in the experimental group were shown a film, 'Ethan has an Operation' which depicts a 7-year-old child encountering the various events associated with surgery including admission, introduction to the surgeon and anesthesiologist, having a blood test, exposure to hospital equipment, separation from mother, and scenes in the operating and recovery room. The child in the film narrated his thoughts and feelings as he coped with the anxiety-provoking stimuli. Children in the control group saw a film unrelated to the hospital. Children who viewed the film exhibited lower anxiety and fewer behavior problems than control subjects, both preoperatively and postoperatively. Such results suggest the efficacy of using filmed modeling in preparing children for surgery and hospitalization. Peterson and Shigetomi [17] found that children who were taught coping techniques in addition to the use of filmed modeling were more calm and cooperative during invasive medical procedures (tonsillectomies) than children who received modeling or coping techniques alone. However, some of this research has also shown that some children do not benefit from modeling and may actually have their fears increased by it.

Identifying such children in advance, so that they could be given either no preparation or preparation of a different type, is an important research task for the future.

4. CHRONIC PAIN

It was previously noted in this chapter that the current authors are considering chronic pain in pediatric cancer patients in the context of pain resulting from progressive malignant disease. The management of chronic pain problems associated with cancer tends to be a somewhat different type of problem with respect to children as compared to adults. Two factors are likely responsible for this difference. The *first* of these factors is that different types of cancers tend to be associated with pediatric and adult populations [4]. Adults most frequently are found to have carcinomas of organ systems such as stomach, breasts, lungs, and ovaries, which are well known to cause prolonged and severe pain. By contrast, the most frequently occurring malignancy in children is acute leukemia, accounting for about 40% of pediatric cancers [45]. Acute leukemia most frequently is accompanied only by mild to moderate pain and then usually only during periods of relapse [4]. Severe pain in children with cancer generally only occurs very late in the development of the disease when it has become rapidly progressive and widespread [46].

The *second* factor which differentiates chronic pain in children with cancer from such pain in adults is that (as noted previously) young children have a substantially different understanding and conception of the 'meaning' of pain associated with their disease. The importance of the meaning assigned to pain and illness was originally highlighted by the classic research of Beecher [47]. A number of investigators have more recently found that a child's level of cognitive development, in a Piagetian sense, can be a key determinate of a child's conception of illness [48–50]. In general, these investigations have found that children's conception of causality progresses in a developmental sequence such that children in the preoperational stage of development (between about the ages of 2 to 7) tend to have very inadequate and illogical conceptions of both illness and healing. Beales [51] further observed that younger children are far more concerned and disturbed by insults to the surface of their bodies because they have relatively little comprehension of their internal make-up and therefore little awareness of the insidious implications of pain which originates from inside their bodies. During the period of concrete operations (approximately the ages of 7 to 11), children begin to form a more logical understanding of pain and illness, but the above research indicates that they remain unable to fully appreciate some of the more abstract concepts of illness and healing.

This situation changes radically for older children entering the stage of *formal* operations which occurs after the age of 11. However, Schultz [52] found that these children still evidenced a virtually universal fear of bodily injury in addition to concerns of losing control, dependency and inability to maintain favorite activities. The issue of 'meaning' was summarized well by Beales [51] who pointed out that younger children tend to become more upset with external, cutaneous injuries because they can see the injury, and thus understand it in a limited, concrete manner. The older child is equally concerned with internal versus external injury because, unlike the younger child, his/her cognitive processes allow the understanding of abstract and invisible bodily changes.

Somewhat related to the factor of children's conceptualization of illness and pain is the role played by depression in regard to pain. A number of investigators have noted that depression is a frequent concomitant of chronic pain [8]. Although a direct cause and effect relationship between chronic pain and depression has not been established, Sternbach's work has suggested that similar neurochemical processes may be involved with both phenomena. In this regard, it is interesting to note that depression in children is generally not considered to be a very common problem relative to adults, except for those investigators who define depression in children in ways that are substantially different from definitions generally employed for adult depression [53]. It is possible that this reduced incidence of depression as well as chronic pain in children is either due to: (a) the previously noted differences between adults and children in cognitive development and meaning systems, given that depression has often been hypothesized to be a result of certain cognitive processes [54], or (b) differences in susceptibility to biochemical changes which have been associated with both depression and pain [8, 55].

4.1. Psychological intervention for chronic pain

Very little in the way of systematic research has been conducted on psychological interventions for the treatment of chronic pain in children. However, four approaches would appear to have particular promise in this regard and will be briefly reviewed. These approaches include: (a) operant conditioning, (b) family systems therapy, (c) stress management techniques, and (d) hypnosis.

Operant conditioning involves the manipulation of environmental events which differentially influence behavior (example: ignoring a child's tantrums which subsequently decrease in frequency). The primary goal of operant conditioning procedures is the reduction of pain-related *behavior*. It has been well documented by Fordyce and his colleagues [56, 57] that pain-related behavior such as grimaces, moans, medication requests, complaints, reduction or termination of activities, etc. are readily influenced by environmental contingencies, especially in chronic pain problems. These contingencies can be in the form of reassurances and sympathy from a child's mother or father, concern and support expressed by medical staff, the avoidance of aversive tasks at school and home, and so on.

While the goal of operant conditioning is to reduce such pain-related behaviors, it should not be assumed that a reduction in physiological arousal cannot also be effected by operant conditioning procedures. For example, Bonica [55] noted that central mediating mechanisms of inhibition can effect both the perception and expression of pain and that both emotional stresses and certain drugs can impair the efficacy of this mechanism. Furthermore, it is quite possible that operant conditioning principles could effect these central mediating mechanisms, as suggested by Pomerleau and Brady [58]. They stated that there is strong support for, 'the notion that whenever one can specify a neurally-mediated response which is pathognomonic, there is a strong possibility that this response can be brought under stimulus control' (p. XXII).

Some of the major principles of operant conditioning which could be applied to pain-related behavior have been reviewed by Bonica and Fordyce [57] and include the following: (a) positive reinforcement which is a technique involving the delivery of a positive stimulus following the occurrence of a desired behavior. In this case, positive reinforcement could be given for behaviors which are incompatible with pain behavior such as exercise; (b) punishment which involves the delivery of a negative or aversive consequence following the occurrence of a behavior designed to decrease the rate of that behavior in the future; and (c) extinction which is a procedure involving the elimination of any positive or negative reinforcement following the occurrence of a behavior. With such elimination, behaviors generally cease to occur. Finally, Bonica and Fordyce noted that the timing of the delivery of such reinforcers is an important ingredient in bringing about behavior change, with prompt delivery of reinforcers being generally preferable to delayed reinforcement. Bonica and Fordyce go on to thoroughly explain how these principles can be applied to common chronic pain problems. Unfortunately, these applications deal exclusively with adult chronic pain problems.

Two case examples exist in the literature utilizing operant conditioning to alter chronic pain behavior in children. The first of these is by Sank and Biglan [59] who utilized a positive reinforcement system to decrease the reported level of chronic recurrent abdominal pains and increase school attendance in a 10-year-old boy and these gains were successfully maintained over a prolonged follow-up period. The second example involved an extensive program for a 3-year-old child who had been exhibiting chronic pain responses ten months following a burn injury [60]. Utilizing a multiple baseline design across three different settings, the authors successfully reduced pain behaviors such as crying, sobbing and screaming, verbal statements of pain, nonverbal expressions of pain, and resistance to physical therapy with the use of contingent social reinforcement. In these cases, it is impossible to determine whether the patient is actually feeling pain or simply displaying pain-related behaviors. It should be noted, however, that even if only behavioral suppression of pain is occurring, this can often be a crucial therapeutic goal. The patient's life functioning, activity level, and school attendance can be vastly improved through such treatment procedures. Furthermore, subsequent research including the use of physiological variables as dependent measures will help clarify whether or not operant conditioning is concomitantly reducing physiological reactions.

Unfortunately, the current authors as well as others [56, 57] have observed that the implementation of operant conditioning procedures for chronic pain problems can entail a number of difficulties. For example, it is sometimes difficult for parents to emotionally 'disengage' from the pain responses in their children. Parents can easily fail to see the relationship between contingencies and their child's pain-related behavior, and they will sometimes accuse nurses and physicians of being 'cruel', insensitive, and incompetent for failing to effectively ameliorate their child's pain problems. As Graner [61] noted, parents often feel that it is their role to take care of their child's pain and provide the '*needed*' nurturance and sympathy for it. Unfortunately, this sympathy and nurturance can be far in excess of what might be considered appropriate empathy and reassurance at essential times. On occasion, this nurturance and sympathy can reach a magnitude whereby it may actually exacerbate the expression of pain-related behavior to the extent that more of the pain behavior is due to the social reinforcement provided by the parents than to nociceptive stimuli *per se*. For these reasons, parents often need much reassurance and support when implementing an operant intervention program. It must be noted also that parents' observations and reactions to their child's pain are an important source of information and should not be automatically discarded under the assumption that they are 'hysterical' or inappropriate.

Three suggestions in particular seem to be appropriate to consider when implementing operant conditioning programs for children's chronic pain behavior. The *first* of these has been advanced by Bonica [55] who suggested that it is important to realize that even if pain behavior is not directly connected to nociceptive stimuli, the 'pain habit' is real. Thus, it is quite important to point out to parents and the child alike that the medical staff is not suggesting that the pain is based upon imagination, but rather it is much like any other habit, such as smoking, etc. which can be changed. The *second* suggestion was made by Graner [61] who pointed out the advantage of having parents keep a log of pain behavior upon which the time of onset, duration, type, location, antecedents, and consequents to pain behavior can be recorded. In this way, patterns may be revealed which can elucidate the variables responsible for the exacerbation and/or alleviation of the pain behaviors. This can give the parents a significant role in the program as well as provide an element of needed objectivity with regard to the problem. Overall, the need to appropriately educate parents, children (according to their ability to understand), and even medical staff concerning the relationship of pain behavior to its consequences cannot be stressed enough in the delivery of an operant conditioning program. Without such careful education and subsequent cooperation, these programs can quite readily be sabotaged.

The *third* suggestion involves the decision as to when operant conditioning is an appropriate psychological intervention for chronic pain. Clearly, the primary goal in the care of the terminally ill child in severe pain is reduction of *experienced* pain, not merely suppression of pain behaviors. Intractable disease-related pain is generally best treated by high doses of narcotic medications. Addiction is generally not a major concern in the terminally ill child; the final days in a child's life should be as comfortable and pain-free as possible regardless of the quantity of pain medications necessary to achieve this goal. With terminally ill children, operant conditioning is warranted only when the child's pain-related behavior is extreme, exceeds the level of what is thought to be caused by the disease, or is inappropriate to the point where the child's medical and emotional care may be compromised. An example involves a 5-year-old terminally ill leukemic child referred to the first author by her physician for behavioral intervention. This child had severe disease-related pain and was being treated with large doses of morphine. However, her behavior (which included high pitched screams every time the physician entered the room, tantrums, excessive screaming at the parents, extreme obstinacy, etc.) became so extreme that the parents and physician alike had become frustrated to the point of anger toward the child. The child's manipulative behavior was being reinforced by parent attention and over-indulgence in relation to her demands. Intervention involved counseling the parents to set limits on her behavior, to be more firm with her, and to ignore her tantrums. The parents were also given much reassurance and support. The child's behavior improved dramatically and the parents were able to maintain a less tense relationship with their child prior to her death.

Thus, psychological intervention in the form of operant conditioning can be an effective supplement to medical approaches in intractable disease-related pain in terminally ill children and generally should not be used alone to suppress pain-related behavior. Also, operant conditioning techniques must be used with much discretion, sensitivity, and skill, as the naive inexperienced clinician can create serious problems if applying operant principles in an inappropriate or unskilled manner.

A second approach to the treatment of chronic pain problems in children can be found in the literature on family systems therapy. Minuchin and his colleagues [62, 63] advocated the combination of family systems therapy with reinforcement strategies. Conceptually, this approach can be supported particularly by the fact that many of the contingencies for pain behavior are commonly found within various interaction sequences within the family. This reinforcement can be derived from sympathy and attention or avoidance of responsibilities, or possibly even from the deflection of parental conflicts that exist within the family. A rather wide variety of specific techniques have been described in the family systems therapy literature. These strategies are not a well-systematized set of techniques from a theoretical and conceptual perspective. Two of the most common techniques in the literature involve: (1) a variety of paradoxical strategies which are aimed at breaking up dysfunctional communication patterns within the family and (2) 'reframing' the meaning of the particular symptom (in this case pain behavior) in a way that will change the motivational set of both the patient and the other family members. Zimmerman and Elliott [64] recently described the successful application of a combined family systems and reinforcement approach to reduce pain behavior and over-utilization of hospital facilities on the part of a female adolescent with hereditary angioneurotic edema. However, the literature currently lacks any systematic controlled outcome studies on the use of family systems therapy for the alleviation for chronic pain problems in either children or adults.

A third potential approach to the treatment of chronic pain problems in children with cancer can be found in the literature on behavioral stress management techniques. This category includes a variety of strategies which also are not necessarily closely linked from a conceptual and theoretical framework. Some of the most common techniques include relaxation, imagery, modeling, various cognitive strategies, reinforcement, and combinations of these. Sanders [2] reviewed a wide body of data indicating quite promising results for various combinations of behavioral stress management techniques with both chronic and acute laboratory-induced pain in adults. In addition, the current authors will review in some detail the use of these techniques in acute pain associated with medical procedures for pediatric cancer patients. However, the literature to date contains no examples of the use of these techniques for *chronic* pain in children. Given their successful use with chronic adult pain however, one would expect that they would also have potential for reducing chronic pain behavior in children.

Though quite speculative at this time, it is possible that subsequent research will demonstrate that stress management designed to reduce pain-related behavior, as well as physiological arousal, may effect actual development of cancer itself, as indicated by research which has demonstrated substantial effects of stress on tumor growth [65].

A fourth psychological approach to the treatment of children's chronic pain problems involves the use of hypnosis. Hypnosis has been reviewed in greater detail by the authors elsewhere in this chapter. It was noted previously that hypnosis has clearly been the most widely used intervention strategy for distress and pain in pediatric cancer patients. The only two studies of a systematic, controlled nature utilizing hypnosis for the reduction of pain-related behavior in children are currently in progress [27, 28]. Unfortunately, neither of these studies involve chronic pain and the use of hypnosis in that regard remains empirically untested. However, a number of investigators [31, 66, 67] have reported anecdotal data suggesting the efficacy of hypnosis for the control of chronic pain in children with cancer. These investigations utilized a variety of induction techniques generally followed by various fantasized scenes that are individualized for each child (e.g., at the beach, on top of a mountain, in one's own bed, etc.). In addition, Keane [66] utilized symbolic imagery such as flipping a switch or removing a fuse to give the pediatric patient a direct method for reducing thc experience of pain associated with their cancer. The current authors speculate that the efficacy of hypnosis with respect to chronic pain will be enhanced if it is combined with substantial reinforcement for its successful use by the child. This speculation is based upon the aforementioned role that reinforcement likely plays in much of chronic pain behavior.

5. MEDICAL APPROACHES TO PAIN

The current chapter is not primarily concerned with medical approaches to the amelioration of children's cancer-related pain. However, a brief mention of some of the major medical strategies is warranted on the basis that it is important to be aware of the various options available to the clinician in the management of such pain problems. In addition, future research comparing medical approaches to the management of children's pain to the psychological strategies reviewed in more detail in this chapter would be highly desirable. Furthermore, various combinations of these two different approaches may hold the greatest promise of all for maximizing the effectiveness of treatment outcomes.

Previously in this chapter it was noted that a recent review revealed very little in the way of systematic controlled research designed to investigate the use of medical approaches to the treatment of *pediatric* pain [1]. Several excellent reviews of such techniques with the management of pain associated with adult cancer have appeared, however [3, 68, 69].

The primary pharmacological agents available for the control of pain associated with cancer can largely be divided into: (a) mild and strong analgesics and (b) psychotrophic medications in the category of tranquilizers and/or anti-depressants. The mild analgesics include a group of chemically diverse agents. Some of the more commonly used agents in this group include the salicylates (including aspirin), Acetaminophen and Phenacetin. These drugs exert their primary effect peripherally and are usually ineffective in producing relief for severe pain [70]. In addition, Codeine and Propoxyphene are substances related to narcotic analgesics but differ primarily with respect to relatively lower potency. However, neither of these drugs has been demonstrated to be substantially more effective than the salicylates. In general, the mild analgesics have the greatest potential to relieve the mild to moderate pain and discomforts that are frequently associated with cancers in pediatric populations. In particular, the most common cancer in children is acute leukemia which is generally not considered to be a highly painful disease, although it is often associated with bone pain, fatigue, and symptoms similar to influenza during conditions of relapse [4].

The strong analgesic drugs include a variety of opium extracts such as Morphine, Oxycodone, and Methadone, all of which are considered to be narcotics. Two strong analgesics not considered to be narcotics are somewhat less potent and include Pentazocine and Methotrimeprazine [70]. The strong analgesics are generally utilized only late in the manifestation of cancer in children when the disease has become quite widespread. Usually it is only at this stage that severe pain is associated with childhood cancer [46].

Psychotropic drugs have received considerable attention in regard to their use for the treatment of cancer-related pain. Unfortunately, there do not appear to have been any controlled investigations demonstrating their efficacy in this application [68]. With respect to anti-depressant psychotropic drugs, these agents have been recommended most often for patients with chronic pain, which as noted previously, occurs somewhat less often with pediatric cancer patients. However, research has documented that the use of these drugs has been quite effective with chronic pain in adults, especially for those patients who are depressed as well [71]. It has even been speculated that anti-depressants are useful not only for their effects on the patient's depression which may exacerbate the pain experience, but also may have properties which potentiate narcotic analgesia [68]. With respect to tranquilizing agents, the Benzodiazephines have demonstrated relatively little efficacy in the treatment of cancer-related pain [72]. However, other anti-anxiety agents such as the sedative antihistamines and the phenothiazines have shown a much greater potential to potentiate narcotic analgesia, in addition to their anti-anxiety effects [72]. Unfortunately, psychotropic drugs are frequently disliked by adolescents with cancer because of a reported feeling of loss of control that can accompany their use.

Medical approaches other than drug therapy include anesthetic procedures (such as peripheral nerve block and subarachnoid) neurosurgery, radiation therapy, and endocrine therapy among others [46, 68]. While these other procedures can sometimes be useful for the control of certain types of pain, they tend to be less effective for most childhood cancers [46].

The actual use of pain medications with pediatric cancer patients varies quite widely from one clinic to the next. For example, Eland and Anderson [1] demonstrated that frequently nurses fail to give prescribed and needed pain medications. In addition, a few clinics utilize total anesthesia before administering critical diagnostic procedures such as lumbar punctures and bone marrow aspirations. On the other hand, other clinics utilize much more limited analgesic agents for these situations due to what they consider to be unwarranted medical risks and expense to the patients.

Clearly, far more in the way of systematic controlled investigations into the use of various kinds of medications for pain associated with pediatric cancer would be desirable. Nitrous oxide in particular is an agent which has received considerable attention as a method for the control of pain and distress associated with dental procedures and would appear to have some promise for the amelioration of pain and distress in response to painful medical procedures. Excellent reviews have recently been presented on the use of nitrous oxide inhalation, although no controlled investigations have been made of its use with highly painful medical procedures [73, 74]. The current authors are conducting a pilot study investigating the efficacy of nitrous oxide in reducing distress of pediatric cancer patients undergoing bone marrow aspirations and spinal taps.

6. CLINICAL APPLICATIONS

The authors have developed a multi-component intervention 'package' designed to teach effective coping skills and to reduce children's distress during painful medical procedures. The five intervention components were developed on the basis of: (a) a pilot study which assessed factors associated with distress [12], (b) clinical experience with and observations of pediatric cancer patients undergoing painful procedures, and (c) the literature on stress and anxiety intervention with children and adults. The rationale for using multidimensional intervention or 'package' approaches is based upon two arguments. First, Turk [75] has noted the importance of providing subjects with a 'smorgasboard' of strategies because different individuals may find different aspects of the intervention package useful. Second, as some investigators have suggested, it is advisable to first develop an intervention package with a maximum probability of effectiveness and then to conduct analytic studies to isolate the effective components, especially when investigating problems which have not been effectively treated by existing approaches [76].

The current treatment package is based, in part, on a 'stress-inoculation' model as described by Meichenbaum and Turk [77]. In their stress-inoculation approach, the subject is first provided with information concerning the nature of the stressful situation. In the second phase, the subject is taught a number of coping skills or techniques such as distractions, relaxation, altering attributions, imagery, etc., and these coping skills are rehearsed. Finally, the subject is given the opportunity to practice his/her coping skills during exposure to a variety of stressors.

The current package of intervention techniques is designed to prepare the pediatric cancer patient for stressful and painful medical procedures – bone marrow aspirations and lumbar puntures. The intervention package consists of five primary components: filmed modeling, reinforcement, breathing exercises, emotive imagery, and behavioral rehearsal. Each component will be described in detail; the rationale of each will be reviewed, and relevant clinical issues will be discussed.

6.1. Filmed modeling

Prior to the procedures, the child is shown a 12-minute film entitled 'Joy Gets a Bone Marrow and Spinal Tap'. The film is about a six-year-old leukemic patient who comes to the clinic for her routine bone marrow and spinal tap. The film proceeds through the following sequences: leaving home, checking into the clinic, sitting in the waiting room, the fingerstick procedure, the intervention session with the psychologist, the actual bone marrow and spinal tap procedures, and finally, leaving the clinic. Joy describes her thoughts and feelings, throughout each step of the procedure on an audio voice overlay. The film is based on a 'coping' rather than a 'mastery' model since coping models have been found to be more effective in facilitating identification with the model and in reducing anxiety [78]. As a coping model, Joy admits she is scared about the procedures, exhibits some signs of distress, but at each stress point models effective coping behaviors and expresses positive coping statements.

The film includes edited segments of the intervention session with the psychologist in which Joy is taught various coping techniques (breathing exercises, imagery, etc.), the rationale being that modeling of the intervention process might also facilitate intervention and facilitate the rapport between the patient and the psychologist.

The film contains a number of additional factors which were designed to reduce children's distress and enhance coping. *Information* is a major element and the rationale for providing such information is based on research reporting that patients receiving preoperative preparation of a specific, rather than general, nature showed less postoperative anger, depression, and negative effects than did those with inadequate information [79]. Thus, edited segments of each step of the actual procedures are shown to the child. Most children have never seen what goes on 'behind their back' and many relate that a major part of their distress is that they 'can't see' what the doctor is doing to their backs.

Joy, the model, also explains *why* she has to get such painful procedures in an attempt to correct any misconceptions children may have concerning the procedures (i.e., punishment, torture, etc.). *Interpersonal* elements are emphasized since the child's trust in the physician has been observed as a crucial variable in successful coping. Joy emphasizes that the doctors and nurses are her friends and that they are just trying to help her get well. *Coping* with the noxious situation is stressed in the film. Joy expresses positive coping statements such as 'I'm a big girl', 'I know I can handle it even if I'm scared', and 'It feels good to be so brave' in order to elicit motivations or 'current concerns' (e.g., Meichenbaum and Butler) [80] of coping rather than fearful avoidance.

6.2. Breathing exercises

The children are taught a simple breathing exercise. The purpose of the breathing exercise is twofold: (1) to induce relaxation as much as is possible in such an aversive situation; and (2) to serve as a distraction for the child. The breathing exercises give the child an active attention-diversion strategy during the procedure and are effective in providing the child a sense of active mastery over pain/anxiety rather than passive submission during the procedures. Most children feel they have more control over the painful situation if they have a specific technique they can utilize. Research has indicated that a subjects' perception of control generally results in higher pain threshold and/or pain tolerance [81–83].

The children are instructed as follows: 'Pretend that you are a big round tire. Take a deep breath and fill the tire with as much air as possible. Then slowly let the air out, making a hissing sound as the air slowly goes out of the tire. Let all the air out very slowly. Then pump it back up again and start over' [84]. The child is shown how to do the breathing exercise and is then instructed to practice it several times.

6.3. Reinforcement

Children are shown a small trophy and are told that the trophies are given to children who act very brave during the medical procedures. It is explained to the child that, to obtain the trophy, he/she has to: (1) lay still during the procedure; and (2) do the breathing exercises which they were taught. These contingencies are based on two rationales: (1) laying still makes it much easier for the physician to conduct the procedure as quickly as possible without complications and (2) the breathing exercises distract the child and generally preclude severe behavioral distress (screaming, kicking, and fighting). These criteria are relatively easy for the child to meet, thus success is likely. Occasionally, a child has not met the criteria; in such cases, the psychologist gives the parent the option of giving or withholding the trophy since non-reinforcement of poor coping behavior can be a sensitive issue in an already-stressful situation.

Again, the reinforcement component tends to elicit current concerns of *mastery* and the child is rewarded for merely attempting to cope with the procedures. The child is told that it is okay to cry or yell; however, the importance of staying still and the usefulness of the breathing exercises are stressed. The purpose of the trophy is to provide the child with a symbol of accomplishment and courage. Self-esteem and self-competence are generally enhanced when the child 'wins' a trophy and a very noxious painful situation can result in a positive, rewarding situation. Children have been observed after the procedures proudly displaying their trophy to others in the clinic and other children have often asked when they can 'win' a trophy, an indication of the reinforcement potency of the trophy.

6.4. Imagery

'Emotive imagery' is used as a cognitive pain-distraction strategy. Emotive imagery was developed by Lazarus and Abramovitz [85] for children who didn't respond to standard desensitization or relaxation procedures. In this technique, 'emotive' images are used to inhibit anxiety. Preferred hero or superhuman images of the child such as Superman, Wonderwoman, or the Incredible Hulk are ascertained and a credible story with positive affective images is made up, weaving together the medical situation with one of these hero images.

The emotive images presumably transform the meaning of pain for the child and elicit 'current concerns' which are related to mastery of pain rather than avoidance. Each child's imagery differs depending upon his/her hero preferences and the extent to which the child can engage in imagery. During the medical procedures, children are reminded of the imagery scenario which has been developed and coached to do the imagery, (e.g., 'Remember Wonderwoman – What would she do right now?' An example of an emotive imagery script is as follows:

> Pretend that Wonder Woman has come to your house and told you that she wants you to be the newest member of her Superpower Team. Wonder Woman has given you special powers. These special powers make you very strong and tough so that you can stand almost anything. She asks you to take some tests to try out these super powers. The tests are called bone marrows and spinal taps. These tests hurt, but with your new super powers, you can take deep breaths and can lie very still. Wonder Woman will be very proud when she finds out that your super powers work and you will be the newest member of her Superpower Team.

6.5. Behavioral rehearsal

After the child is shown the trophy, taught the breathing exercises, and briefed on emotive imagery, the procedure is practiced three different times. First, the child is allowed to play doctor and to give a doll the bone marrow or lumbar puncture. The medical kits which are used in actual procedures by physicians are used by the child in the doll play. The child is shown the cleansing materials and the various needles, and is instructed step-by-step in the administration of the bone marrow aspiration or lumbar puncture. As the child administers the procedure, the doll is coached to stay still and to do her breathing exercises.

The child is then allowed to practice administering the procedure on the psychologist (without the use of needles!). The psychologist models coping behaviors as the child plays doctor. For example, when the child pretends to be cleansing the back for the procedure, the psychologist might model coping statements such as. 'I'm feeling scared now but I know I can handle it. I'll pretend I'm Wonderwoman's assistant and I'll do my breathing exercises so I won't be so scared. It will be over fast if I lay still'. Finally, the psychologist has the child practice undergoing the procedure. The child is coached to lay still and to do the breathing exercises while the psychologist pretends to administer the procedure.

The practice sessions contain several important behavioral components which may be helpful in alleviating distress. The child is provided with *information* concerning how the procedure is administered, what behaviors are expected, and the importance of coping behaviors in the successful administration of the procedure. For example, when the child is playing doctor, the psychologist can demonstrate how difficult it is for the physician to puncture the exact site on the child's back when he/she is writhing and kicking by pretending the doll is flailing and have the child try to get the needle in the small hole on the doll's back. In this sense, the rehearsal may help to facilitate *identification* with the physician. Other components which may be helpful in the behavioral rehearsal phase include *modeling* of coping behaviors and *in vivo desensitization* through graded exposure to the needles and cleansing materials. The child is given the opportunity to confront the situation with maximum psychological distance initially (playing doctor with the doll) and then gradually confronting the most stressful aspect (personal involvement through actual rehearsal). Finally, the rehearsal gives the child the opportunity to 'try out' his/her new coping techniques and generally is helpful in getting the child 'psyched up' and mentally ready for the actual procedure.

6.6. Intervention procedures

The sequence in the intervention process is as follows: showing the film; showing and explaining the trophy, teaching the breathing exercises, discussing possible imagery scripts, and behavioral rehearsal. The intervention session is held on the day of the procedures after the child checks into the clinic, the rationale being that modeling has been shown to be most effective immediately prior to the impending event [84], especially for young children [39]. Parents accompany their children during the intervention session and are encouraged to act as 'coaches' for their children during the procedures. The inclusion of parents in the intervention is essential since a strong relationship between parental anxiety and children's distress during medical procedures has been documented [12]. Regardless of the direction of causation of anxiety, the involvement of parents minimizes the 'contagious' effect of anxious anticipation and distress which develops between parent and child.

Preliminary data has indicated that the intervention package described is effective in reducing children's distress during bone marrow aspirations and spinal taps [37]. The majority of children showed dramatic (at least 40%) decreases in distress levels after the intervention session as compared to baseline levels of distress. Additional studies are being conducted to further explore the efficacy of the intervention package.

6.7. Problems in clinical application

Treatment outcome research in an applied setting such as an oncology clinic is often difficult due to a number of potential problems. The intervention described previously is very expensive in terms of professional manpower and time. An observer and a professional to conduct the intervention session are necessary and must cover all clinic days so that no data are missed. Observer bias can be a problem since it is impossible to 'coach' a child during the procedures without the observer being aware that intervention has occurred. There are ways to circumvent observer bias, but such procedures often require even more manpower or may not be as effective in reducing children's distress. Maintaining positive effects of intervention can be difficult; differences in whether or not children maintain lower distress levels appear to be related to individual coping styles and individual differences in suggestibility and expectancy factors [37]. The authors are currently experimenting with methods to increase the longterm maintenance of positive intervention effects.

Research in any clinical, applied situation will include a certain number of uncontrolled variables or unanticipated problems. Examples of such problems include scheduling changes, unforeseen changes in the child's medical procedures, changes in the child's physical condition, serious negative side effects of medical procedures which may negate effects of the psychological intervention, and lack of cooperation of medical staff. The cooperation of medical personnel is absolutely essential in conducting any type of research in a clinical setting and in minimizing uncontrolled variance. Medical staff must be informed of all details of the research study and, ideally, must see the benefits of the study. The authors have found that the cooperation and flexibility of medical personnel increase as a function of the observed effectiveness on their part of the psychological intervention. Thus, psychologists have, in some ways, a built-in accountability to medical personnel which, ideally, serves to enhance intervention effectiveness and collaborative efforts between psychologists and medical staff.

7. SUMMARY AND CONCLUSIONS

The child with cancer must deal with numerous painful as well as frightening experiences during the course of cancer treatment including frequent vena punctures, bone marrow aspirations, lumbar punctures, biopsies, surgeries, and severe side effects of chemotherapy such as nausea, vomiting, and hair loss. Such experiences may challenge the emotional adjustment of pediatric cancer patients as they attempt to adapt to repeated experiences of pain and fear. Psychological intervention may facilitate positive adaptation and may prevent the development or exacerbation of phobias, conditioned anxiety responses, and regressive behavior which sometimes occur as a result of repeated aversive experiences. Psychological intervention involves teaching specific coping techniques which children can utilize in aversive situations, reinforcing positive coping skills, and giving emotional support and reassurance as needed.

The purpose of this chapter was to review the literature on pain management in pediatric oncology, discuss current methods of assessment and intervention, and to delineate methods, issues, and problems in clinical application. Unfortunately, the medical and psychological literature in the area of pediatric pain is almost nonexistent. The reports that do exist are almost exclusively anecdotal or case study reports with little or no empirical data concerning efficacy. The need for controlled studies in this area is certainly demonstrated by a review of the literature. A few investigators are currently conducting controlled studies which will contribute to the literature in pediatric pain intervention.

Various methods of assessing pain in children were reviewed (behavioral, physiological, self-report) and other mediating factors such as cognitive development, individual coping styples, and parental behavior were discussed as they relate to children's perceptions of pain. Psychological methods of intervention which can be used in acute and chronic pain were reviewed including hypnosis, behavior therapy, preparation, operant conditioning, family therapy, and stress management. Medical approaches to pediatric pain were reviewed very briefly. Finally, a 'package' of behavior therapy techniques designed to reduce children's distress during painful medical procedures was presented in detail and issues in clinical application were discussed.

Much work remains to be done in the area of pediatric pain intervention. The adaptation of the child with cancer to his/her disease and the treatment regimen may be dependent upon careful preparation, education, and intervention in relation to painful and traumatic procedures. Psychologists, as integral members of the medical treatment team, can provide useful and necessary intervention to children with cancer which may offset future adjustment difficulties and emotional problems.

REFERENCES

1. Eland JM, Anderson JE: The experience of pain in children. In: Pain: A source book for nurses and other health professionals, Jacox A (ed). Boston: Little, Brown and Co., 1977, pp 453–473.
2. Sanders SH: Behavioral assessment and treatment of clinical pain: Appraisal and current status. In: Progress in behavior modification, Hersen M, Eisler RM, Miller PM (eds). New York: Academic Press, 1979, pp 249–291.
3. Bonica JJ: Introduction to management of pain of advanced cancer. In: Advances in pain research and therapy, Vol 2, Bonica JJ, Ventafridda V (eds). New York: Raven Press, 1979b, pp 115–130.
4. Varni JW, Katz ER, Dash J: Behavioral and neurochemical aspects of pediatric pain. In: Behavioral pediatrics: Research and practice, Russo DC, Varni JW (eds). New York: Plenum Press, 1982, pp 177–224.
5. Jay SM, Elliott CH, Ozolins M, Doan R: Assessment of distress in children undergoing painful medical procedures: Paper presented at American Psychological Association Convention, Washington, DC, August, 1982.

6. Katz ER, Kellerman J, Siegel S: Behavioral distress in children undergoing medical procedures: developmental considerations. J Consult Clin Psychol 48(3):356–365, 1980.
7. Fordyce W: Behavioral methods for chronic pain and illness. St. Louis: Mosby, 1976.
8. Sternbach RA: Pain patients: Traits and treatments. New York: Academic Press, 1974.
9. Varni JW: Self-regulation techniques in the management of chronic arthritic pain in hemophilia. Behavior Therapy 12:185–194, 1981.
10. Huskisson E: Measurement of pain. Lancet ii:1127–1131, 1974.
11. Katz ER, Kellerman J, Siegel SE: Self-report and observational measurement of acute pain, fear, and behavioral distress in children with leukemia. Paper presented at 3rd Annual Meeting of Society of Behavioral Medicine, Chicago, March, 1982.
12. Jay SM, Ozolins M, Elliott C, Caldwell S: Assessment of children's distress during painful medical procedures. Health Psychology: 2 (2):133–148, 1983.
13. Sternbach R: Pain: A psychophysiological analysis. New York: Academic Press, 1968.
14. Epstein L: Psychophysiological measurement in assessment. In: Behavioral assessment: A practical handbook, Hersen M, Bellack AS (eds). New York: Pergamon, 1976, pp 207–232.
15. Lang P: The application of psychophysiological methods. In: Handbook of psychotherapy and behavior change, Bergin A, Garfield S (eds). New York: Wiley, 1971.
16. Melamed BG, Siegel LJ: Reduction of anxiety in children facing hospitalization and surgery by use of filmed modeling. J Consult Clin Psychol 43(4):511–521, 1975.
17. Peterson L, Shigetomi C: The use of coping techniques to minimize anxiety in hospitalized children. Behavior Therapy 12:1–14, 1981.
18. Shaw EG, Routh DK: Effect of mother presence on children's reaction to aversive procedures. J Pediatr Psychol 7(1):33–42, 1982.
19. Willis D, Elliott CH, Jay SM: Psychological effects of physical illness and its concomitants. In: Handbook for the practice of pediatric psychology, Tuma J (ed). New York: John Wiley, 1982, pp 28–66.
20. Simeonsson RJ, Buckley L, Monson L: Conceptions of illness causality in hospitalized children. J Pediatr Psychol 4:77–84, 1979.
21. Sheridan M: Talk time for hospitalized children. Social Work 20:40–44, 1975.
22. Korsch BM: Psychologic reactions to physical illness in children. 107th Annual Session of the Medical Association of Georgia, Atlanta, 50:519–523, 1961.
23. Gardner GG, Olness K: Hypnosis and hypnotherapy with children. New York: Greene & Stratton, 1981.
24. Neuhauser C, Amsterdam B, Hines P, Steward M: Children's concepts of healing: Cognitive development and locus of control factors. Am J Orthopsychiatry 48:334–341, 1978.
25. Lipowski ZJ: Physical illness, the individual, and the coping process. Psychiatric Medicine 1:91–102, 1970.
26. Miller SM: Coping with impending stress: Psychophysiological and cognitive correlates of choice. Psychophysiology 16:572–581, 1979.
27. Kellerman J: Pain and anxiety in children with acute leukemia. National Institute of Health study in progress.
28. Zeltzer L, LeBaron S: A controlled study of hypnosis for pain and anxiety during bone marrow aspirations and lumbar punctures in children with cancer. Pediatr Res 16(4):219A, 1982. (Abstract)
29. Hilgard JR, Morgan AH: Treatment of anxiety and pain in childhood cancer through hypnosis. Paper presented at the 7th International Congress of Hypnosis and Psychosomatic Medicine, Philadelphia, 1976.
30. Hilgard JR, LeBaron S: Relief of anxiety and pain in children and adolescents with cancer: Quantitative measures and clinical observations. Int J Clin Exp Hypn 30(4):417–442,

1982.
31. Olness K: Imagery (self-hypnosis) as adjunct therapy in childhood cancer: Clinical experience with 25 patients. Am J Pediatr Hematol Oncol 3:313–321, 1981.
32. LaBaw W, Holton C, Tewell K, Eccles D: The use of self-hypnosis by children with cancer. Am J Clin Hypn 17(4):233–238, 1975.
33. Redd WH, Andresen GV, Minagawa RY: Hypnotic control of anticipatory emesis in patients receiving cancer chemotherapy. J Consult Clin Psychol 50(1):14–19, 1982.
34. Burish TG, Lyles JN: Effectiveness of relaxation training in reducing the aversiveness of chemotherapy in the treatment of cancer. Journal of Behavior Therapy and Experimental Psychiatry 10:357–361, 1979.
35. Cangello VW: Hypnosis for the patient with cancer. Am J Clin Hypn 4:215–226, 1962.
36. Jay SM, Elliott CH, Ozolins M, Olson R: Behavioral management of children's distress during painful medical procedures. Behavior Research and Therapy, In press, 1983.
37. Elliott CH, Olson R: Management of children's behavioral distress in response to painful medical treatment for burn injuries. Paper submitted for publication, 1982.
38. LeBaron S, Zeltzer L: Behavioral treatment for control of chemotherapy-related nausea and vomiting in children and adolescents with cancer. Pediatr Res 16(4):208A, 1982.
39. Melamed BG, Siegel LJ: Behavioral medicine. New York: Springer Publishing Co., 1980.
40. Vernon DT, Foley JM, Sipowicz RR, Schulman JL: The psychological responses of children to hospitalization and illness. Springfield, Ill.: Charles C. Thomas, 1965.
41. Peterson L, Ridley-Johnson R: Pediatric hospital response to survey on prehospital preparation for children. J Pediatr Psychol 5:1–7, 1980.
42. Johnson BH: Before hospitalization: A preparation program for the child and his family. Child Today 3:18–26, 1974.
43. Cassell S: Effects of brief puppet therapy upon the emotional responses of children undergoing cardiac catherization. J Consult Clin Psychol 29:1–8, 1965.
44. Dimock HG: The child in the hospital: A study of his emotional and social well-being. Philadelphia: Davis, 1960.
45. Kellerman J (ed): Psychological aspects of childhood cancer. Springfield, Ill.: Charles C. Thomas, 1980.
46. Lane DM: Principles of total care—psychological support. In: Clinical pediatric oncology, (2nd ed.), Sutow WW, Vietti TJ, Fernbach DJ (eds). St. Louis: C.V. Mosby, 1977, pp 238–263.
47. Beecher HK: Relationship of significance of the wound to the pain experienced. JAMA 161:1609–1613, 1956.
48. Carandang MSA, Folkins CH, Hines PA, Steward MS: The role of cognitive level and sibling illness in children's conceptualizations of illness. Am J Orthopsychiatry 49:474–481, 1979.
49. Perrin E, Gerrity S: There's a demon in your belly: Children's understanding of illness. Pediatrics 67(6):841–849, 1981.
50. Whitt K, Dykstra W, Taylor CA: Children's conceptions of illness and cognitive development. Clin Pediatr 18:327–334, 1979.
51. Beales JG: Pain in children with cancer. Advances in Pain Research and Therapy 2:89–98, 1979.
52. Schultz NV: How children perceive pain. Nursing Outlook 19(10):670–673, 1971.
53. Wright L, Schafer A, Solomons G (eds): Encyclopedia of pediatric psychology. Baltimore: University of Pennsylvania Press, 1979.
54. Beck AT, Rush AJ, Shaw BF, Emery G: Cognitive therapy of depression. New York: The Guilford Press, 1979.
55. Bonica JJ: Important clinical aspects of acute and chronic pain. In: Mechanisms of pain and

analgesic compounds, Beers RF, Bassett EG (eds). New York: Raven Press, 1979, pp 15–30.
56. Fordyce WE: Operant conditioning: An approach to chronic pain. In: Pain: A source book for nurses and other health professionals, Jacox AK (ed). Boston: Little, Brown and Co., 1979, pp 275–284.
57. Bonica JJ, Fordyce WE: Operant conditioning for chronic pain. In: Recent advances on pain, Bonica JJ, Procacci P, Pagni CA (eds). Springfield: Charles C. Thomas, 1974, pp 299–312.
58. Pomerleau OF, Brady JP: Behavioral medicine: Theory and practice. Baltimore: The Williams and Wilkins Co., 1979.
59. Sank LI, Biglan A: Operant treatment of a case of recurrent abdominal pain in a 10-year-old boy. Behavior Therapy 5:677–681, 1974.
60. Varni JW, Bessman CA, Russo DC, Cataldo MF: Behavioral management of chronic pain in children: Case study. Arch Phys Med Rehabil 61:375–379, 1980.
61. Graner A: The effects of pain on child, parent, and health professional. In: Home care for the dying child: Professional and family perspectives, Martinson IM (ed). New York: Appleton-Century-Crofts, 1976.
62. Minuchin S, Rosman B, Baker L: Psychosomatic families. Cambridge: Harvard University Press, 1978.
63. Minuchin S: A conceptual model of psychosomatic illness in children: Family organization and family therapy. In: Psychosomatic medicine, Wittkower ED, Warnes H (eds). Hagerstown, MD: Harper & Row, 1977.
64. Zimmerman JL, Elliott CH: The relationship of stress to angioneurotic edema: Implications for improved management. Submitted for publication, 1982.
65. Sklar LS, Anisman H: Stress and cancer. Psychol Bull 89(3):369–406, 1981.
66. Keane WM: Hypnosis with pediatric cancer patients: Giving control in an uncontrollable situation. Paper presented at the annual meeting of the APA, Montreal, September, 1980.
67. Miller JA: Hypnosis in a boy with leukemia. Am J Clin Hypn 22(4):231–235, 1980.
68. Noyes R: Treatment of cancer pain. Psychosom Med 43(1):57–70, 1981.
69. Twycross RG: Overview of analgesia. In: Advances in pain research and therapy, Vol. 2, Bonica JJ, Ventafridda V (eds). New York: Raven Press, 1979, pp 617–633.
70. Carruthers SG: Clinical pharmacology of pain. In: Pain, meaning and management, Smith WL, Mersky H, Gross SC (eds). New York: Spectrum Publications, 1980, pp 89–104.
71. Ward NG, Bloom VL, Friedal ROL: The effectiveness of tricyclic anti-depressants in the treatment of coexisting pain and depression. Pain 7:331–341, 1979.
72. Sadone MD, Albrecht RF: Sedatives and tranquilizers in the treatment of pain. Med Clin North Am 52(1):47–53, 1968.
73. Simon JF, Vogelsberg GM: Use of nitrous oxide-oxygen inhalation sedation for children. In: Behavioral management in dentistry for children, Wright G (ed). Toronto: W.B. Saunders Co., 1975, pp 178–196.
74. Griffin GC, Campbell VD, Jones R: Nitrous-oxygen sedation for minor surgery: Experience in a pediatric setting. JAMA 245(23):2411–2413, 1981.
75. Turk D: Cognitive behavioral techniques in the management of pain. In: Cognitive behavior therapy, Foreyt JP, Rathjen DP (eds). New York: Plenum Press, 1978, pp 199–227.
76. Mahoney MJ: Self-reward and self-monitoring techniques for weight control. Behavior Therapy 5:48–57, 1974.
77. Meichenbaum D, Turk D: The cognitive-behavioral management of anxiety, anger, and pain. In: The behavioral management of anxiety, depression, and pain, Davidson PO (ed). New York: Brunner/Mazel, 1976, pp 1–34.
78. Meichenbaum DM: Examination of model characteristics in reducing avoidance behavior. J

Pers Soc Psychol 17:298–307, 1971.
79. Johnson JE, Leventhal H: Effects of accurate expectations and behavioral instructions on reactions during a noxious medical examination. J Pers Soc Psychol 29:710–718, 1974.
80. Meichenbaum D, Butler L: Cognitive ethiology: Assessing the streams of cognition and emotion. In: Advances in the study of communication and affect. Assessment and modification of emotional behavior, Blankenstein K, Pliner D, Pollivey J (eds). New York: Plenum Press, 1979.
81. Bandler R, Madras G, Bem D: Self-observation as a source of pain perception. J Pers Soc Psychol 9:205–209, 1968.
82. Bowers K: The effects of VCS temporal uncertainty on heart rate and pain. Psychophysiology 8:382–389, 1973.
83. Geer J, Davison G, Gathel R: Reduction of stress in humans through nonveridical perceived control of aversive stimulation. J Pers Soc Psychol 16:731–738, 1970.
84. Elliott C, Ozolins M: Imagery and imagination in the treatment of children. In: Handbook of child clinical psychology, Walker C, Roberts M (eds). New York: John Wiley & Sons, in press.
85. Lazarus A, Abramovitz A: The use of emotive imagery in the treatment of children's phobias. Journal of Mental Science 68:191–192, 1962.
86. Flanders J: A review of research on imitative behavior. Psychol Bull 69:316–337, 1968.

7. The Role of Ultrasonography, Computed Tomography, Scintigraphy and Angiography in the Localization of Adrenal Disease

MILTON D. GROSS, RICHARD A. BOWERMAN, KURT W. MORI and KYUNG J. CHO

1. INTRODUCTION

The introduction of sensitive biochemical tests for the measurement of adrenal hormones and their metabolites has presented the clinician with powerful tools to investigate adrenal function and disease. Adrenal abnormalities can now be identified at times that precede the onset of significant clinical symptoms of disease. The extreme sensitivity of such tests is a mixed blessing, for once abnormal function has been demonstrated, successful management is dependent upon the localization of the site(s) of dysfunction. In a fashion parallel to the rapid development of sensitive hormonal analyses, modalities for the localization of adrenal disease have also experienced significant advances. The proliferation of diagnostic techniques for the localization of adrenal disease forces those involved physicians to acquire the knowledge for their appropriate utilization. Non-invasive studies are now available that demonstrate extremely high spatial resolution, i.e., computed tomography and ultrasonography. In addition, there are studies that combine both functional and localization analysis such as scintigraphy and selective venous hormone sampling procedures. Adrenal venography with sampling, however, remains the mainstay in the localization of adrenal cortical disease once the diagnosis of functional abnormality has been made.

The following chapter will review the various modalities in the localization of adrenal gland tumors and emphasize their roles in the management of pediatric adrenal disease. Such abnormalities are uncommon (Table 1) and necessitate extensive clinical evaluation for proper diagnosis prior to their localization [1]. An effort has been made to compare and contrast each modality in order to place them into a logical schema in the evaluation of adrenal disease.

G. Bennett Humphrey et al. (eds), Adrenal and Endocrine Tumors in Children.

Table 1. Adrenal disorders in children [a].

Adrenocortical Hyperfunction	*Adrenocortical Hypofunction*
Cushing's Syndrome	Primary
1. Adrenocortical carcinoma	1. Hypoplasia
2. Bilateral adrenal hyperplasia	2. Infection
3. Adrenocortical adenoma	3. Injury
4. Iatrogenic	4. Iatrogenic
Aldosteronism	5. Idiopathic
1. Bilateral adrenal hyperplasia	Secondary
2. Adenoma	1. Hypopituitarism
Adrenogenital Syndromes	2. Idiopathic
1. Congenital virilizing hyperplasia	
2. Adrenocortical adenoma	*Adrenal Medulla Hyperfunction*
3. Adrenocortical carcinoma	1. Pheochromocytoma
Feminizing Syndromes	2. Neuroblastoma
1. Tumors	
Metastatic Tumors	

[a] Adapted from Moses DC and Beierwaltes WH (1) used with permission of the publisher.

2. MODALITIES OF LOCALIZATION

2.1. Ultrasonography

Recent advances in gray scale ultrasound instrumentation and image processing have greatly facilitated ultrasonic examination of the adrenal glands. New scanning techniques have allowed successful visualization of up to 85% of normal adrenal glands [2, 3]. The efficacy in detecting adrenal mass lesions is now well established [3–13]. Improved resolution and availability of real-time sector scanners have contributed to the improvement in sensitivity, thus increasing its acceptance as an important diagnostic tool.

Ultrasonography is a logical initial imaging procedure when clinical and laboratory findings suggests an adrenal lesion. It is particularly appealing in the pediatric population, for ultrasound is non-invasive and independent of ionizing radiation. Ultrasound examinations can be performed rapidly and real-time scanning allows the study of the generally less cooperative pediatric patient.

2.1.2. Technique. Evaluation of adrenal masses is accomplished with currently available commercial gray scale ultrasound equipment. Depending on body habitus, the examination is performed with a transducer of the highest possible frequency, either 3.5 or 5.0 mHz. Improved resolution results from higher frequency transducers at the expense of decreased tissue penetration, but in neonates and small infants a 5.0 mHz transducer can generally be employed. Similarly, a short or medium depth focused transducer is used in smaller infants, whereas a medium focus transducer is necessary in larger patients.

Real-time ultrasonography employs rotating or sequentially firing transducers to produce rapidly changing images for evaluation of moving structures and rapid survey scanning of the abdomen. Real-time scanning of the upper abdomen and high retroperitoneum is possible as bulky linear array transducers have been supplemented with small head sector scanners that facilitate examination between the ribs or beneath the costal margins. While the resolution of real-time scanners is now comparable to that of static gray scale scanners, limitations in field of view and positional information pose some problems with image documentation and reproducibility.

Patient preparation is not required for an adrenal ultrasound examination. Generally, immobilization is not necessary except for an occasional neonate and younger infant. Feeding a hungry infant can have a quieting effect, and a calm scanning atmosphere is recommended. Parents are encouraged to be present during scanning, and if necessary, to help in holding the child. This makes sedation rarely necessary.

When evaluating a child with a suspected adrenal lesion, initial sequential supine transverse and longitudinal scans are obtained throughout the abdomen. The right adrenal gland is located cephalad, anterior and medial to the right kidney, and adrenal masses in this region are usually well seen on supine transverse sonograms. The liver acts as a sonic 'window' through which the sound beam readily passes to image adrenal masses bounded

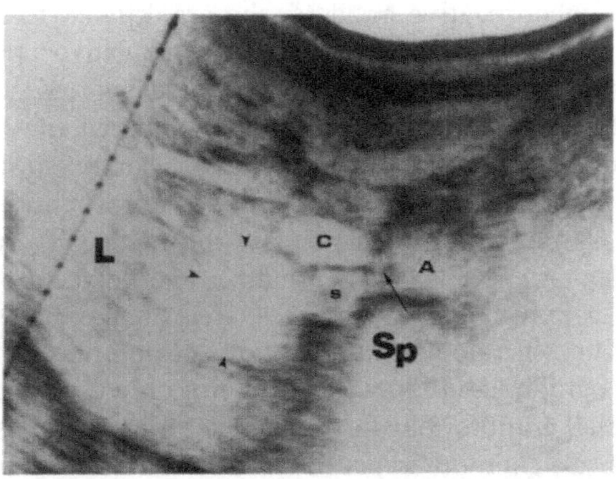

Figure 1. Supine transverse sonogram shows bilobed pheochromocytoma with a solid retrocaval component(s) lateral to the right diaphragmatic crus (arrow) and large cystic component (arrows). (L = liver; C = inferior vena cava; A = aorta; Sp = spine).

laterally by the liver, anteriorly by the inferior vena cava, and medially by the crus of the diaphragm (Figure 1).

The left adrenal is similarly located cephalad to the left kidney, but lies more anterior and medial to the upper pole than the right adrenal. Frequently, masses of the left adrenal will be obscured on supine scans by overlying stomach and bowel gas, and necessitate alternative views. Either prone longitudinal or transverse scans, and coronal oblique scans in the lateral decubitus position can image adrenal masses without intervening gas and help delineate their spatial relationships to adjacent organs and vascular structures.

Real-time scanning has added another dimension to the sonographic evaluation of adrenal tumors, allowing rapid clarification of the nature of upper abdominal masses, a particularly vexing problem in the left upper quadrant due to splenic, gastric, pancreatic and colonic 'pseudomasses' [14, 15].

2.1.3. Indications. Both ultrasonography and computed tomography (CT) are cross-sectional imaging modalities with comparable accuracy in diagnosing adrenal masses [3, 4, 8, 16–18]. Clinical guidelines should be used to select the optimum initial imaging modality. Ultrasound cannot penetrate gas or bone, so if gas obscures an area to be examined and alternate planes would traverse bone, CT would be recommended. In cases where transducer-skin contact is limited, such as postoperative patients with extensive surgical wounds, CT might be required. Fat attenuates the ultrasound beam and degrades ultrasound images, but aids in CT imaging. However, as most children are not obese and have little retroperitoneal fat, ultrasonography may be superior for imaging adrenal masses. Real-time ultrasound can be employed with uncooperative patients who are difficult to scan with CT or static ultrasound scans. Real-time examinations can be performed at the bedside for those patients who cannot be transported to the radiology department. Radiation exposure is a major concern in the pediatric age group, and ultrasound should be considered as a first step in the evaluation of an adrenal lesion. The inherent flexibility of ultrasound permits scanning in multiple planes and positions not possible with CT and allows better definition of cleavage planes between masses and adjacent organs [6, 12, 13] (Figure 2). As a non-invasive procedure free of ionizing radiation, ultrasound examination has no contraindications or complications and, as such, makes ultrasonography a unique modality, not only for initial diagnosis and staging of adrenal tumors, but also for longitudinal studies evaluating the success of surgical, chemotherapeutic, and/or radiation therapy.

2.1.4. Interpretation. The identification of small adrenal masses by ultrasound is accomplished by identifying contour changes that are different

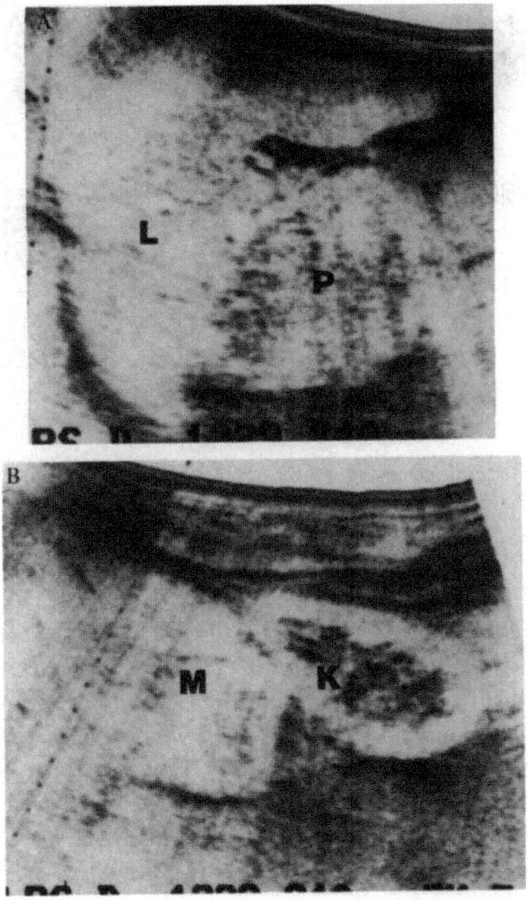

Figure 2. (A) Supine longitudinal sonogram shows an echogenic, heterogeneous right adrenal pheochromocytoma (P) located posterior to the right lobe of the liver (L). Pathologically, this tumor had extensive non-coalescent areas of hemorrhage and necrosis. (B) Prone longitudinal scan shows cleavage plane between the mass (M) and right kidney (K).

from the normal adrenal gland. Masses as small as 1.3 cm [3] can be identified by a focal rounding of adrenal contours. Generalized enlargement of both adrenals in adrenal hyperplasia is a difficult sonographic diagnosis, but may be suggested by convex adrenal surfaces [4]. Larger masses are more readily seen, frequently with an adjacent remnant of normal adrenal tissue. Uncomplicated smaller adrenal neoplasms of all types are sonographically solid, homogeneous and hypoechoic. Solid masses can be identified sonographically by their internal echoes, sound attenuation without distal acoustic enhancement, and less well-defined posterior margins than cystic masses (Figure 3). As tumors enlarge and outgrow their vascular supply, central necrosis and hemorrhage may occur, rendering variable patterns of internal

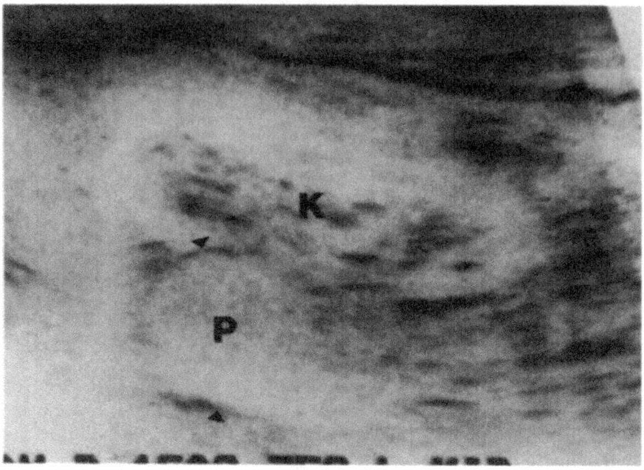

Figure 3. Prone longitudinal sonogram shows homogeneous, solid, well-marginated pheochromocytoma (P) located anterior to the left renal hilum. Pathologically, only microscopic hemorrhage and necrosis were present. The echogenic tumor margin (arrowheads) is a result of a well-defined fibrous capsule (K = kidney).

hyper- and hypoechogenicity (Figure 2). Necrosis procedes from an initial solid state to a homogeneous, acellular, gelatinous consistency which gradually liquifies and ultimately becomes fibrotic. Sonographically, these stages appear differently, ranging from initial hyperechoic foci to sonolucent areas without enhanced acoustic transmission (Figure 4), to fluid-filled cystic areas with enhanced acoustic transmission (Figure 5), and finally variable hyper- and hypoechoic centra. Hemorrhage and necrosis can be microscopic and not alter the homogeneous sonographic nature of smaller solid masses

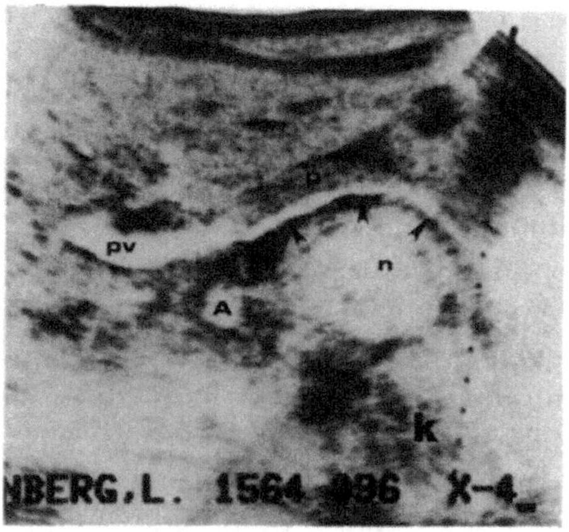

Figure 4. Supine transverse sonogram shows heterogeneous solid left adrenal pheochromocytoma displacing the splenic vein (arrowheads) anteriorly. Note anechoic center due to liquifactive necrosis (n) within the tumor. (p = Pancreas; A = aorta; PV = Portal vein; K = kidney).

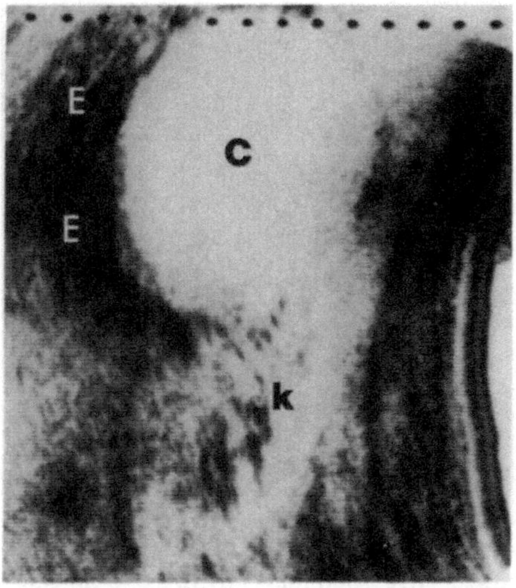

Figure 5. Upright longitudinal sonogram of a cystic left adrenal pheochromocytoma (C) located cephalad and anterior to the left kidney (K). The anechoic nature, well defined posterior wall, and enhanced distal acoustic transmission (E) indicate the cystic character of the mass.

(Figure 3). Macroscopic hemorrhages appear as echogenic foci (Figure 2). Focal calcifications will appear sonographically as densely echogenic foci, frequently with marked distal acoustic shadowing (Figure 6).

As adrenal masses enlarge, characteristic displacements of adjacent organs and vascular structures are observed [12, 19]. Caudal displacement of the ipsilateral kidney is frequently observed, often with lesser degrees of poster-

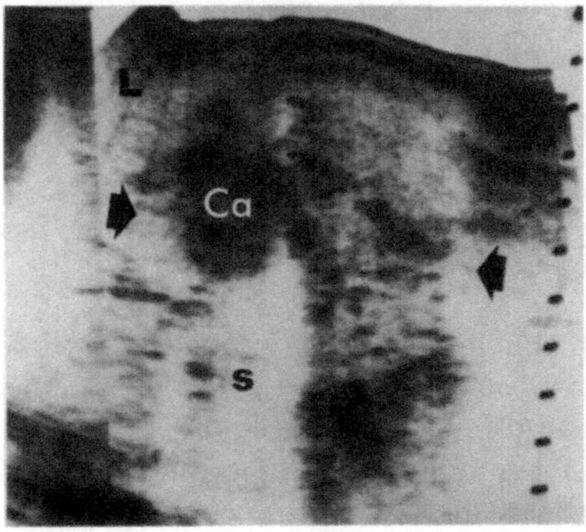

Figure 6. A one year old female with a densely calcified neuroblastoma. Left lateral decubitus coronal sonogram shows a large, solid mass (arrows) caudal to the liver (L). Strong central echos (Ca) represent calcium deposits reflecting the acoustic beam with resultant distal acoustic 'shadowing' (S).

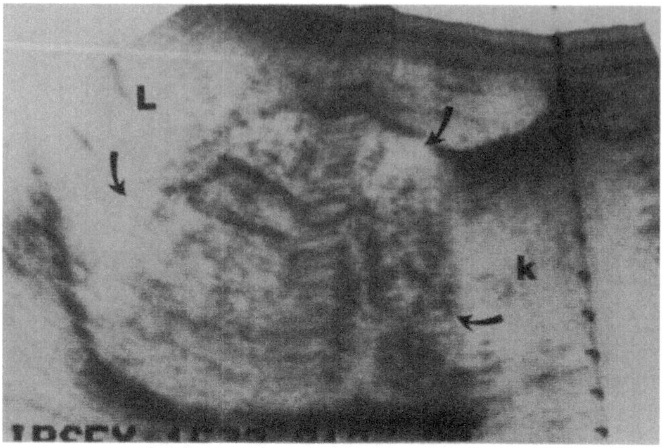

Figure 7. A two year old female with a nonfunctioning right adrenocortical adenoma. Supine longitudinal sonogram shows a large, solid mass (arrows) compressing the posterior aspect of the liver (L). The upper pole of the right kidney is displaced caudally (K).

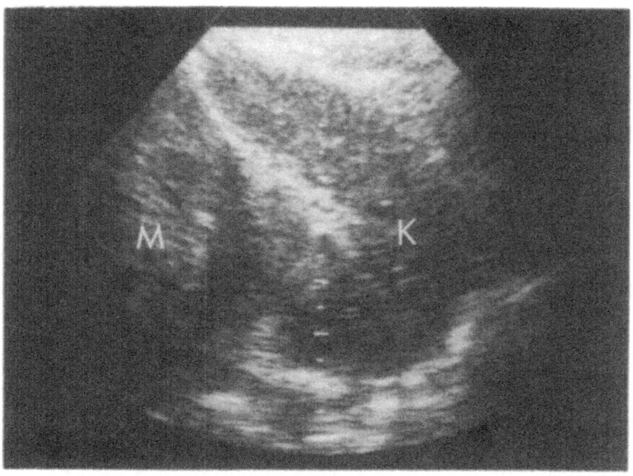

Figure 8. An eighteen month old male with a right adrenal neuroblastoma. A left lateral decubitus coronal real-time sonogram demonstrates a cleavage plane between mass (M) and displaced kidney (K), excluding a renal mass.

ior and lateral shift (Figures 7 and 8). Left adrenal tumors may lie anterior to the left kidney with only posterior renal displacement, simulating pancreatic tail masses on prone scans. On supine scans, the characteristic position of left adrenal masses posterior to the splenic vein helps to differentiate them from distal pancreatic lesions (Figure 4). The right adrenal is closely associated with the inferior vena cava and frequently posterior impression or anterior displacement of that vessel is noted with right adrenal masses (Figure 9). The distinction of adrenal masses from the spleen, pancreas and gastric fundus, the caudate lobe of the liver and the upper pole of the kid-

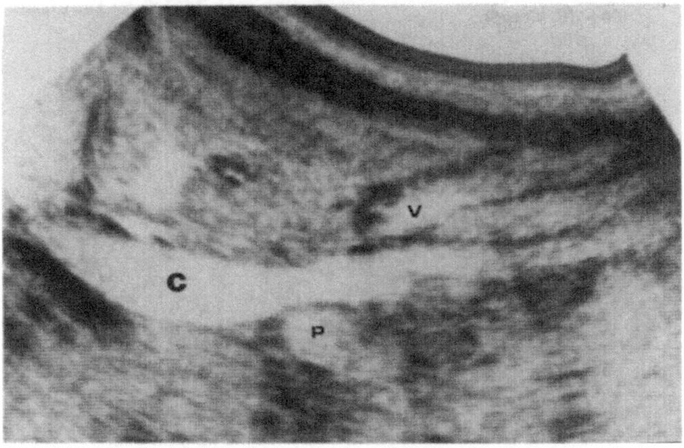

Figure 9. A supine longitudinal sonogram of a right adrenal pheochromocytoma (P) posterior to, and mildly indenting, the inferior vena cava (C), located cephalad to the main portal vein (V).

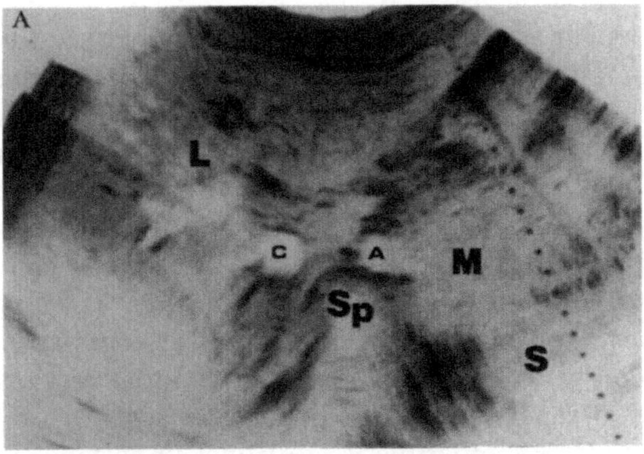

Figure 10. (A) Supine transverse sonogram 1 cm below the xyphoid shows homogeneous solid gastric 'pseudomass' (M) in the left upper quadrant anteromedial to the spleen (S) and lateral to the aorta (A). (L = liver; C = Inferior vena cava; Sp = Spine.).

neys can generally be accomplished with meticulous scanning technique in multiple positions and planes (Figures 8 and 10).

2.2. Computed tomography

Since its introduction by Hounsfield [20] in 1972, computerized tomography (CT) has rapidly evolved. Scanning times have been reduced from four minutes per tomographic cut to under five seconds per cut. Initially limited to the head, technological advancements have allowed for widespread applications throughout the body. A thinly collimated x-ray beam is passed

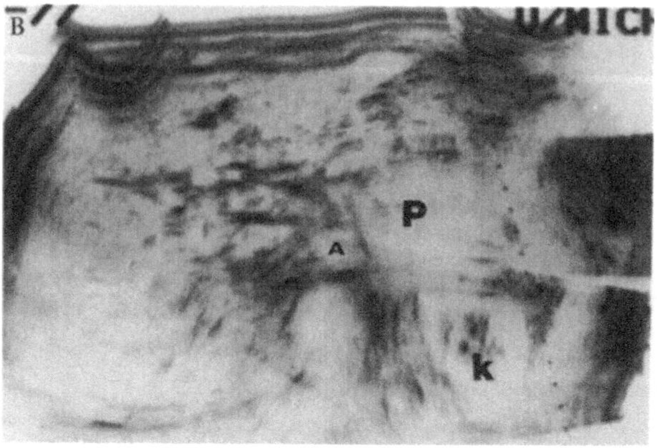

Figure 10. (B) Supine transverse sonogram 5 cm below the xyphoid shows a similar homogeneous solid pheochromocytoma (P) anteromedial to the left kidney (K) and lateral to the aorta (A).

through the patient and a series of two-dimensional axial plane images are generated. Computer processing of the x-ray density information is necessary in order to produce CT images. This system allows for a detailed evaluation of tissue density characteristics and anatomic visualization.

The major advantages of CT are lack of invasiveness and clarity of anatomic display. Disadvantages include equipment costs and radiation exposure. Brasch [22] has described the radiation dosimetry characteristics for a variety of scanners, and calculated skin exposures that range from 0.63 to 4.7 rads. Other risks of CT include reactions to contrast media and hypothermia in neonates. Contrast reactions in children are less common than adults with five reported major reactions in a series of 12,419 contrast examinations [22]. Hypothermia is of distinct importance in neonates, particularly in prematures, as this condition predisposes to intraventricular hemorrhage. Different systems have been devised to ensure proper temperature control, including warming blankets and heat lamps. In our institution a special isolette unit has been adapted which can fit into the CT scanning gantry permitting adequate temperature control and less handling of the neonate.

In general, ultrasound is recommended as the initial examination, considering the lack of radiation, cost, and portability. However, many situations arise in which CT is needed for a more precise delineation of abnormalities or as a result of a technical failure of ultrasound due to tubes, drains, surgical wounds, or bowel gas. Because of its densitometric capabilities, CT is preferred for evaluation of calcifications within lesions.

Another disadvantage of CT in children, particularly neonates, is the relative lack of tissue fat planes, which are helpful in defining adult anatomy. Because of motion artifacts, children between the ages of two and six will likely require sedation, i.e., intramuscular pentobarbital (6 mg/kg), oral chloral hydrate (50 mg/kg) or rectal thiopental.

The patient should not have ingested food for 4 hours prior to scanning to reduce the likelihood of aspiration related to vomiting after contrast administration. Intravenous contrast is generally employed, but is not always necessary. The dosage of these agents should be the same as for pediatric excretory urography.

2.2.1. Technique. Routine adrenal CT scanning is performed as follows: starting at the crus of the diaphragm, 0.5 cm contiguous scans are made to the level of the renal hilus, usually after a bolus of intravenous contrast. Oral contrast material is given prior to the examination to identify the duodenum on the right and jejunal loops on the left, both of which can simulate adrenal masses. For a thorough examination the entire length of the adrenal glands must be visualized. If the study is performed for localization of a hormonally active adrenal tumor, which is not identified initially, the examination should be continued cephalad to the dome of the liver and caudally to the symphysis pubis at 1.0 cm intervals.

For routine abdominal examinations, 1.0 cm contiguous slices are used, scanning from the top of the diaphragm to the symphysis pubis, after intravenous contrast. If hepatic metastasis is a consideration, a non-contrast study of the liver is obtained initially. Adequate opacification of bowel loops with oral contrast material is essential for all examinations. Oral hypaque or a diluted mixture of barium (1–5% w/v) can be used depending on the type of scanner. The barium concentrations used for fluoroscopic studies such as upper gastrointestinal series or barium enema are too dense for CT scanning and create unacceptable reconstruction artifacts.

A radiograph of the abdomen after contrast examinations should be obtained, particularly if the patient has not had a recent excretory urogram. Whenever a mass lesion is encountered the entire mass should be included in the study, as occasionally they can cross the diaphragm to involve the thorax. This occurs with some frequency in neuroblastoma, other neural crest-derived tumors, and sarcomatous tumors.

Using CT, the normal adrenal gland can be accurately visualized in approximately 95% of patients [25]. Usually the length of the gland varies from 3-5 cm and can be approximated by summing the slice thicknesses showing the gland. Measurements of normal glands are almost always less than 2.5 cm for AP diameter and less than 1.0 cm for thickness [17, 23–25] (Figure 11). The adrenal glands are variable in size and shape. Each gland may have a linear, Y, V, or triangular configuration [26–28]. Visualization

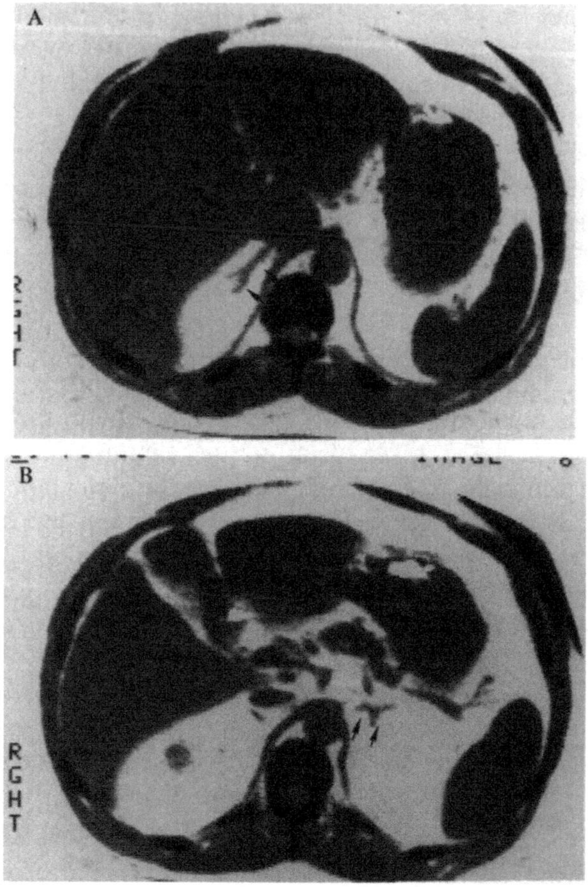

Figure 11. CT scan of normal right (A) and normal left (B) adrenal glands.

may be more difficult in those patients with poor fat planes, or with metallic clips from previous surgical procedures.

Further technical refinements in scanners have permitted reconstruction of the axial images into coronal, sagittal, or oblique planes which can be helpful in selected cases. With a cooperative patient, imaginative positioning and gantry tilting capability, images may be obtained in direct or near-direct coronal planes (Figure 12).

2.3. Adrenal scintigraphy

Adrenal imaging has been clinically available for the past 10 years. In this interval it has demonstrated efficacy in the localization of adrenal cortical disease. Unlike the other modalities utilized in the localization of adrenal gland tumors, adrenal scintigraphy reflects adrenal function in addition to anatomy. As a biochemical probe of adrenal function, the scintigraphic

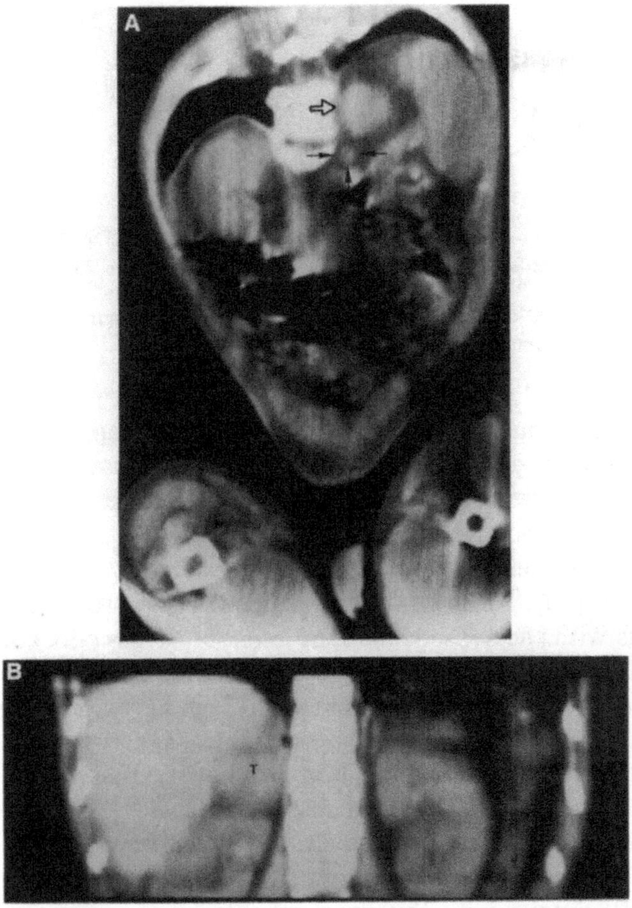

Figure 12. (A) CT scan (direct coronal section) demonstrating two left sided pheochromocytomas. One tumor is intra-adrenal (large arrow) and the other is extra-adrenal (small arrows). (B) CT scan (coronal reconstruction) from contiguous 5 mm thick axial slices demonstrating a pheochromocytoma arising in the right adrenal gland (T = Tumor).

approach is unique. Although other studies provide greater spatial resolution than scintigraphy, information from the functional aspects of the procedure are at times more important than the localization or delineation of abnormal adrenal anatomy.

The iodocholesterols in clinical use today were not the first compounds used to image the adrenal cortex. A host of other radiolabeled steroids, steroid precursors and adrenal enzyme inhibitors have been proposed as adrenal imaging agents [29, 30]. However, the iodocholesterols and in particular ^{131}I-6β-iodomethyl-19-norcholesterol (NP-59) are the only radiotracers in routine clinical use at this time (Figure 13) [31].

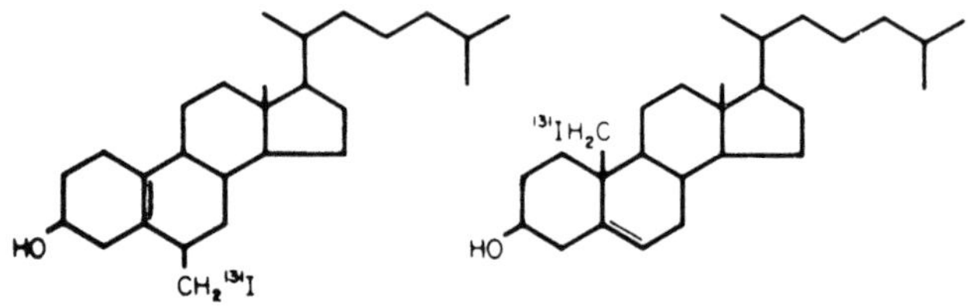

^{131}I-NP-59 ^{131}I-19-IODOCHOLESTEROL

(6β-^{131}I-IODOMETHYL-19-NOR CHOLEST-5(10)-EN-3β-OL) (^{131}I-19-IODOCHOLEST-5(6)-EN-3β-OL)

Figure 13. The structural configurations of the adrenal cortical imaging agents ^{131}I-19-iodocholesterol and ^{131}I-6β-iodomethyl-19-norcholesterol.

The cholesterol analogs were chosen for adrenal imaging agents as a result of their importance as precursors of steroid biosynthesis. As a direct result, uptake of these agents is observed in tissues that metabolize cholesterol, i.e. the adrenals, ovaries, and testes [32].

^{14}C-cholesterol was the first derivative to demonstrate selective adrenal cortical uptake [33]. This prompted further investigation into other cholesterol analogs with the subsequent synthesis of ^{131}I-19-iodocholesterol (NM-145) [34]. The demonstration of successful adrenal localization with NM-145 sufficient for imaging in a patient with Cushing's syndrome in 1970 was predicted from previous animal investigations [35]. Although not an ideal agent for adrenal cortical imaging, NM-145 has been demonstrated useful in the localization of adrenal cortical disease processes [36]. The second generation adrenal cortical imaging agent ^{131}I-6β-iodomethyl-19-norcholesterol (NP-59) was noted to be a contaminant produced during the synthesis of NM-145 [37]. Studies with this agent revealed it to possess a 5- to 20-fold increased avidity for the adrenal cortex, and as a result NP-59 has supplanted NM-145 as the agent routinely used for adrenal cortical scintigraphy [38].

An understanding of the transport, adrenal uptake, and metabolism of cholesterol is critical to the interpretation of the adrenal scintiscan. Dietary sources provide most of the circulating cholesterol. Solubilization of dietary cholesterol is achieved by transport lipoproteins [39]. The lipoproteins originate from the liver and circulate to the gut to allow transport of cholesterol to target tissues [39]. The lipoproteins responsible for cholesterol transport to the adrenal glands are species specific [40]. In man, low density lipoproteins (LDL) represent the major mode of conveyance of cholesterol to the adrenal glands [39]. Previous studies indicate that the iodocholesterol derivatives are also conveyed in LDL, and approximately 20% of an administered dose of iodocholesterol can be found within the LDL fraction of the plasma lipoproteins [41].

Complex mechanisms exist to provide an adequate supply of cholesterol for adrenal steroidogenesis. The adrenal cortical uptake of LDL-derived cholesterol is dependent upon the prevailing levels of adrenocorticotrophic hormone (ACTH) circulating LDL-cholesterol and intra-adrenal cholesterol levels [39]. A specialized portion of the adrenal cortical cell membrane, the LDL receptor, is a high affinity binding site for LDL-cholesterol and facilitates the movement of cholesterol into the adrenal cell for esterification, storage, and steroid hormone biosynthesis [39, 40, 43]. Extensive investigations have shown that the LDL receptor modulates cholesterol uptake into the adrenal cell [40]. The level of both intra- and extra-adrenal cholesterol and ACTH have been shown to effect adrenal gland cholesterol uptake. A lowering of the serum cholesterol results in increased LDL receptor activity and increased *de novo* cholesterol synthesis within the adrenal. Elevated serum cholesterol levels result in a diminution of the LDL receptor activity (receptor-down-regulation) [43]. Although direct evidence of LDL-receptor effects upon iodocholesterol adrenal gland uptake is lacking, studies of NP-59 uptake in hypercholesterolemic patients suggests that iodocholesterol uptake is dependent upon LDL-receptor activity [44].

Once sequestered within the adrenal cortical cell, NP-59 and NM-145 are felt to be enzyme inhibitors. Little, if any, ^{131}I labeled steroids or their metabolites are found after radiotracer administration [45]. The low level of metabolism of these compounds explains the extended times at which adrenal images can be collected. It thus appears that the mechanisms of uptake of radiolabeled cholesterols and native cholesterol are similar.

2.3.1. Adrenal dosimetry. Debate has existed over the actual adrenal gland radiation exposure from the iodocholesterol adrenal imaging agents. High estimates have been obtained using data from animals and human patients with disease [46]. In a recent re-evaluation of adrenal uptake of NP-59, Carey *et al.* [47] have shown that the absorbed dose to the adrenals in nor-

Table 2. Absorbed dose of ^{131}I from ^{131}I-6β-Iodomethyl-19-norcholesterol*.

Tissue	Absorbed dose (Rads/mCi)
Whole body	1.4
Adrenals	25 ± 7.2 [a]
Testes	1.7
Ovaries	3.8
Liver	7

From Carey *et al.* [47].
[a] Range 12–39 Rads/mCi.

mals is 25 ± 7.2 RADS/mCi (range 12-39 RADS/mCi). In patients with Cushing's syndrome a mean of 57 ± 25 RADS/mCi (range 17–160 RADS/mCi) has been found (Table 2). This reflects a considerable reduction from previous estimates and places the radiation exposure in the same order of magnitude as other radiographic procedures. Moreover, it has recently been shown that the adrenal uptake of NP-59 can be decreased approximately 50% with dexamethasone suppression, and a considerable reduction in the radiation exposure during suppression studies would be anticipated [48].

2.3.2. Technique. Table 3 outlines the present method of adrenal scintiscanning. The usual dose of NP-59 is 1 mCi/1.73 m^2. The agent is formulated in ethanol and Tween-80 to pH of 5.5. A technique of slow intravenous injection of up to 1.0 cc of injectate is used. This contains 2–4 mg of cholesterol base. A few immediate reactions to injection have occurred and these have been ascribed to the histamine-releasing qualities of Tween-80 [31]. No delayed reactions have been recorded. All patients are given Lugol's solution or other suitable iodine preparations 2–3 days prior to radiotracer injection. This is done to block the thyroidal uptake of free ^{131}I [31]. Standard images are collected 4–6 days post tracer administration. This provides for a decrement of background activity and more favorable target to background ratios.

Table 3. Adrenal scintigraphy.

1. All medications that influence adrenal function are stopped 6 weeks prior to imaging.
2. Lugol's solution, 1–2 drops twice daily, is started 48 hours prior to for 7 days after the completion of the study.
3. 1.OmCi/1.73 m^2 ^{131}I-6β-iodomethyl-19-norcholesterol (NP-59) is given intravenously.
4. Images are collected at 72 or 96 hours post injection for studies on DS*, 5–6 days post injection for studies not on DS.
5. Posterior and left lateral images are performed on an Anger Camera (parallel hole, high energy collimator, 50,000 counts/image).
6. Uptake is estimated by a semioperator-independent-computer algorithm.

* DS: 4 mg dexamethasone (1 mg 4× daily) for 7 days prior to and throughout the imaging sequence.

Images are collected using a standard gamma camera interfaced to a dedicated mini-computer. A parallel hole collimator is routinely used for a collection of images. The 364 KEV peak of iodine is selected with a 20% window. 50,000 counts are obtained. The studies require approximately 20 minutes per image. The computer is used for information storage, image enhancement, and quantitative assessment of iodocholesterol uptake [31].

2.3.3. Normal adrenal scintiscan. The adrenal images produced with iodocholesterol can be used to study the anatomical and functional aspects of the adrenal glands. The interpretation of these studies is dependent not only upon an understanding of the biochemical functions involved but also upon the normal adrenal anatomy. The adrenal gland weight averages 2–3 gms, with variable size, shape and position [49]. In the majority of studies the right adrenal appears triangular in shape; the left is usually crescentic or elongate [50] (Figure 14). Left adrenal is usually encountered on the anteromedial aspect of the left kidney. The right adrenal is generally located more cephalad and posterior in comparison to the left and is usually found at the superior pole of the right kidney (Figure 15) [51].

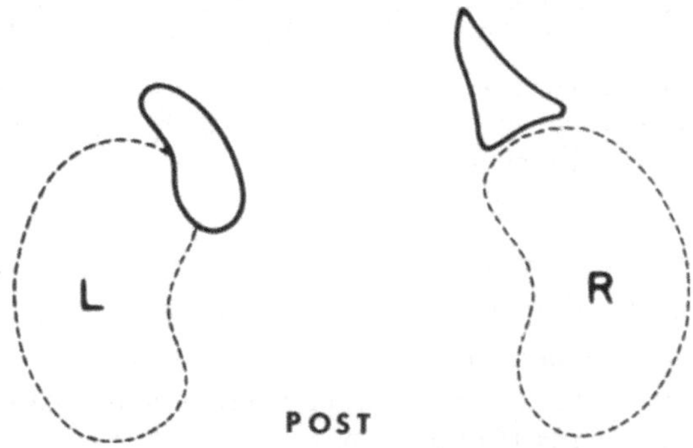

Figure 14. The normal position and configuration of the adrenal glands.

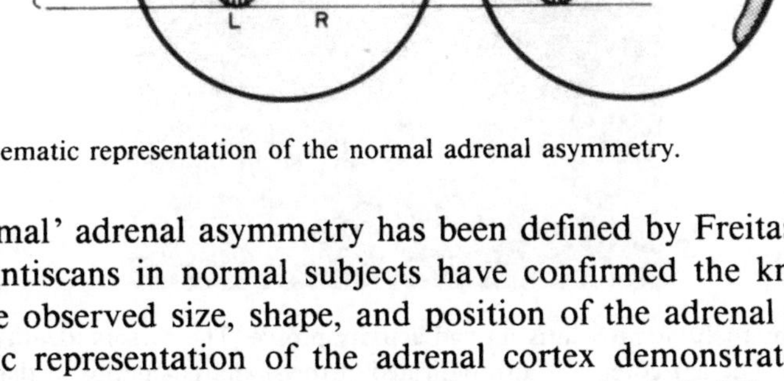

Figure 15. Schematic representation of the normal adrenal asymmetry.

The 'normal' adrenal asymmetry has been defined by Freitas *et al.* [52]. Adrenal scintiscans in normal subjects have confirmed the known differences in the observed size, shape, and position of the adrenal glands. The scintigraphic representation of the adrenal cortex demonstrates the right adrenal to be more cephalad and posterior than the left (Figure 16). The

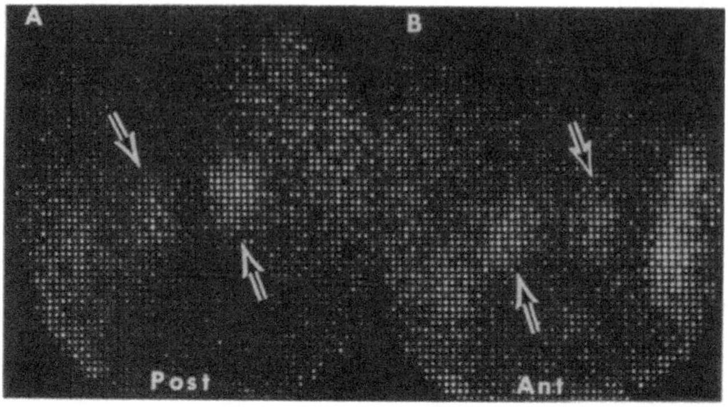

Figure 16. Normal posterior (A) and anterior (B) adrenal scintiscans. There is an apparent increase in right adrenal gland activity as compared to that of the left in the posterior view. This can be reversed in the anterior projection.

anteroposterior adrenal asymmetry causes the right adrenal to appear to have more ^{131}I activity than that of the left on the posterior scintiscan. The lateral scintiscan assists in distinguishing these differences in depth and in discriminating other areas of abdominal activity such as gallbladder or bowel from the adrenal glands (Figure 17).

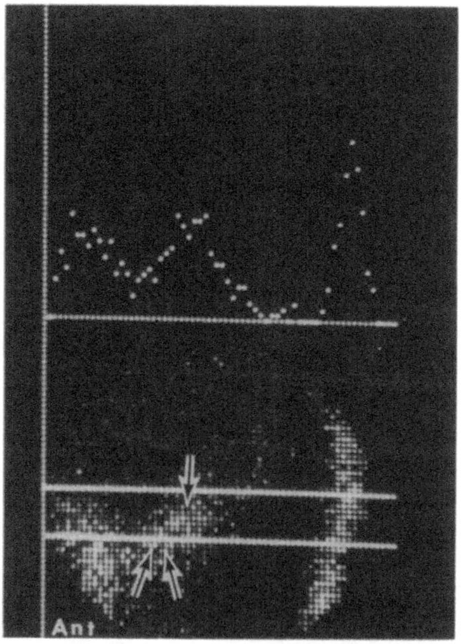

Figure 17. Normal left lateral scintiscan and activity profile. The cursors identify right adrenal activity (arrow). The left adrenal is also indicated (arrows) and is anterior to the right adrenal. The linear band of activity is a ^{133}Ba marker placed on the lumbar spine.

2.3.4. In vivo adrenal uptake calculations. In a manner similar to the measurement of ^{131}I uptake in the thyroid, NP-59 adrenal gland uptake can be quantitated. The method developed by Koral *et al.* [53] allows consistent and reproducible estimations of ^{131}I adrenal activity using a semioperator-independent-computer algorithm. The algorithm provides a background, depth, and decay corrected estimation of adrenal gland uptake. The normal range of uptake is 0.07 to 0.26 %/dose with a mean of 0.16 %/dose per gland. There is a consistent right-to-left ratio of 0.9 to 1.2 if the anteroposterior adrenal asymmetry is not considered [55]. The measurement of adrenal depth provides a correction for the anteroposterior asymmetry and produces left-to-right uptake ratios that approach 1.

The introduction of dexamethasone suppression to adrenal scintigraphy results in a fall of adrenal ^{131}I uptake with higher background activity and lower target to background ratios [31, 54]. Uptake calculations under these conditions are somewhat more difficult. The modification of the original uptake algorithm by Reader *et al.* [55] provides improved discrimination of adrenal activity from continguous areas of uptake, i.e., bowel and liver.

2.4. Angiography

Various radiologic methods have been used in the localization of adrenal lesions and their role in localization of adrenal tumors is changing. Most of the previous radiologic studies including excretory urography, nephrotomography and retroperitoneal pneumography, have a small role in the evaluation of adrenal tumors. Likewise, the role of angiography has been reduced and, in many institutions, its use has greatly diminished during the past several years. However, for certain adrenal lesions, angiography continues to assume an important role in the preoperative evaluation.

2.4.1. Vascular anatomy. Thorough knowledge of the arterial and venous anatomy of the adrenal gland is a prerequisite for the proper execution of angiographic studies. The adrenal gland is highly vascular and the adrenal arterial origins and their distribution within the gland are complex with considerable variation. The following classification of the adrenal arteries into superior, middle and inferior arteries is generally used and suffices for the purposes of angiographic studies. The superior adrenal artery arises from the inferior phrenic artery, a branch of either the aorta or celiac artery. The middle adrenal artery arises from the aorta, inferior phrenic or renal artery, and the inferior adrenal artery generally arises from the renal artery.

The venous blood from the cortex drains into the central vein in the adrenal medulla and emanates from the hilus as an adrenal vein. The right adrenal vein, shorter in length, enters the inferior vena cava at the level of the 12th thoracic vertebra, posteriorly. The left adrenal vein, immediately after uniting with the inferior phrenic vein, opens into the cranial aspect of the left renal vein, opposite to the gonadal vein. Venous blood from the adrenal capsule drains toward the capsular veins, connected by the renal capsular, phrenic, and retroperitoneal veins. Although the central venous drainage system described above is constant, occasional variations do occur. An awareness of possible variations in the venous drainage patterns is important for the expeditious performance of adrenal venography and for the precise interpretation of blood samples obtained for hormonal assays.

2.4.2. Technique. Adrenal arteriography and venography in children is performed as in adults using the Seldinger percutaneous technique [56, 57]. The cut-down method is rarely necessary. Different sizes of puncture needles and catheters are used depending on the weight and age of the child. A 20-gauge needle and a catheter of 3–4 French (Fr.) size may be used in children under the age of 6 months, a 19-gauge and 5 Fr. catheter for 6 months to 5 years, and over 5 years of age, either a 19- or 18-gauge needle with a 5–6 Fr. catheter is used. Premedication which has been commonly used is a 'cocktail' consisting of meperidine, promethazine, and chlorpromazine, mixed in the ratio of 1:1:1. The dosage is determined by the weight of the patient. Local anesthesia is performed with 1% lidocaine. General anesthesia may be used if necessary.

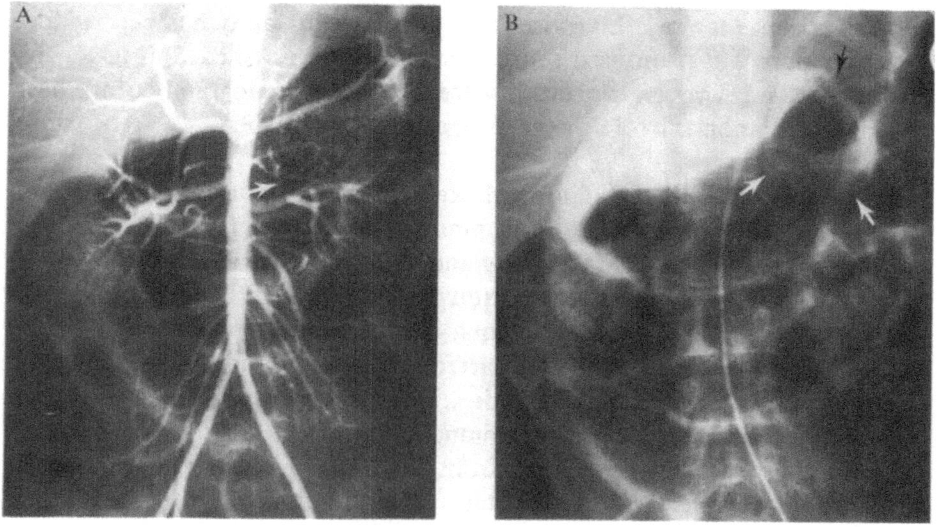

Figure 18. An aortogram of a 6-year-old girl with a left adrenal pheochromocytoma.
(A) Arterial phase. The left inferior adrenal artery (arrow) arises from left renal artery and supplies the tumor.
(B) Capillary phase. There is a homogeneous tumor stain in left suprarenal area (arrows).

The preferred puncture site for the percutaneous catheterization technique is the femoral artery or vein below the inguinal ligament. Anticoagulation is performed with either an intra-arterial bolus of heparin, a heparinized flushing solution, or both.

Arteriographic study usually begins with a flush aortogram. This provides a general picture of the vascular anatomy (Figure 18). Additional study frequently requires selective opacification of superior, middle, and inferior adrenal arteries. The initial aortogram furnishes a useful guide for identification of small aortic branches. Superior and inferior adrenal arteries, when arising from celiac and renal arteries, can be visualized with celiac and renal arteriograms, respectively. Selective injections of epinephrine (6–10 μg for renal and 10–15 μg for celiac artery) enhances visualization of the adrenal arteries. The middle adrenal artery commonly arising from the aorta, if dilated, can be easily catheterized using a curve-tipped catheter.

The photographic subtraction technique of aortography is essential for the complete evaluation of the patient with a suspected pheochromocytoma. Arteriographic study of the neck, thorax and pelvis may be performed if extra-adrenal pheochromocytomas are suspected. Proper preangiographic preparation of such a patient with adrenergic blocking agents should be instituted to alleviate potential hypertensive crises during injections of contrast media. Equally important are the availability of intravenous phentolamine (Regitine) and continuous monitoring of blood pressure and heart rate.

Adrenal venography is performed through a percutaneous transfemoral route. The catheterization technique has been previously described [58]. Catheterization of the left adrenal vein can be performed without difficulty. However, in most instances it has been more difficult to catheterize the right adrenal vein. Using a preformed catheter, Farah [59] was successful in catheterization of the right adrenal vein in over 90% of patients. In the hands of experienced angiographers, both adrenal veins can be successfully catheterized in approximately 90% of cases. Adrenal vein catheterization is safe if catheter wedging and forcible injections of contrast are avoided. The most serious complications include adrenal hemorrhage with subsequent adrenal insufficiency, and adrenal vein thrombosis.

Successful adrenal venography with magnification techniques, is one of the most sensitive means of demonstrating intra-adrenal pathologic lesions [58, 60]. Blood samples obtained from the adrenal veins before venography provide important information concerning the functional status of adrenal lesions. Dilution of adrenal venous blood can result in erroneously low concentrations of adrenal hormones. Such errors may be avoided by analyzing the blood for other hormones secreted by the adrenal glands. A correction for dilution can be made by determining the aldosterone/cortisol ratio from each adrenal vein, and this is particularly useful if there is a consideration of aldosterone excess [61].

2.4.3. Complications. The specific complications of adrenal angiography include hypertensive crisis in pheochromocytoma and adrenal hemorrhage. Hypertensive crises have been usually associated with adrenal arteriography and rarely with venography in patients with pheochromocytoma [62, 63]. Lecky *et al.* [64] reported a 22.7% hypertensive response in their literature review of 198 patients with pheochromocytomas who underwent arteriography (181 cases) or venography (17 cases). Most patients recovered spontaneously; a few required intravenous phentolamine but suffered no permanent sequelae. Three deaths were, however, reported after translumbar aortography [65]. In recent years, preangiographic preparation with alpha and beta adrenergic blocking agents and the use of less toxic contrast agents in conjunction with close monitoring of blood pressure and heart rate have significantly reduced the incidence of serious hypertensive crises [60, 66].

Adrenal hemorrhage has been the most common specific complication of adrenal venography. Adrenal venous rupture causes immediate pain persisting about 12 hours and disappearing in 24–30 hours (Figure 19) [67]. Bilateral hemorrhage may result in adrenal insufficiency. Furthermore, a hematoma produced by intra-adrenal contrast extravasation may mimic a tumor and make localization difficult during surgical exploration [67]. The incidence of adrenal hemorrhage during venography has dropped significantly

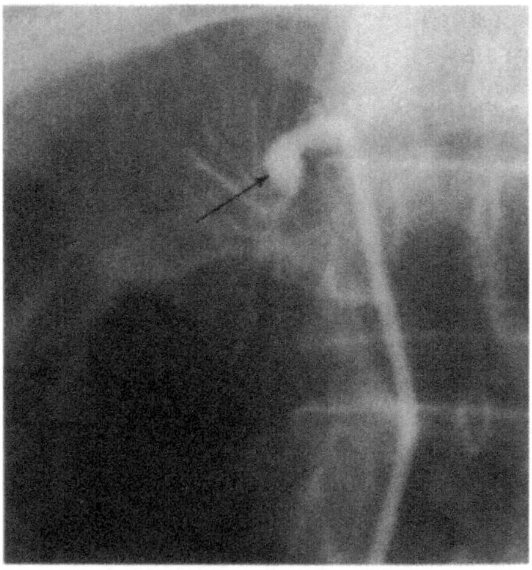

Figure 19. Adrenal vein rupture during right adrenal venography. There is a rounded collection of contrast medium (arrow) representing a ruptured adrenal vein with extravasation of contrast. The intra-adrenal venous branches are unremarkable. Adrenal hemorrhage also occurred in the opposite gland, resulting in adrenal insufficiency.

during the past 10 years. Avoidance of catheter wedging and the use of short-tipped catheters have been primarily responsible for improved venographic technique and a reduced risk of adrenal rupture.

3. ADRENAL DISEASE

3.1. Cushing's syndrome

When the classic signs of Cushing's syndrome appear in an adult, the cause is usually due to adrenal hyperplasia [68]. The clinical findings and hormonal laboratory data usually provide the diagnosis. Commonly this syndrome results from prolonged administration of steroids. If the laboratory data point to pituitary origin (ACTH dependent), the cause is most likely a functioning pituitary adenoma or microadenoma, and transphenoidal hypophysectomy is the procedure of choice [69]. However, when Cushing's syndrome occurs in a child the most common cause is adrenal carcinoma [68].

Adrenal carcinomas in children are frequently large and readily localized using ultrasonography. Internal hemorrhage, necrosis and occasionally calcification can sonographically appear as markedly heterogeneous solid masses with characteristic organ and blood vessel displacements localizing the tumor to the adrenal gland (Figure 20).

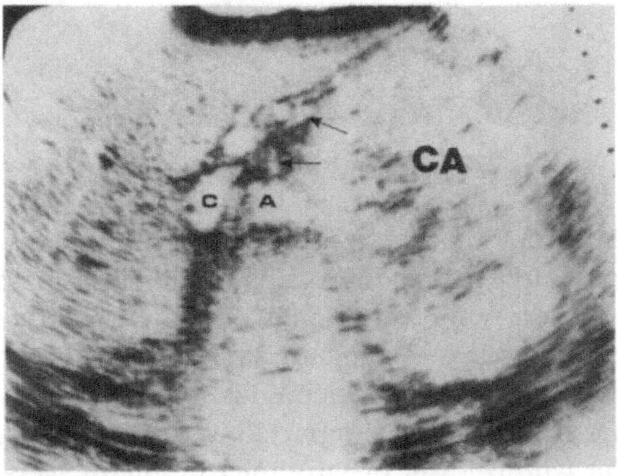

Figure 20. Supine transverse sonogram scan of an adrenocortical carcinoma (CA) with central hemorrhage and necrosis. The aorta (A) and celiac vessels (arrows) are displaced medially by the mass. (C = inferior vena cava).

The clinical, endocrinologic, and radiographic features of carcinoma of the adrenal cortex have previously been summarized [68]. While differentiation of benign from malignant neoplasms is often impossible, one of the advantages of CT is the ability to detect metastatic disease, either by direct

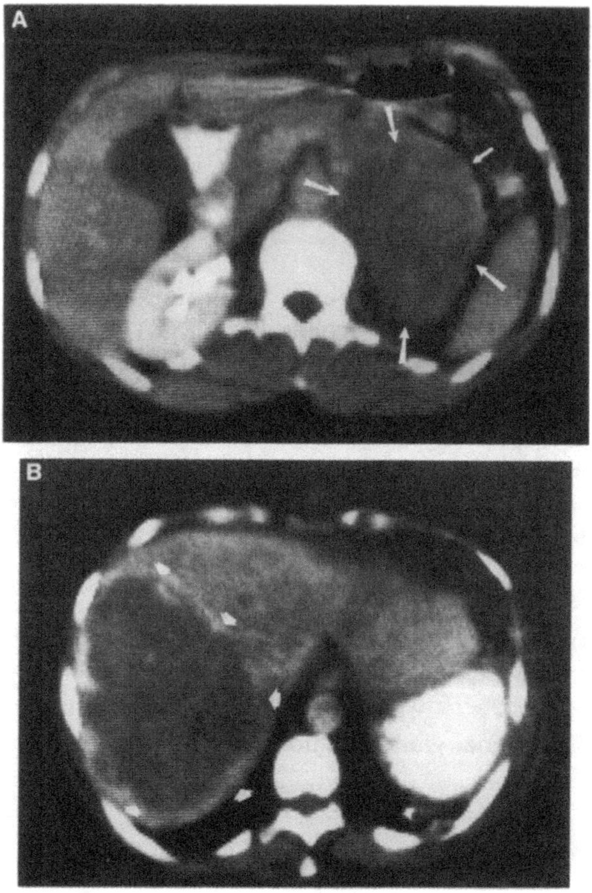

Figure 21. CT scan of left adrenal carcinoma (A) metastatic to liver (B).

extension into the liver, adjacent vessels, or to lymph nodes (Figure 21). The CT scan usually identifies these tumors as round solid masses replacing the normal adrenal gland. While carcinoma of the adrenal gland usually presents as a solitary adrenal mass, it may be bilateral in as many as 10% of cases [70]. Calcification is rare in adenomas, but more common in carcinomas [23]. Schaner *et al.* [71] have reported a series of patients with adrenal cortical tumors in whom lower density measurements were obtained, ranging from 16–34 Hounsfield units (HN) instead of the expected range of 60–80 HN units. This may be due to unusually high concentrations of fat within some tumors. Other causes for unusually low density measurements can include hemorrhage, necrosis, or gas formation after embolization therapy [68, 72].

Since adrenal carcinoma is the most common cause of Cushing's syndrome in children, adequate CT evaluation of the adrenals in these patients must be obtained. If an adrenal carcinoma can be excluded, most of the remaining cases are due to bilateral adrenal hyperplasia. In adults, adrenal hyperplasia may be seen as bilaterally enlarged or normal glands, but little data is available in children. In approximately 15% of cases of childhood Cushing's syndrome, a benign adenoma is found, and rarely a non-adrenal ACTH secreting tumor (ectopic ACTH syndrome) will be found [70]. Cushing's syndrome is not present in all patients with adrenal cortical tumors. Depending on the hormonal activity of the tumor, there may be minimal symptoms of glucocorticoid excess with either signs of masculinization or feminization. The sonographic appearance of such tumors depends on their size and presence of calcification, hemorrhage and/or necrosis (Figure 22).

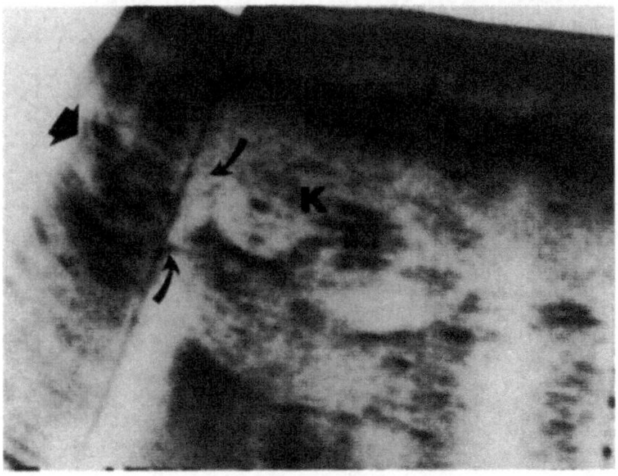

Figure 22. 30 month old male with precocious puberty due to an adrenal adenoma. The prone longitudinal sonogram shows a densely echogenic calcified solid mass (arrows) cephalad to the left kidney (K).

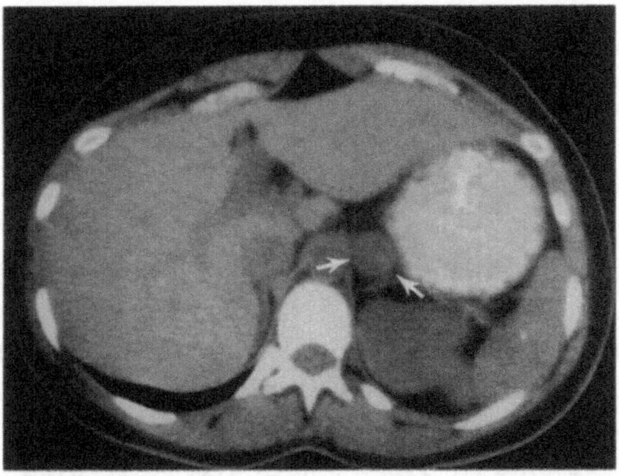

Figure 23. CT scan of a left adrenal adenoma in a female with virilization. A remnant of normal adrenal gland is seen adjacent to the tumor.

Most adrenal tumors of 1.0 cm or greater size will be visualized by the current generation of sub-5 second CT scanners (Figure 23). Tumors of smaller size may not be identified so that in the face of compelling biochemical data, adrenal venous sampling or scintigraphy may be required.

Adrenocortical carcinomas manifest as large intra-abdominal masses with little or no ^{131}I-adrenal activity noted on scintiscans. The uptake per gram of iodocholesterol in adrenal cortical carcinoma is low and does not allow sufficient activity for visualization in the face of excessive glucocorticoid secretion from generally large tumors. This results from suppression of both pituitary ACTH and contralateral adrenal uptake of iodocholesterol (Table 4). Although the presence of bilateral nonvisualization on an adrenal scintiscan provides information concerning the etiology of the disease, further localization using other modalities is necessary for complete evaluation.

Table 4. Interpretation of scintiscans in Cushing's syndrome

Scan pattern	% uptake	Diagnosis
Bilateral symmetrical	Normal [a]	Non-diagnostic [b]
	Elevated [c]	Hyperplasia
Bilateral asymmetrical	Elevated [a,d]	Hyperplasia
	Elevated [a,e]	Nodular hyperplasia
Unilateral	Normal	Adrenal infarction
	Normal	Contralateral-nonfunctioning Tumor
	Elevated	Adenoma
Bilateral nonvisualization		Adrenal carcinoma (functioning)

[a] Normal = 0.16%/dose/gland [52].
[b] Serum cholesterol may be responsible for low adrenal gland uptake [44].
[c] Greater than $0.52 \pm .07$%/dose [74].
[d] <50% difference.
[e] >50% difference [31].

Adrenal cortical adenomas result in unilateral patterns of imaging (Table 2). The uptake of iodocholesterol is then lateralized to the tumor which suppresses pituitary ACTH and contralateral adrenal iodocholesterol uptake (Figure 24). Studies indicate that this application of the adrenal scintigram is most efficacious in the diagnostic localization and confirmation of this form of Cushing's syndrome in over 95% of cases [31, 73]. In Cushing's syndrome, as the result of either excessive or autonomous ACTH secretion, bilateral elevated iodocholesterol uptake is observed [31] (Figure 25). Pre-

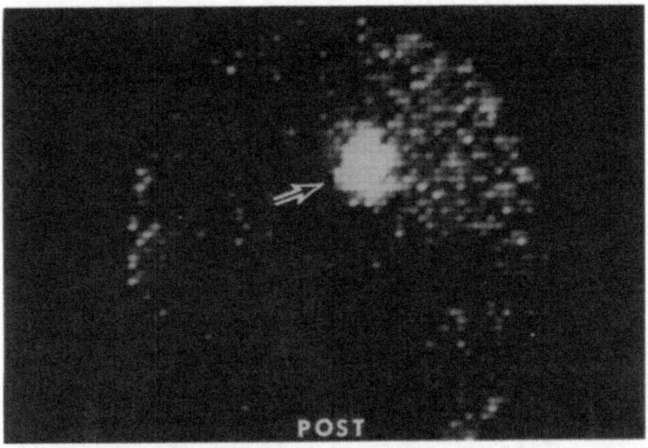

Figure 24. Posterior adrenal scintiscan in a patient with an adrenal adenoma (arrow) resulting in Cushing's syndrome.

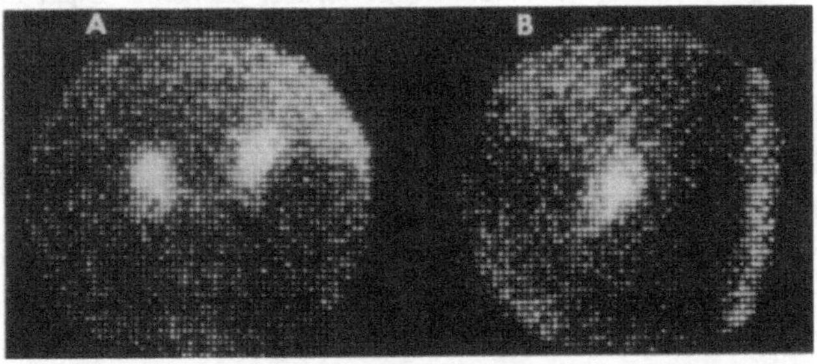

Figure 25. (A) Posterior adrenal scintiscan demonstrating bilateral visualization in a 16 year old patient with ACTH dependent Cushing's syndrome. (B) The left lateral scintiscan shows the activity to be posterior.

vious studies indicate that the pattern and degree of iodocholesterol uptake can be used to confirm the diagnostic impression and assess the disease activity in Cushing's syndrome [31]. The level of calculated ^{131}I uptake can be used to separate normal from abnormal adrenal activity, as it has recently been shown that patients with Cushing's syndrome exhibit generally higher adrenal iodocholesterol uptake than normals [74].

Although differentiation between adrenal hyperplasia and adenoma resulting in Cushing's syndrome is possible by adrenal scintigraphy and CT, adrenal vein catheterization with blood sampling for cortisol is the method for definitive diagnosis. Venographically, an adenoma appears as a rounded mass with dilated circumferential veins and a reticular venous network within the mass (Figure 26). The size and vascularity of an adenoma determines the venographic findings. The adenoma is generally hypervascular or slightly vascular on arteriograms with a homogeneous stain in the parenchy-

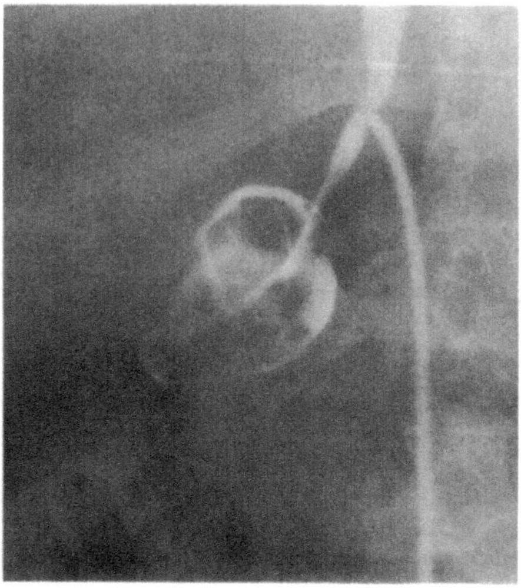

Figure 26. Cushing's syndrome due to adrenal cortical adenoma. Right adrenal venogram demonstrates arcuate stretching of dilated adrenal vein with sinusoidal accumulation of contrast typical of a cortical adenoma.

mal phase [75]. Larger and more vascular tumors generally have prominent venous patterns on adrenal venography. Venography is not useful in differentiating benign from malignant tumors.

The venographic appearance of adrenal hyperplasia is nonspecific, including generalized enlargement of the gland and spreading of adrenal vein branches. It should be noted that there is no correlation between venographic size and function of the gland. The absence of a tumor in the venogram of patients with Cushing's syndrome generally indicates adrenal hyperplasia.

3.2. Primary aldosteronism (Conn's syndrome)

Primary aldosteronism is produced by autonomous adrenal hypersecretion of aldosterone. The syndrome is characterized by elevated blood pressure, weakness, polyuria, polydipsia, and hypokalemic alkalosis. While usually due to a functioning adrenal adenoma, other etiologic considerations are adrenal hyperplasia or carcinoma. Aldosterone secreting tumors are extremely rare in children [70]. They can be bilateral and multiple, and may measure 0.5 cm or less in diameter [76]. A critically important problem in diagnosis of aldosterone excess is whether the disease is unilateral (tumor) or bilateral (hyperplasia). The presence of hyperplasia is more common in the pediatric age group than adrenal adenoma. The successful treatment of primary aldosteronism due to bilateral adrenal hyperplasia is medical whereas adrenalectomy is the treatment of choice for unilateral adrenal cortical adenomas [77].

As the sonographic identification of adrenal tumors is primarily size dependent, aldosterone secreting tumors of less than 2 cm in diameter may not be consistently imaged. However, with a flexible scanning approach in multiple planes, and by incorporating real-time examination, aldosteronomas can be imaged (Figure 27).

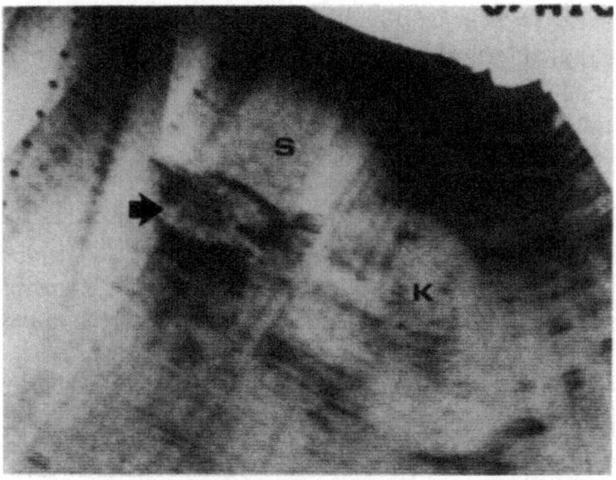

Figure 27. Right lateral decubitus coronal sonogram of a 2 cm left adrenal aldosteronoma located (arrow) cephalad to the left kidney (K) and medial to the spleen (S).

Ganguly *et al.* [78] have reported CT visualization of 4 of 6 proven aldosterone secreting tumors. The tumors were visualized by adrenal venography or venous sampling in all 6. In a different series of nine patients, Linde *et al.* [79] report that CT failed to identify three aldosterone secreting tumors, each measuring 1.0 cm or less in diameter. In the same series, adrenal venous sampling was shown to be of equal accuracy. Since adrenal adenomas secreting aldosterone are generally of small size many of these tumors will be missed by both CT and ultrasound. Ganguly *et al.* [80] emphasize that in aldosteronomas CT scanning should not be the sole technique of localization. In two patients with primary aldosteronism, both adrenals were clearly seen on the CT scan, but the tumors were missed. Both of these had been identified by adrenal vein catheterization and were subsequently proven surgically.

Studies indicate that the scintigraphic approach is variable with regard to the sensitivity and accuracy in primary aldosteronism [77, 81]. Standardization, however, of the scintigraphic approach with consideration of prior dexamethasone suppression (DS) and the intervals of optimal imaging has been shown to provide an accurate and sensitive assessment of adrenal anatomy and function in patients with primary aldosteronism [82].

DS is used to amplify abnormal mineralocorticoid secretion in primary aldosteronism. Previous studies have shown that the normal adrenal cortex will image while on DS [54, 83]. Using a standardized dose and duration of DS (4 mg daily for seven days prior to and throughout the imaging intervals) it has been shown that the normal adrenal cortex will image at 120 hours (5 days post-injection) after iodocholesterol (NP-59) administration [54]. With these parameters in mind, scanning protocols can be devised to provide imaging at optimal intervals and to distinguish normal from bilateral hyperplasia and adrenal adenoma (Table 5). Figure 28 (A-B) illustrates adrenal imaging in primary aldosteronism.

Table 5. Interpretation of dexamethasone suppression scintiscans[a].

Scan pattern	Days after NP-59 injection	Diagnosis
Unilateral	3–5 days	Adenoma
Bilateral	5	Hyperplasia
Unilateral	5	Non-diagnostic

[a] From Gross *et al.* [111] adapted from Freeman L, Weissman H, Nuclear Medicine Annual 1980 Raven Press, New York used with permission.

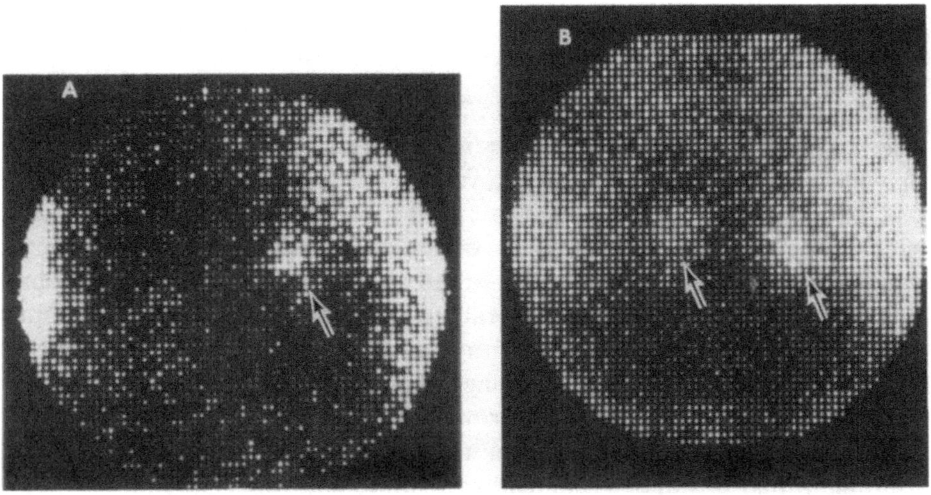

Figure 28. Adrenal scintigrams in primary aldosteronism. (A) Unilateral tracer uptake in a patient with an aldosterone-secreting adrenal adenoma. (B) Bilateral adrenal activity in a patient with primary aldosteronism due to bilateral adrenal hyperplasia.

Adrenal vein catheterization with blood sampling for aldosterone determinations remains an important method for diagnosis and localization of disease in primary aldosteronism [61]. Unilateral elevated levels of aldosterone from an adrenal vein confirms the diagnosis of adenoma, whereas bilateral elevations indicate hyperplasia. Injection of contrast media demonstrates a mass, however, the technique has been frequently avoided for fear of adrenal hemorrhage. Adrenal vein catheterization is complementary to scintigraphy and plays a definite role in the evaluation of patients with non-diagnostic scintiscans.

Venographically, an adenoma presents arcuate stretching of intra-adrenal veins. A dilated venous network and sinusoidal accumulation of contrast may be present (Figure 29). Adrenal hyperplasia may increase the overall

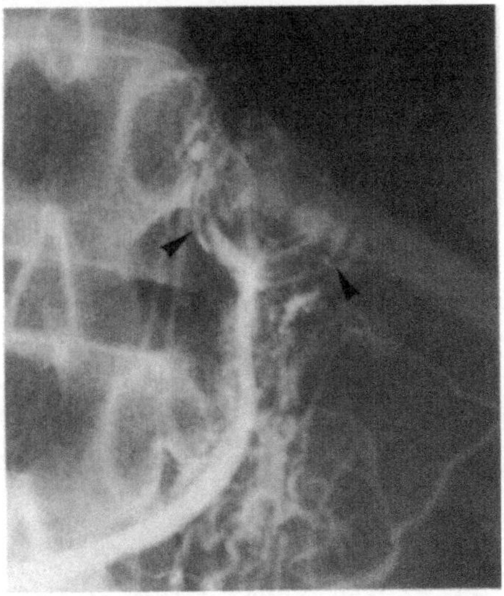

Figure 29. Left adrenal venogram of an aldosteronoma (X2) demonstrates stretching and displacement of adrenal veins in an arcuate pattern in the upper part of the adrenal gland (arrows). pituitary adenoma and excessive ACTH secretion.

gland size and diffuse arcuate stretching may be present in nodular hyperplasia (Figure 30). Because most adenomas are small, less than 3 cm, arteriorgraphic demonstration is difficult without superselective adrenal injections. Adrenal vein catheterization and blood sampling are the most commonly used angiographic tests for localization in patients with aldosteronism. Dilution of adrenal blood with caval blood during sampling may cause an erroneous interpretation of hormonal analysis. Thus, determination of the aldosterone/cortisol ratio has been useful. This is based on the fact that cortisol secretion is not influenced by an aldosteronoma and thereby corrects for differences caused by sampling errors and dilution of the adrenal vein blood. Aldosterone determinations after ACTH stimulation also assists in localization of adenomas. Dunnick *et al.* [61] recently studied 14 patients with primary aldosteronism with determinations of adrenal vein aldosterone/cortisol ratios. In 10 patients with histologically proven adenomas, 9 had localizing aldosterone elevations in the adrenal vein effluent. In 2, ade-

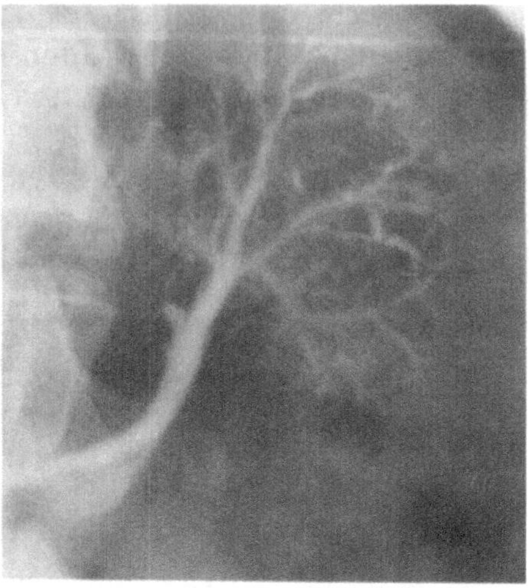

Figure 30. Primary aldosteronism due to nodular adrenal hyperplasia. Left adrenal venogram demonstrates general enlargement of the gland with stretching and displacement of adrenal vein secondary to numerous cortical nodular hyperplasia.

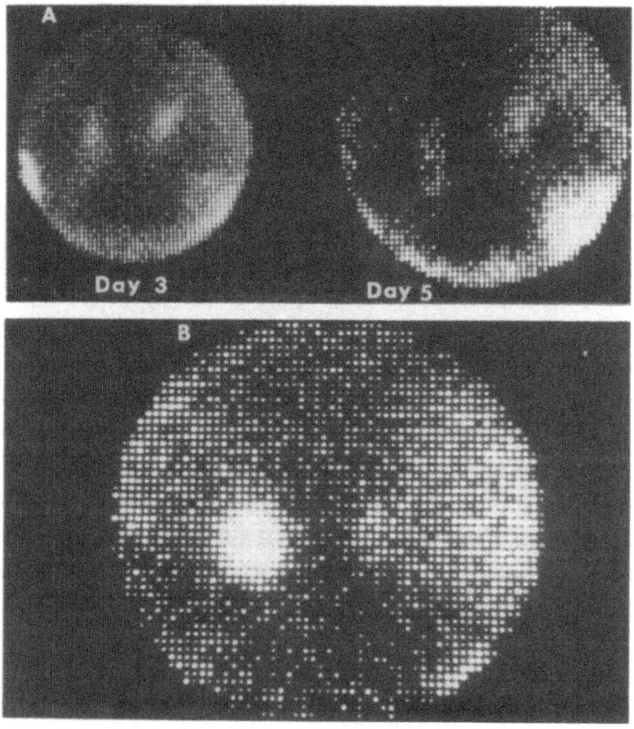

Figure 31. Posterior adrenal scintiscans in hyperandrogenism. (A) Bilateral adrenal hyperplasia with sequential images on Day 3 and Day 5 post-tracer injection. (B) Unilateral adrenal activity in a patient with an androgen-secreting adrenal adenoma.

nomas could not be definitely localized, while in 3 other patients the aldosterone/cortisol ratios were useful in establishing tumor localization.

3.3. Hyperandrogenism

The most frequent cause of hyperandrogenism in children is congenital adrenal hyperplasia (CAH). Adrenal imaging procedures in this disorder are performed primarily to exclude adrenal tumors; a complete biochemical evaluation, however, generally makes imaging unnecessary. In later adolescence the emergence of hyperandrogenism with irregular menses and hirsutism can present diagnostic problems. Studies indicate that adrenal scintiscanning procedures can be used to identify patients with an adrenal component to their hyperandrogenism [84]. These studies, performed on dexamethasone suppression, identify those patients with adrenal hyperplasia (bilateral imaging) and patients with adrenal adenoma (unilateral imaging) (Figure 31 A-B). Patients with CAH while on replacement doses of dexamethasone have normal adrenal scintiscans (Figure 32).

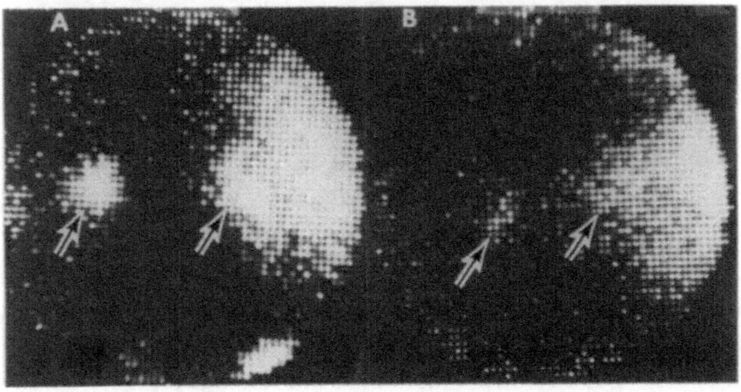

Figure 32. Posterior adrenal scintiscan of a 16 year old female with CAH. Excessive bilateral activity is observed (A) while on suppressive steroid therapy the adrenal activity is normal (B).

3.4. Neuroblastoma

Neuroblastoma is the most common solid abdominal tumor of childhood, and a complete radiologic evaluation is essential in the evaluation of any child suspected of having a neuroblastoma [85]. This insidious tumor often grows to a large size and metastasizes widely prior to diagnosis. Approximately three-fourths of all patients will have metastases before diagnostic confirmation (Figure 33). Moreover, two-thirds of all neuroblastomas arise in extra-adrenal locations, such as the organ of Zuckerkandl, or in locations where neural crest cell derivatives can be found.

The sonographic findings in neuroblastoma are variable. Usually the tumor is large, solid and heterogeneous with multiple internal echoes (Fig-

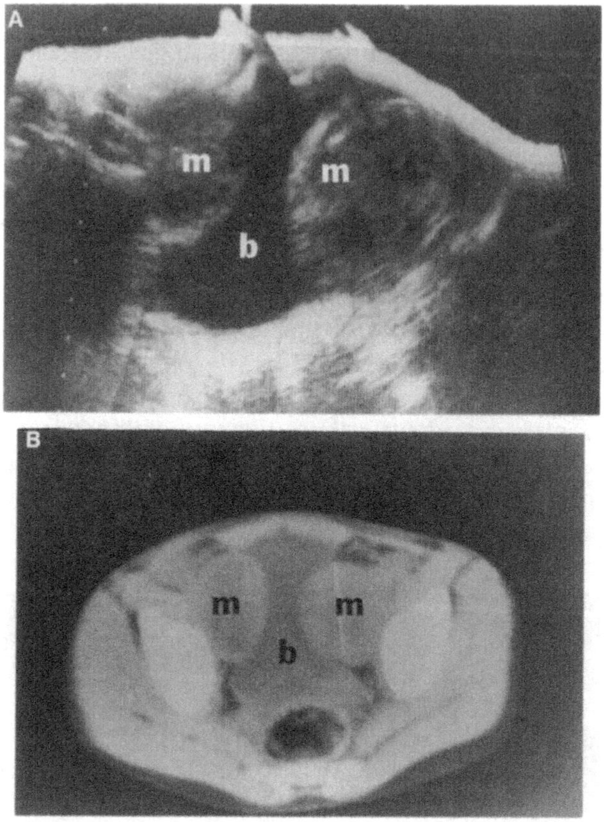

Figure 33. (A) A transverse sonogram of the urinary bladder in a 5 year old child demonstrating bilateral solid masses impinging on the bladder.
(B) CT section of this region confirms the ultrasound findings on metastatic lymphadenopathy from neuroblastoma (courtesy of D.R. Kirks, M.D.).

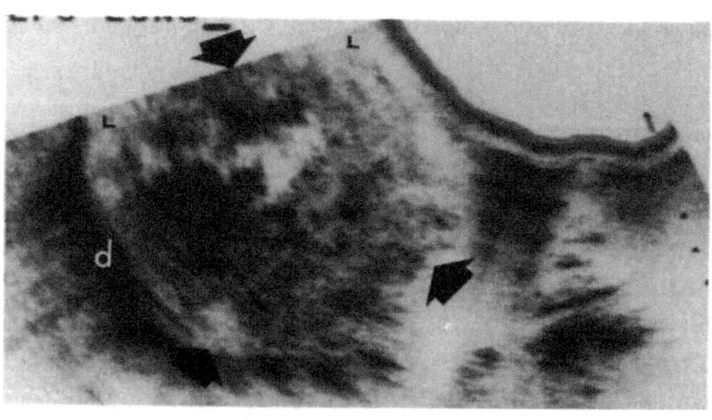

Figure 34. Eighteen month old male with a right adrenal neuroblastoma. The supine longitudinal sonogram demonstrates the characteristic large, solid, echogenic mass (arrows) in the right upper quadrant. (L = liver; d = diaphragm).

ure 34). A complex sonographic pattern results from tumor necrosis and hemorrhage. Mass effects can be striking and some difficulty may arise in attempting to exclude invasion of the kidney or liver even when well-defined cleavage planes are seen [13] (Figure 35). Fifty to 60% of these

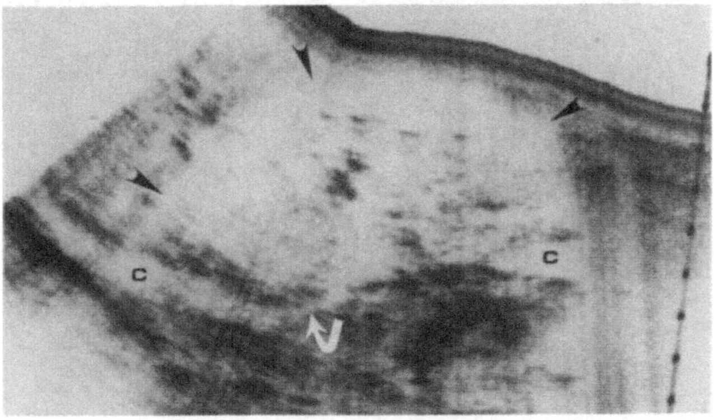

Figure 35. A five year old female with a right upper quadrant neuroblastoma. The supine longitudinal sonogram shows a solid mass (arrowheads), anterior to the inferior vena cava (C) A portion of the tumor displaces the inferior vena cava anteriorly (arrow) and suggests adrenal involvement, but the extensive infiltrative nature of the tumor obscures its primary adrenal origin.

tumors calcify, a feature that can be identified sonographically (Figure 6). Liver metastases from neuroblastoma are frequent and sonography is ideal for their delineation. Occasionally in neonates only a small primary tumor is identified (Figure 36). Ultrasound can also assist in evaluation of tumor extent and distal spread. The less malignant ganglioneuroblastomas and benign ganglioneuromas are sonographically solid, can be quite echogenic, occasionally calcify, but tend to necrose less frequently than neuroblastomas (Figure 37).

The CT scan will usually demonstrate the presence and extent of tumor masses (Figure 38). CT will often demonstrate tumor extension into the spinal canal or adjacent bones. While as many as one half of neuroblastomas demonstrate calcifications within the tumor on plain radiographs, the sensitivity of density measurements afforded by CT demonstrates calcifications in a higher number of cases. Berger *et al.* [86] studied children with proven neuroblastoma and found that CT added valuable clinical and diagnostic information in 10 of 15 patients. Other adrenal neoplasms can mimic neuroblastoma. If fat and calcification are demonstrated within a lesion, a dermoid tumor or teratoma should be considered as other diagnostic possibilities [87].

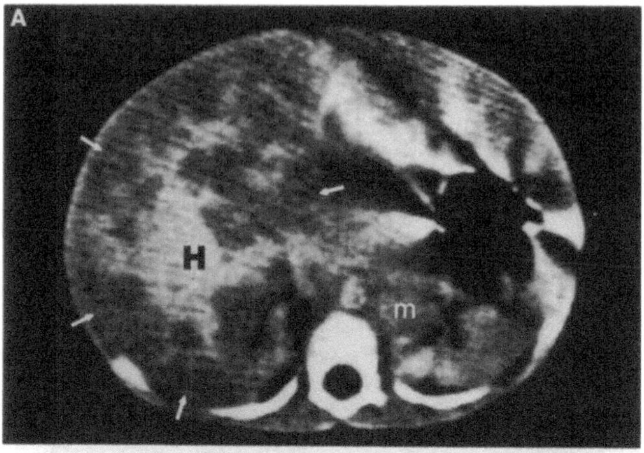

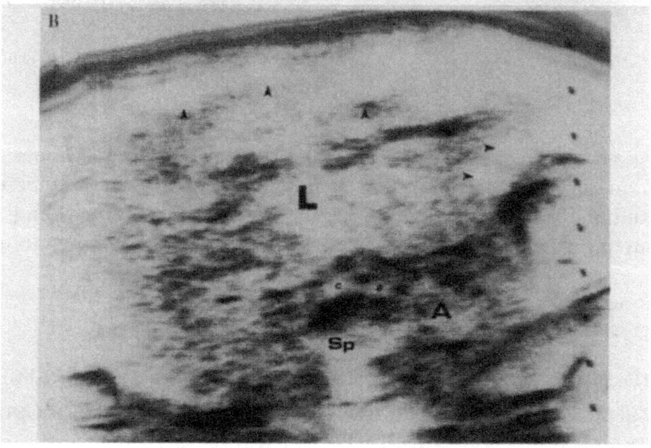

Figure 36. (A) A two month old female with hepatomegaly. CT scan shows hepatomegaly (H) with multiple lesions exhibiting decreased attenuation (arrows) and a small left adrenal mass (M). (B) Transverse supine sonogram confirms an enlarged liver (L) with multiple discrete hypoechoic, solid masses (M) from metastatic neuroblastoma. A small, solid left adrenal neuroblastoma (A) was confirmed surgically. (Sp = spine; a = aorta; c = inferior vena cava).

The contribution of angiography to the evaluation of children with suspected neuroblastoma has greatly diminished in recent years. Angiographically, neuroblastoma is vascular with numerous pathologic vessels and accumulation of contrast within the tumor (Figure 39). The extent of tumor and invasion of adjacent organs can be precisely assessed by arteriographic study and may be helpful in determining resectability. Inferior vena cavography should be performed before surgical exploration. Complete surgical extirpation of tumor may not be possible when the vena cava is displaced or obstructed [56]. If necessary, an adequate vena cava examination can be obtained with injection of contrast medium into an ankle or femoral vein.

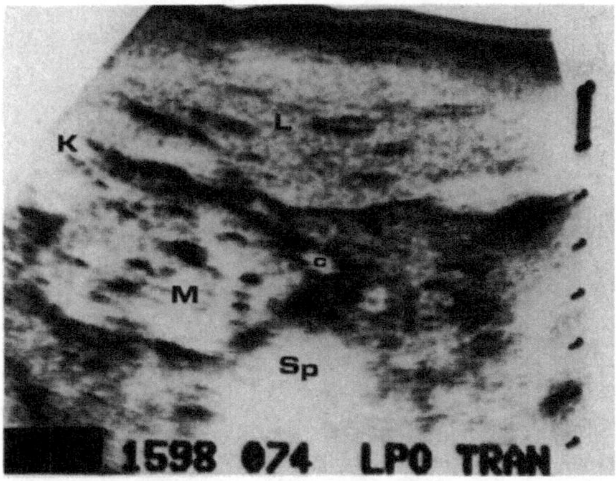

Figure 37. A two year old female with prior resection of a right paraspinal ganglioneuroblastoma. The left posterior oblique transverse sonogram shows a right retroperitoneal mass with several dense echogenic foci (M) compressing the kidney laterally (K). (L = liver; Sp = spine; C = inferior vena cava).

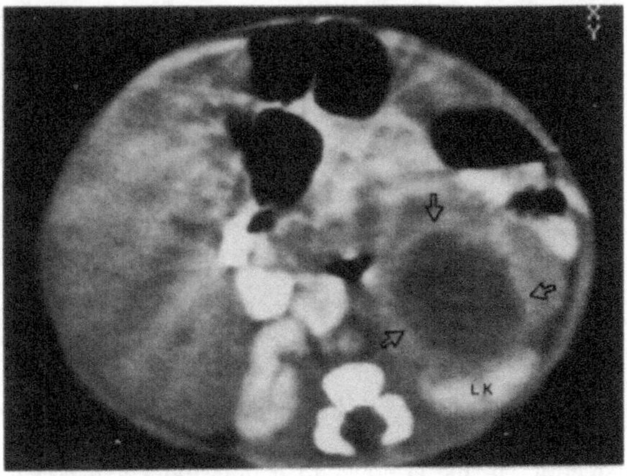

Figure 38. CT scan of a neuroblastoma in a 2 day old infant arising in the left adrenal gland. There is lateral displacement of the left kidney and poor tissue plane definition.

3.5. Pheochromocytoma

Until recently, nephrotomography and angiographic studies have been the most commonly used radiologic methods for localization of pheochromocytomas. The capability of CT in demonstrating slight tissue density differences has made it the most sensitive screening method for tumors of the adrenal medulla (Figure 40). Although CT and gray scale ultrasound have become important imaging modalities, angiography continues to play an

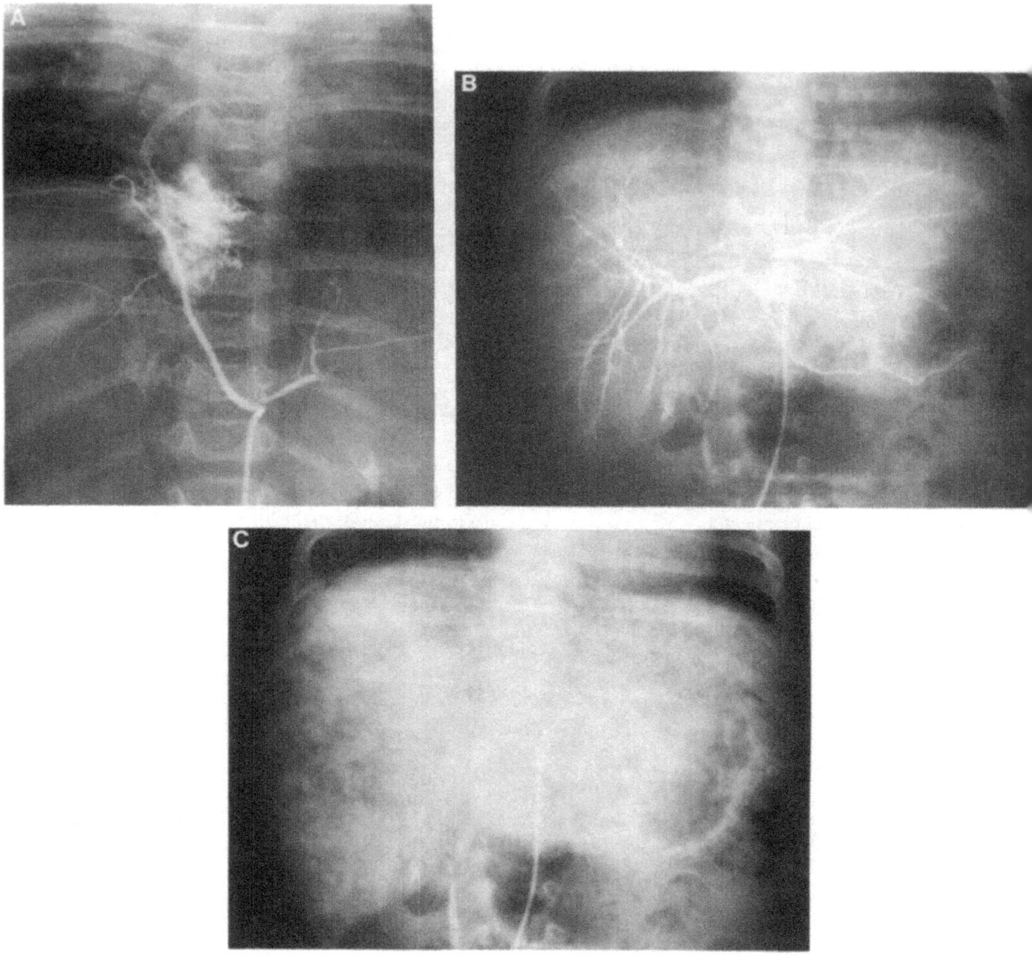

Figure 39. A neuroblastoma of the right adrenal gland with hepatic metastases in a 4-month-old infant.

(A) Selective right inferior phrenic arteriogram demonstrates a hypervascular mass in right suprarenal region.

(B) Selective hepatic arteriogram (arterial phase) showing hepatomegaly and stretching of intrahepatic arteries.

(C) Parenchymal phase of same angiogram demonstrates numerous hypervascular metastatic nodules scattered throughout the entire liver.

important role in the evaluation of patients with suspected pheochromocytomas.

Extra-adrenal pheochromocytomas, or paragangliomas, arise from the chromaffin cells of sympathetic ganglia from the neck to the pelvis. The incidence of paraganglioma in children has been reported in up to 32% of

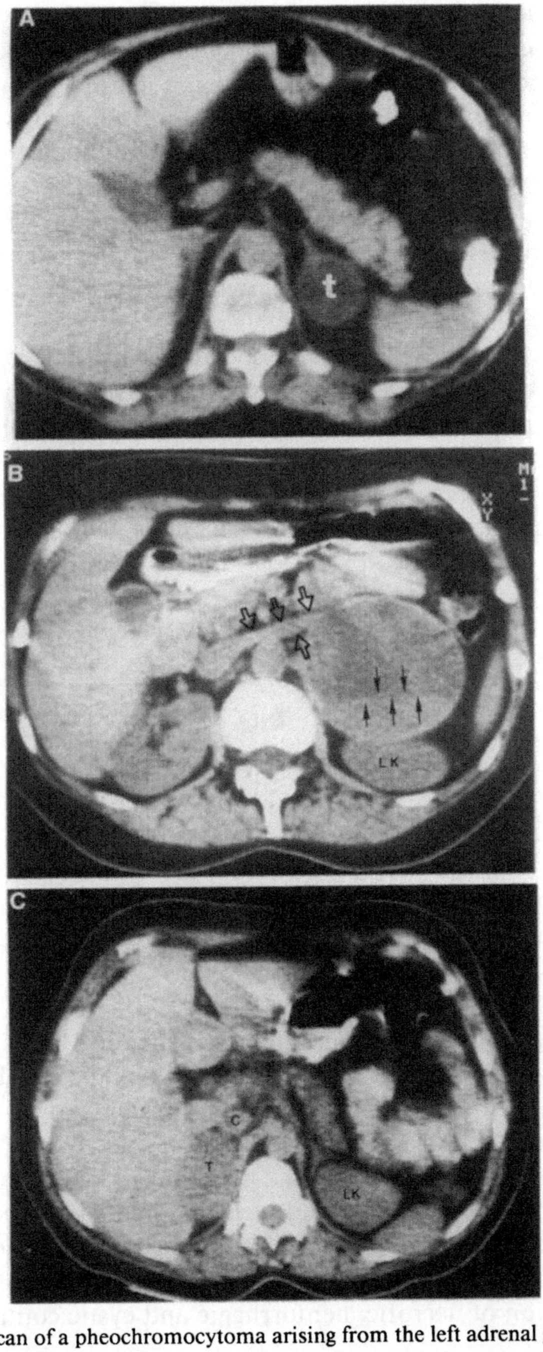

Figure 40. (A) CT scan of a pheochromocytoma arising from the left adrenal gland. (B) Pheochromocytoma with internal hemorrhage and displacement of the left renal vein. (C) Pheochromocytoma (T) arising in the right adrenal gland. Same patient as Figure 12B (C = inferior vena cava; LK = left kidney).

cases [88, 89] while in adults paraganglioma are reported in 10% of cases [64]. About 10% of pheochromocytomas are multiple. Most extra-adrenal pheochromocytomas arise within the abdomen and common sites are the renal pedicle, the organ of Zuckerkandl, the origin of iliac arteries, and in the area of the bladder [63, 90, 91]. In childhood the tumor is more common in males, while the reverse is true in adults. Over 90% of children with pheochromocytomas have sustained hypertension, which is present in about one-half of cases in adults. Additional features seen more commonly in children include visual complaints, nausea, vomiting, weight loss, polyuria, and polydipsia.

Pheochromocytomas have been associated with neurofibromatosis and medullary thyroid carcinoma [60]. Familial pheochromocytoma associated with medullary thyroid carcinoma and parathyroid hyperplasia is known as multiple endocrine neoplasia II (MEN-II) syndrome [92, 93]. In a recent institutional review of eight cases of MEN II seven of the eight patients had bilateral adrenal pheochromocytomas and none had extra-adrenal tumors (Table 6) [60].

Table 6. Patients with pheochromocytoma at University[a] of Michigan Medical Center, 1966–1978.

	Sporadic pheochromocytoma	Pheochromocytomas associated with MEN-II	Total
No. patients	40	8	48
Bilateral adrenal	2	7	9
Extra-adrenal	10	0	10
Malignant	3	0	3

[a] Cho KJ, *et al.* [60] reproduced with permission.

Suspicion of pheochromocytoma may be generated by any of a wide variety of clinical symptoms, but scanning should be preceded by definite laboratory evidence of disease such as elevated plasma and/or urine catecholamines or their metabolites.

Preoperative localization by ultrasonography is useful in most cases as these tumors are generally large and well marginated. A spectrum of sonographic features has been described with pheochromocytomas, including homogeneous and variably heterogeneous solid masses, the latter dependent on the distribution of necrotic, hemorrhagic and cystic components (Figures 1–5, 41) [94].

CT has been shown to be efficacious in the localization of pheochromocytomas [18, 95–99]. In a patient with laboratory data suggesting pheochro-

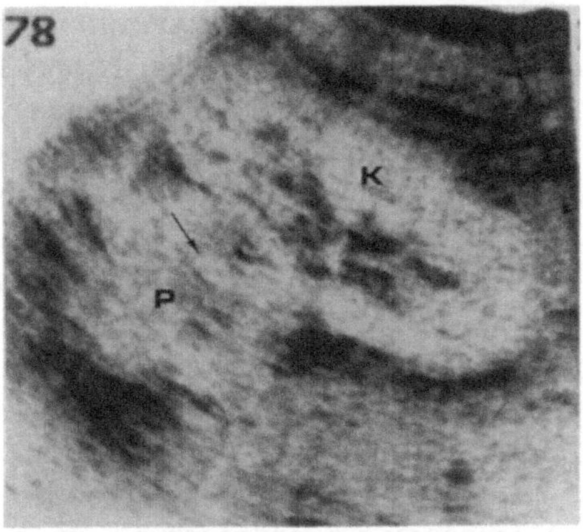

Figure 41. Prone longitudinal scan of a six year old hypertensive female shows a well defined solid mass (P) anterior to and compressing the left kidney (K). Tumor was largely composed of central hemorrhage and foci of necrosis (arrow).

mocytoma the initial examination is limited to the adrenal glands, by scanning contiguous 5 mm thick slices from the level of the diaphragmatic crus to the level of the renal hilum. The most common error in adrenal CT scanning is not to include the entire length of the adrenal gland. A pedunculated tumor attached to the limb of an adrenal may be missed if the examination is terminated at the slice which shows a normal appearing gland. If the tumor is not clearly identified initially, the scan should be extended to include the entire abdomen and pelvis, which can be performed as a series of 1.0 cm thick contiguous slices. Close attention should be given to areas such as the organ of Zuckerkandl, the renal hilus and the bladder. Intravenous contrast can be helpful in these extra-adrenal locations. In patients with pheochromocytoma, glucagon should not be used as an adjunct in scanning because of the possibility of precipitating a hypertensive crisis. With slower CT scanners propantheline may be used for bowel paralysis. The use of intravenous contrast is not essential but may be helpful in separating normal vascular structures which can abut the adrenal, particularly on the left, simulating a tumor. Contrast studies may require premedication of the patient, but a recent article by HessEl and Adams [100] suggests that premedication may not be useful.

Angiography, venography, and adrenal vein sampling have been traditionally helpful in tumor localization. If non-invasive modalities cannot localize the tumor, these studies may be the appropriate next step and can direct more specific CT examinations in less common areas such as the neck and mediastinum.

Awareness of the clinical syndromes such as MEN-II (multiple endocrine neoplasia, type II) [60] and their association with bilateral pheochromocytomas is helpful in interpreting CT scans. Pheochromocytomas can also occur in association with neurofibromatosis and von Hippel-Lindau disease.

The CT scan cannot predict benignancy or malignancy of pheochromocytoma unless there is local invasion or distant metastasis. In fact, histologic differentiation is quite difficult and the determination must often be made by the clinical behavior of the tumor [101, 102]. In addition, recurrence of benign tumors can also occur [18]. Laursen and Damgaard-Pederson [95] recently published a series of 26 patients in which pheochromocytoma was found in 14, and proven in 12. Of the remaining 12, all had negative CT scans and tumor was not identified by any other means in this group. There are numerous reports of CT localization of pheochromocytomas in a variety of locations and occasionally those not found by other modalities [78, 97, 98, 102, 103]. The angiographic approach to patients with suspected pheochromocytomas has differed from institution to institution. Zelch *et al.* [63] advocated sequential angiographic injections of contrast medium as a provocative test for localization. There is no difference in the arteriographic or venographic appearance between the tumors of adults and children. Although adrenal pheochromocytomas present as nonspecific angiographic abnormalities, demonstration of such vascular masses in patients with clinical and laboratory evidence of pheochromocytoma should establish the diagnosis. The angiographic study can be a safe and reliable procedure in children provided that proper preparation with adrenergic blocking agents and careful patient monitoring is performed.

The arteriographic study is performed with a selective sequential injection of right and left renal arteries, and followed by high and low aortograms. Adrenal venography is reserved for those patients in whom arteriograms are non-diagnostic [104]. Catecholamine sampling from the inferior vena cava and right atrium may be necessary for localization of extra-adrenal pheochromocytomas [104].

The arteriographic appearance of pheochromocytomas is nonspecific including hypervascularity with dilated feeding arteries and numerous neovascularities (Figures 18A and 42). In the parenchymal phase, homogeneous accumulation of contrast medium is present [66] (Figure 18B). Frequently, hemorrhage and subsequent necrosis of the tumor produces a central lucency within the tumor stain giving the appearance of a so-called 'ring sign' (Figure 42). About 30% of pheochromocytomas are hypovascular and may escape detection by arteriographic study [63, 105]. In a retrospective review of 14 patients with pheochromocytomas by Christenson *et al.* [66], arteriographic abnormalities were present in all but one tumor. Subtraction methods in the arteriographic evaluation of extra-adrenal pheochromocytomas are important for demonstration of those tumors overlying the spine.

The venographic appearance of pheochromocytomas, like other adrenal

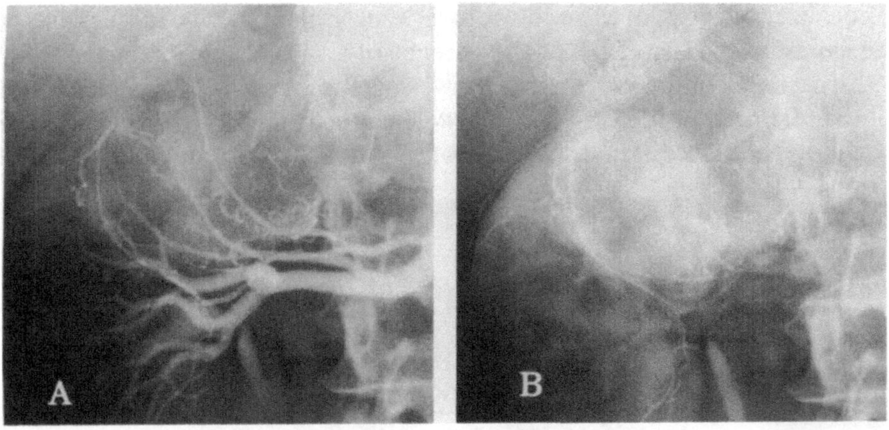

Figure 42. Pheochromocytoma associated with neurofibromatosis.
(A) A selective right renal arteriogram (arterial phase) demonstrates hypertrophy of inferior adrenal arteries and numerous tumor vessels.
(B) The parenchymal phase of same angiogram demonstrates tumor stain in the periphery of a large pheochromocytoma with a central lucency ('ring sign'). The central lucency represents necrosis secondary to hemorrhage. A small rounded soft tissue density overlying midportion of the right kidney represents a neurofibroma present on the skin surface.

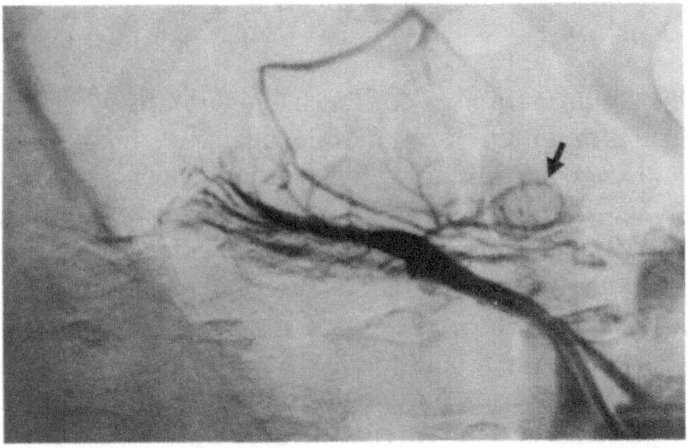

Figure 43. Bilateral multiple pheochromocytomas associated with left adrenal venogram (subtraction X2) showing a 6 mm pheochromocytoma in the lower portion of the adrenal gland (arrow). There is stretching and spreading of intra-adrenal veins due to nodular medullary hyperplasia.

masses, includes stretching and displacement of veins in an arc-like manner (Figure 43). In large vascular pheochromocytomas, dilated tortuous veins are visible with amorphous accumulations of contrast medium within the mass.

Localization of pheochromocytomas by scintigraphic techniques has not been satisfactory as a result of the absence of a suitable radiopharmaceutical with specific affinity for catecholamine-secreting tissues. The iodocholesterols can be used to identify intra-adrenal pheochromocytomas [106] (Figure 44); however, the high incidence of multiple, recurrent and metastatic

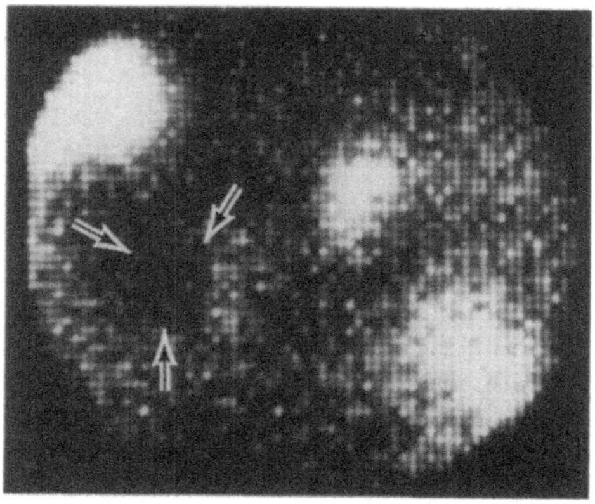

Figure 44. Posterior adrenal scintigram in a patient with a left adrenal pheochromocytoma. The area of decreased activity (arrows) corresponds to the tumor mass.

tumors in this condition makes cortical agents unsatisfactory, as functioning adrenal cortex is required for tumor localization. Numerous attempts at imaging the adrenal medulla have failed using catecholamines or their precursors, although definite adrenal medulla uptake of these agents can be demonstrated [107]. Recent success, however, with guanethidine derivatives has been achieved in the production of imaging agents for the adrenal medulla [108]. These agents have demonstrated selective localization within intra-adrenal, extra-adrenal, and metastatic pheochromocytomas [109]. It is anticipated that these agents may make it possible to localize and functionally characterize disorders of adrenal medulla.

3.6. Non-functioning tumors

About one-half of adrenal carcinomas are non-functioning tumors [110]. Occasionally such tumors become sufficiently large to present as an adrenal mass on routine fluoroscopic examination or at excretory urography. Sonographically, these tumors are similar to those with documented function. The larger tumors tend to demonstrate central necrosis and occasionally calcification (Figure 45). In children, adrenal metastases are rare. Lymphoma or other retroperitoneal soft tissue neoplasms may however, involve the adrenal by direct extension. Metastatic adrenal lesions may be found inci-

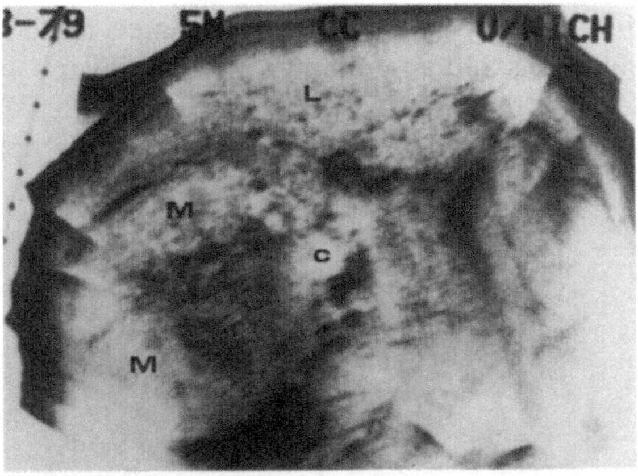

Figure 45. A 30 month old female with a non-functioning benign adrenocortical adenoma. Transverse supine scan shows a large adrenal mass (M) posterior to the liver (L), and postero-lateral to the inferior vena cava (C).

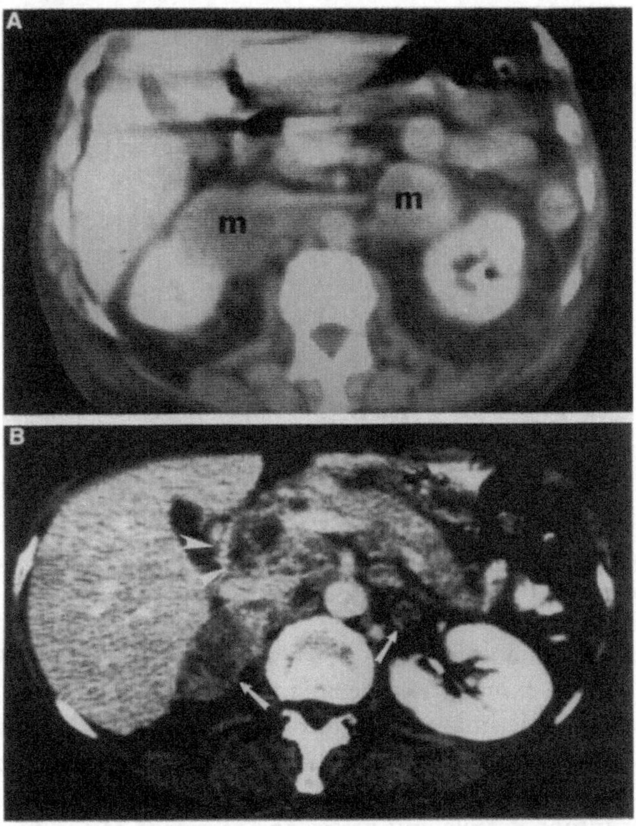

Figure 46. (A) Bilateral adrenal (arrows) and peripancreatic (arrowheads) metastases from an ovarian carcinoma. (B) Bilateral adrenal metastases from a primary lung carcinoma.

dentally on examinations performed for unrelated reasons, or in patients with known metastases and an unknown primary (Figure 46). Whether unilateral or bilateral, adrenal metastases are seen by both CT and ultrasound as diffuse gland enlargement. When larger, they may appear cystic with central necrosis (Figures 47 and 48).

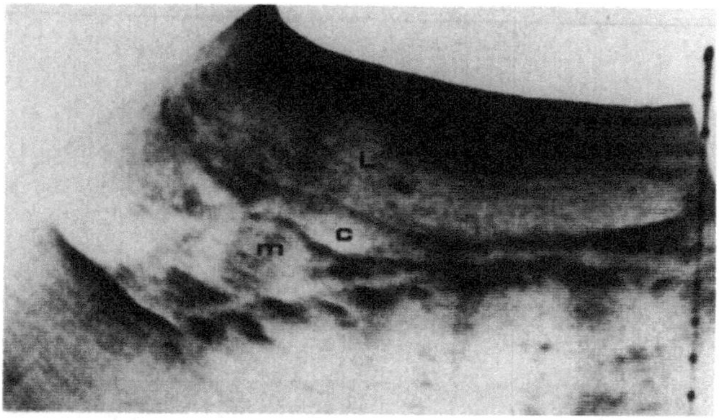

Figure 47. Supine longitudinal sonogram in an eleven year old female shows solid retrocaval mass (M), surgically confirmed to be metastatic hepatocellular carcinoma adjacent to but not definitely arising from the right adrenal. (C = inferior vena cava; L = liver)

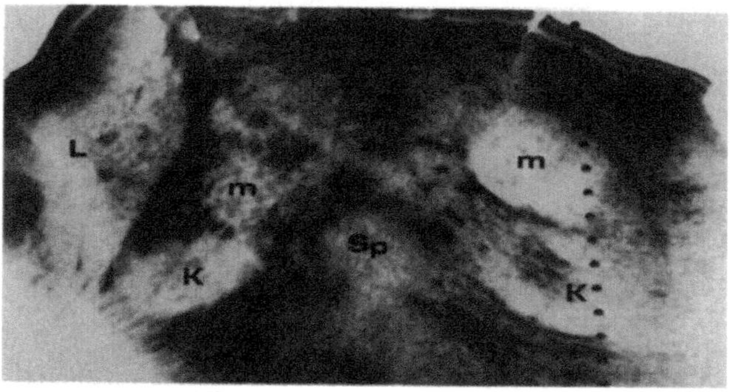

Figure 48. Supine transverse sonogram shows solid right and cystic left adrenal masses (M) anterior to the kidneys (K). (Sp = spine; L = liver)

Gray scale ultrasound and CT are generally performed for the evaluation of adrenal cortical tumors. Replacement of the adrenal cortex by neoplasm presents scintigraphic images with intra-adrenal defects. Intra-adrenal cysts, lymphoma, and metastatic disease all provide scans with decreased focal or absent adrenal cortical activity [111]. Arteriography remains useful in demonstrating tumor vessels and assessing the extent of the tumor. Selective celiac and hepatic arteriograms are usually performed to evaluate invasion of the liver and to exclude hepatic metastases [112].

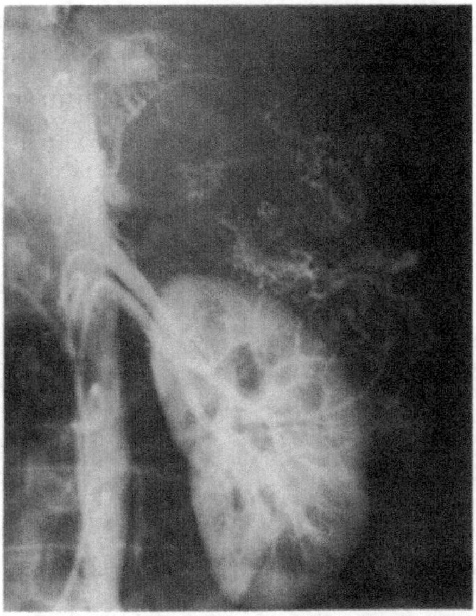

Figure 49. Left adrenal carcinoma. Simultaneous arteriograms of the left renal arteries demonstrate a large tumor in left suprarenal area with numerous neovascularities arising from middle adrenal and left renal capsular arteries.

Adrenal carcinomas are usually large with dilated feeding arteries and prominent neovascularities on arteriographic study (Figure 49). Arteriovenous shunting may be present, but tumor stain is generally absent [75]. Differentiation between an adrenal carcinoma and an upper pole hypernephroma may be difficult. A recent review of angiographic vascular patterns in 9 adrenal carcinomas and 45 renal cell carcinomas by Fritzsche *et al.* [113] indicated that differentiation between these two tumors was possible.

Other rare tumors are particularly well suited for CT imaging due to their unusual tissue components. In myelolipoma CT will demonstrate an adrenal mass with fatty components [18, 114, 115]. The differential diagnosis can include lipoma, liposarcoma, and renal angiomyolipoma. Sonographically, tumors of high fat content are markedly echogenic [116, 117]. Teratomas and dermoids will show the presence of both fat and bone within the tumor. Cystic components may also be present [86]. Rarely stromal tumors such as fibromas, neurofibromas, hemangiomas, lymphangiomas, and their sarcomatous counterparts are encountered; usually these tumors remain asymptomatic unless significant mass effects are present [117].

3.7. Miscellaneous

In neonates, particularly those subjected to stress, such as sepsis, hypoxia, maternal diabetes, or birth trauma, massive bilateral adrenal hemorrhage can occur [118]. Adrenal hemorrhage can also occur in the clinical setting of dehydration and renal vein thrombosis. Although neuroblastoma may be considered in the differential, it is much less common than hemorrhage in the neonatal period. Furthermore, there is usually prompt resolution over a period of weeks, followed by the appearance of rim-like calcification [118]. Idiopathic adrenal calcifications may be found and represent residua of previous undocumented hemorrhages. Sonographically, adrenal hemorrhage appears as either a cystic or complex suprarenal mass (Figure 50) [119].

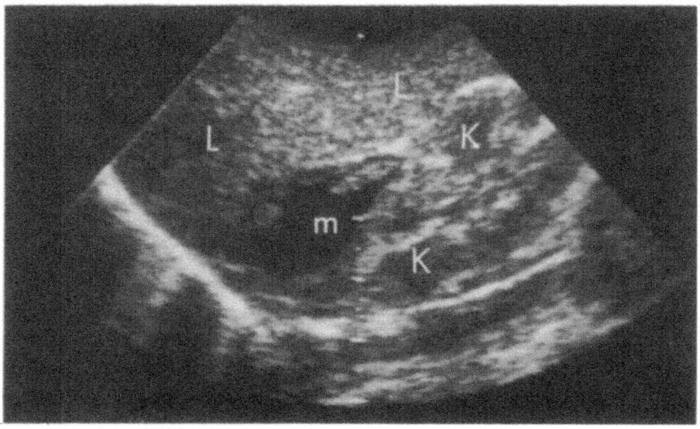

Figure 50. 3 day old female with birth asphyxia, and bilateral adrenal hemorrhages. A real-time oblique longitudinal sonogram of the right upper quadrant shows a cystic mass with scattered internal echos (M) cephalad and anterior to the right kidney (K) and posterior to the liver (L).

These masses can be confused with necrotic or cystic neuroblastomas although the clinical setting is frequently suggestive of this entity as adrenal hemorrhages gradually decrease in size, a feature not characteristic of neuroblastomas. Adrenal cysts are rare, occasionally calcified lesions that may present as mass lesions on a plain abdominal radiograph or excretory urograms, however, ultrasound examination readily defines their cystic thin-walled nature [120] and should differentiate them from 'cystic' adrenal masses which have solid components or shaggy, irregular walls. The CT scan in these instances will usually show a thin-walled lesion with a water-like density (Figure 51).

Occasionally an adrenal abscess or duplicated upper pole renal collecting system will present as a mass on plain radiographs or excretory urograms, and ultrasound helps in differentiating these from adrenal neoplasms. The characteristic CT findings of an abscess is a mass with an enhancing rim. Granulomatous lesions may also occur in association with tuberculosis or histoplasmosis. Calcifications may be noted. Lymphomatous involvement

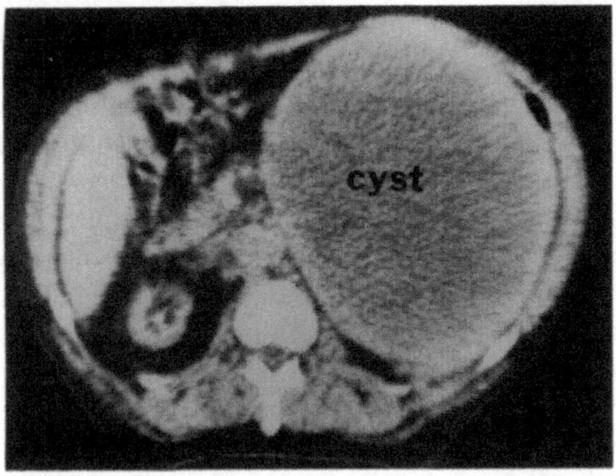

Figure 51. CT scan of a large left adrenal cyst.

of nodes in the adrenal region can be differentiated by demonstration of other areas of adenopathy.

4. CONCLUSION

The preceding discussion has dwelled at length with the modalities utilized in the localization of adrenal disease. The choice of any particular study over another must be made with the following considerations: (1) contraindications to the study, (2) radiation exposure, (3) preparation, (4) technical difficulties, (5) morbidity, (6) individual preference and (7) institutional experience. The analyses used to describe the statistical results for any given test need to be determined for each institution, for there is considerable variation from center to center. Individual bias is another important factor in the selection of a series of diagnostic tests. It is critically important that a diagnosis be clearly defined prior to attempted localization. A logical schema must first include biochemical and clinical evidence of disease. Studies of localization without such confirmatory tests cannot be adequately interpreted, can lead to diagnostic delays, increased costs, morbidity and in rare instances mortality.

As a screening modality or 'first look' test, ultrasound is best suited as a result of the lack of patient preparation and radiation exposure. This would be particularly true for large lesions such as adrenal carcinomas, neuroblastomas or pheochromocytomas. Computed tomography can be used in an identical fashion with cooperative patients, and would add improved spatial resolution. CT has been demonstrated efficacious, particularly in the study of pheochromocytomas and primary aldosteronism. Adrenal scintigraphy, if readily available, can also be used to advantage in Cushing's syndrome due to ACTH independent etiologies, in primary aldosteronism and possibly pheochromocytomas using the newer adrenal medullary imaging agents. The requirement for pretreatment with dexamethasone in the study of primary aldosteronism and hyperandrogenism, the necessity to remove such patients from intradiagnostic medications and multiple scanning procedures may not be possible in some cases. Angiography, venography and adrenal vein sampling are important in demonstrating vascular anatomy immediately prior to operative procedures and remain as tests for the definitive diagnostic confirmation of the non-invasive studies.

The development of sophisticated modalities for the localization of adrenal disease continues. The modification of present generation scanners to include real-time ultrasound and thin slice computed tomography have made marked improvements in spatial resolution. Digital acquisition of angiographic studies promises improved images as data can be optimally manipulated. The synthesis of new radiopharmaceuticals and improvements in gamma camera and computer technology continues to provide improved Nuclear Medicine approaches to adrenal gland dysfunction. Continued development of all these modalities should provide newer approaches to the localization of tumors and in particular in the evaluation of adrenal gland disorders.

ACKNOWLEDGEMENT

The authors wish to acknowledge the secretarial and editorial assistance of G. Gonzales and P. Hedlesky.

REFERENCES

1. Anderson DC, Beierwaltes WH: Adrenal Imaging in Children. In: Pediatric Nuclear Medicine, AE James, HH Wagner, RE Cook (eds) Philadelphia, W.B. Saunders, 1974, p 400.
2. Sample WF: A new technique for the evaluation of the adrenal gland with gray scale ultrasonography. Radiology 124:463–469, 1977.
3. Yeh HC: Sonography of the adrenal glands: normal glands and small masses. AJR 135:1167–1177, 1980.
4. Sample WF: Adrenal ultrasonography. Radiology 127:461–466, 1978.
5. Birnholz JC: Ultrasound imaging of adrenal mass lesions. Radiology 109:163–166, 1973.
6. Yeh HC, Mitty HA, Rose J, Wolf BS, Gabrilove JL: Ultrasonography of adrenal masses; usual features. Radiology 127:467–474, 1978.
7. Yeh HC, Mitty HA, Rose J, Wolf BS, Gabrilove JL: Ultrasonography of adrenal masses: unusual manifestations. Radiology 126:475–483, 1977.

8. Sample WF, Sarti DA: Computed tomography and gray scale ultrasonography of the adrenal gland: a comparative study. Radiology 128:377–383, 1978.
9. Pertsemlidis D, Gitlow SE: Diagnosis of pheochromocytoma by computed axial tomographic scan and other methods. N Engl J Med 299:1469, 1978.
10. Kehlet H, Blichert-Toft M, Hancke S: Comparative study of ultrasound ^{131}I-19-iodocholesterol scintigraphy, and aortography in localizing adrenal lesions. Br Med J 2:665–667, 1976.
11. Davidson JK, Morley P, Hurley GD, Holdford NGH: Adrenal venography and ultrasound in the investigation of the adrenal gland: an analysis of 58 cases. Br J Radiol 48:435–450, 1975.
12. Forsythe JR, Gosink BB, Leopold GR: Ultrasound in the evaluation of adrenal metastases. JCU 5:31–34, 1976.
13. Bernardino ME, Goldstein HM, Green B: Gray scale ultrasonography of adrenal neoplasms. AJR 130:741–744, 1978.
14. Rao AKR, Silver TM: Normal pancreas and splenic variants simulating suprarenal and renal tumors. AJR 126:530–537, 1976.
15. Berger M, Smith EH, Bartrum RJ, Holm HH, Mascatello V: False-positive diagnoses of pancreatic tail lesions caused by the colon. JCU 5:343–345, 1977.
16. Stewart BH, Bravo EL, Haaga J, Meaney TF, Tarazi R: Localization of pheochromocytoma by computed tomography. N Engl J Med 299:460–461, 1978.
17. Karsteadt N, Sagel SS, Stanley RJ, Melson GL, Levitt RG: Computed tomography of the adrenal gland. Radiology 129:723–730, 1978.
18. Korobkin M, White EA, Kressel HY, Moss AA, Montague JP: Computed tomography in the diagnosis of adrenal disease. AJR 132:231–238, 1979.
19. Bernardino ME, Lipshitz HI, Green B, Goldstein HM: Ultrasonic demonstration of inferior vena caval involvement with right adrenal gland masses. JCU 6:167–169, 1978.
20. Hounsfield GN: Computerized transverse axial scanning (tomography) I. Description of system. Br J Radiol 46:1016–1022, 1973.
21. Brasch RC: Integrated imaging of the pediatric abdomen. In: Interventional radiologic techniques: computed tomography and ultrasonography 1981. Moss AA, Goldberg HI (eds), New York, Academic Press, 1981.
22. Kirks DR, Harwood-Nash DCF: Computed tomography in pediatric radiology. Pediat Ann 9:66–76, 1980.
23. Reynes CJ, Churchill R, Mosscada R, Lobe L: Computed tomography of adrenal glands. Radiol Clin North Am 17:91–103, 1979.
24. Heitoff KB: Computerized tomography of the adrenals. J Belge Radiol 61:383–398, 1978.
25. Montagne J, Kressel HY, Korobkon M, Moss AA: Computed tomography of the normal adrenal glands. AJR 130:963–966, 1978.
26. Brownlie K, Kreel L: Computer assisted tomography of normal suprarenal glands. J Comput Assist Tomogr 2:1–10, 1978.
27. Wilms G, Baert A, Marchal G, Goddeeris P: Computed tomography of normal adrenal glands: correlative study with autopsy specimens. J Comput Assist Tomogr 3:467–469, 1979.
28. Heuck F, Buck J, Reiser U: Die gesunde und kranke Nebenniere im rontgen-computertomogramm. Radiologie 20:158–171, 1980.
29. DiGiulio W, Beierwaltes WH: Tissue localization studies of a DDD analogue. J Nucl Med 9:634–637, 1968.
30. Beierwaltes WH, Weiland DM, Yu T, Swanson D, Mosley S: Adrenal Imaging Agents: Rationale synthesis, formulation and metabolism. Semin Nucl Med 8:5–21, 1978.

31. Thrall JH, Freitas JE, Beierwaltes WH: Adrenal scintigraphy. Semin Nucl Med 8:23–41, 1978.
32. Goodman DS: Cholesterol ester metabolism. Physiol Rev 45:747–760, 1965.
33. Applegren CE: Sites of steroid hormone formation. Autoradiographic studies using labeled precursors. Acta Physiol Scand 71 Supp 301:1–107, 1967.
34. Blair RJ, Beierwaltes WH, Lieberman LM, Boyd CM, Counsell RE, Weinhold PA, Varma VM: Radiolabeled cholesterol as an adrenal scanning agent. J Nucl Med 12:176–182, 1971.
35. Beierwaltes WH, Lieberman LM, Ansari AN, Nishiyama H: Visualization of human adrenal glands *in vivo* by scintillation scanning. JAMA 216:275–277, 1971.
36. Beierwaltes WH, Sturman MF, Ryo U, Ice RD: Imaging functional nodules of the adrenal glands with ^{131}I-19-Iodocholesterol. J Nucl Med 15:246–251, 1973.
37. Basmajdian GP, Hetzel KR, Ice RD, Beierwaltes WH: Synthesis of a new adrenal cortex imaging agent 6β-^{131}I-Iodomethyl-19-norcholest-5(10)-EN-3B-ol (NP-59). J Label Cpds 11:427–434, 1975.
38. Sarkar SD, Cohen EL, Beierwaltes WH, Ice RD, Cooper R, Gold EN: A new and superior adrenal imaging agent ^{131}I-6β-iodomethyl-19-norcholesterol (NP-59) evaluation in humans. J Clin Endocrinol Metab 45:353–362, 1977.
39. Brown M, Goldstein J: Receptor-mediated control of cholesterol metabolism. Science 91:150–154, 1976.
40. Guywne J, Hess B, Roundtree R: Enhancement of steroidogenesis by serum lipoproteins in human, rats and mouse adrenal cells. Abstract #294. The Endocrine Society, June 14-16, 1970.
41. Fukushi K: Adrenal affinity and plasma lipoprotein binding of radiohalogen derivatives of cholesterol. J Label Cpd Radiopharm 16:49–51, 1979.
42. Balsubramaniam S, Goldstein JL, Faust JR, Brunschede GY, Brown MS: Lipoprotein-mediated regulation of 3-hydroxy-3-methylglutaryl co-enzyme A reductase activity and cholesterol ester metabolism in the adrenal gland of the rat. J Biol Chem 152:1771–1779, 1977.
43. Balsubramaniam S, Goldstein JL, Brown MS: Regulation of cholesterol synthesis in the rat adrenal gland through coordinate control of 3-hydroxymethylglutaryl coenzyme A synthesase and reductase activities. Proc Natl Acad Sci 74:1421–1425, 1977.
44. Valk TW, Gross MD, Freitas JE, Swanson DP, Schteingart DE, Beierwaltes WH: The relationship of serum lipids to adrenal gland uptake of 6β(^{131}I) iodomethyl-19-norcholesterol in Cushing's syndrome. J Nucl Med 21:1069–1072, 1980.
45. Fukuchi S, Nakajima K, Miura T, Haruyama K, Kida T, Saito M, Nakamura M: Comparative study of adrenal scanning agents, 6β-iodomethyl-19-norcholest-5(10)-EN-3B-ol-^{131}I (NCL-6-^{131}I) and ^{131}-19-cholesterol (CL-19-^{131}I). Jap J Nucl Med 13:775–779, 1976.
46. Ice RD, Kircos LT, Coffey JL: Radiation dosimetry of I^{131}-6β-iodomethyl-norcholesterol. J Nucl Med 17:540 (Abst.) 1976.
47. Carey JE, Thrall JH, Freitas JE, Beierwaltes WH: Absorbed dose to the human adrenals from iodomethyl-norcholesterol (I-131) 'NP-59'. J Nucl Med 20:60–62, 1979.
48. Gross MD, Grekin RJ, Brown LR, Marsh DD: The relationship of adrenal gland iodocholesterol uptake to zona glomerulosa function. J Clin Endocrinol Metab 52:612–615, 1981.
49. Kahn PC: Adrenal Arteriography. In Angiography, HL Abrams (Ed), Little Brown and Co, Boston 1971 (2nd Edition) p 929–940.
50. Symington T: Functional pathology of the human adrenal gland. ES Livingstone Co, London 1969, p 13–21.
51. Symington T: Functional pathology of the human adrenal gland. ES Livingstone Co, Lon-

don 1969, p 30.
52. Freitas JE, Thrall JH, Swanson DP, Rifazi A, Beierwaltes WH: Normal Adrenal Asymmetry-Explanation And Interpretation. J Nucl Med 19:149–154, 1978.
53. Koral KF, Sarkar SD: An operator-independent method for background subtraction in adrenal uptake measurements concise communication. J Nucl Med 18:925–928, 1977.
54. Gross MD, Freitas JE, Swanson DP, Brady T, Beierwaltes WH: The normal dexamethasone suppression adrenal scintiscan. J Nucl Med 20:1131–1135, 1979.
55. Reeder M, Koral K, Gross M, Beierwaltes W: Improved calculation of iodomethylnorcholesterol (NP-59) adrenal gland uptake. J Nucl Med Tech 8:7, 1980 (Abst.)
56. McDonald P, Hiller HG: Angiography in abdominal tumors in childhood with particular reference to neuroblastoma and Wilm's tumor. Clin Radiol 19:1–18, 1968.
57. Seldinger SI: Catheter replacement of the needle in percutaneous arteriography: a new technique. Acta Radiol 39:368, 1953.
58. Reuter SR, Blair AJ, Schteingart DE, Bookstein JJ: Adrenal venography. Radiology 89:805–814, 1967.
59. Farah J: New preformed catheter shape for right adrenal venography. Radiology 101:274, 1971.
60. Cho KJ, Freier DT, McCormick TL: Adrenal medullary disease in multiple endocrine neoplasia type II. AJR 134:23–29, 1980.
61. Dunnick NR, Doppmann JL, Mills SR, Gill JR Jr: Preoperative diagnosis and localization of aldosteronomas by measurement of corticosteroids in adrenal venous blood. Radiology 133:331–333, 1979.
62. Gold RE, Wisinger BM, Geraci AR, Heinz LM: Hypertensive crisis as a result of adrenal venography in a patient with pheochromocytoma. Radiology 102:579–580, 1972.
63. Zelch JV, Meaney TF, Belhobek GH: Radiologic approach to the patient with suspected pheochromocytoma. Radiology 111:279–284, 1974.
64. Lecky JW, Wolfman NT, Modic CW: Current concepts of adrenal angiography. Radiol Clin North Am 14:309–352, 1976.
65. Rossi P, Young IS, Panke WF: Techniques, usefulness and hazards of arteriography of pheochromatocytoma: review of 99 cases. JAMA 205(8):547–553, 1968.
66. Christenson R, Smith CW, Burko H: Arteriographic manifestations of pheochromocytoma. AJR 126:567–575, 1976.
67. Bookstein JJ, Conn J, Reuter SR: Intra-adrenal hemorrhage as a complication of adrenal venography in primary aldosteronism. Radiology 90:778–779, 1968.
68. Richie JP, Gittes RF: Carcinoma of the adrenal cortex. Cancer 45:1957–1964, 1980.
69. Wilson CB: Sellar and parasellar lesions. In: Interventional radiologic techniques: computed tomography and ultrasonography 1981. Moss AA, Goldberg HI (eds), New York, Academic Press, 1981, p 223–228.
70. Clayton GW, Holcombe JH: Tumors of the endocrine glands. In: Clinical pediatric oncology. Sutow WW, Vietti TJ, Fernbach DJ (eds), St. Louis, Mosby, 1977 p 691.
71. Schaner EG, Dunnick NR, Doppman JL: Adrenal cortical tumors with low attenuation coefficients: a pitfall in CT diagnosis. J Comput Assist Tomogr 2:11–15, 1978.
72. Long JA, Dunnick NR, Doppman JL: Non-inflammatory gas formation following embolization of adrenal carcinoma. J Comput Assist Tomogr 3:840–841, 1979.
73. Freitas JE, Gross MD, Swanson DP, Beierwaltes WH: Cost effectiveness of adrenal imaging in cushing's syndrome. J Nucl Med 20:677, 1979 (Abst.)
74. Gross MD, Valk TW, Freitas JE, Swanson DP, Schteingart DE, Beierwaltes WH: The relationship of adrenal iodomethylnorcholesterol uptake and cortisol secretion in Cushing's syndrome. J Clin Endocrinol Metab 52: , 1981.
75. Hoevels J, Ekelund L: Angiographic findings in adrenal masses. Acta Radiol Diagn

20:337–352, 1979.
76. Kreel L: Great vessels and retroperitoneal space-computed tomography In: Alimentary tract radiology, vol. 3. Margulis AE, Burhenne HJ (eds), St. Louis, CV Mosby, 1979, p 409–412.
77. Weinberger MH, Grim CE, Holifield JW, Kem DC, Ganguly A, Kramer NJ, Yun HY, Wellman H: Primary aldosteronism: Diagnosis, localization and treatment. Ann Intern Med 90:386–395, 1979.
78. Ganguly A, Pratt J, Yune H, Grim C, Weinberger M: Detection of adrenal tumors by computerized tomographic scan in endocrine hypertension. Arch Intern Med 139:589–590, 1979.
79. Linde R, Coulam C, Battino R, Rhamy R, Gerlock J, Hollifield: Localization of aldosterone-producing adenoma by computed tomography. J Clin Endocrinol Metab 49:642–645, 1979.
80. Ganguly A, Pratt J, Yune H, Grim C, Weinberger M: Computerized tomographic scanning and primary aldosteronism. N Engl J Med 301:558, 1979.
81. Freitas JE, Grekin RJ, Thrall JH, Gross MD, Swanson DP, Beierwaltes WH: Adrenal imaging with iodomethyl-norcholesterol (I-131) in primary aldosteronism. J Nucl Med 20:7–10, 1979.
82. Conn JW, Cohen EL, Herwing KR: The dexamethasone-modified adrenal scintiscan in hyporeninemic aldosteronism (tumor vs hyperplasia). A comparison with adrenal venography and adrenal venous aldosterone. J Lab Clin Med 88:841–855, 1976.
83. Seabold JE, Cohen EL, Beierwaltes WH: Adrenal imaging with ^{131}I-19-Iodocholesterol in the diagnostic evaluation of patients with aldosteronism. J Clin Endocrinol Metab 42:41–51, 1976.
84. Gross MD, Freitas JE, Swanson DP, Beierwaltes WH: Dexamethasone suppression (DS) adrenal scintigraphy in hyperandrogenism. J Nucl Med 21:12–17, 1981.
85. Fernbach DS, Williams TE, Donaldson MH: Neuroblastoma. In: Clinical pediatric oncology. Sutow WW, Vietti TJ, Fernbach DJ (eds), St. Louis, CV Mosby 1977, p 506–537.
86. Berger PE, Juhn JP, Munschauer RW: Computed tomography and ultrasound in the diagnosis and management of neuroblastoma. Radiology 128:663–667, 1978.
87. Gooding CA: Pediatric imaging: quo vadis? In: Computed tomography ultrasound, and x-ray: an integrated approach. Moss AA, Goldberg HI (eds), New York, Academic Press 1980, p 403.
88. Stackpole RH, Melicow MM, Uson AC: Pheochromocytoma in children. Report of 9 cases and review of the first 100 published cases with follow-up studies. J Pediatr 63:315–330, 1963.
89. Weber AL, Janower ML, Griscom NT: Radiologic and clinical evaluation of pheochromocytoma in children: report of 6 cases. Radiology 88:117–123, 1967.
90. Cornell SH: Pheochromocytomas of the lumbar sympathetic chain demonstrated by angiography. AJR 115:175–178, 1972.
91. Reuter SR, Talner LB, Atkin T: The importance of subtraction in the angiographic evaluation of extra-adrenal pheochromocytomas. AJR 117:128–131, 1973.
92. Sipple JH: The association of pheochromocytoma with carcinoma of the thyroid gland. Am J Med 31:163–166, 1961.
93. Steiner AL, Goodman AD, Powers SR: Study of a kindred with pheochromocytoma, medullary thyroid carcinoma, hyperparathyroidism and Cushing's disease: multiple endocrine neoplasia, type II. Medicine 47:371–409, 1968.
94. Bowerman RA, Silver TM, Jaffe MH, Stuck KJ, Hinerman DL: Sonographic spectrum of adrenal pheochromocytomas. Presented at the 81st Annual Meeting of the American Roentgen Ray Society, San Francisco, Cal., March 23–27, 1981.

95. Laursen K, Damgaard-Pedersen K: CT for pheochromocytoma diagnosis. AJR 134:277–280, 1980.
96. Thomas JL, Bernardino ME, Samaan NA, Hickey RC: CT of pheochromocytoma. AJR 135:477–482, 1980.
97. Joyce DA: Localization of pheochromocytoma by computerized axial tomography. Med J Aust 1:540–541, 1980.
98. Johnson LW, Ciccantelli MJ: A non-invasive approach to the diagnosis of pheochromocytoma. Wis Med J 78:30–31, 1979.
99. Ganguly A, Henry DP, Yune HY: Diagnosis and localization of pheochromocytoma. Am J Med 67:21–25, 1979.
100. Hessel SJ, Adams DF, Abrams HL: Complications of angiography. Radiology 138:273–281, 1981.
101. Carney JA, Sizemore GW, Tyce GM: Bilateral adrenal medullary hyperplasia in multiple endocrine neoplasia, type 2. The precursor of bilateral pheochromocytoma. Mayo Clin Proc 50:3–10, 1975.
102. Bradley EL, Bishop B: Non-invasive localization of pheochromocytomas. Am Surg 44:440–444, 1978.
103. Hahn LC, Nadel NS, Bernstein NM, Satya KL: Localization of pheochromocytoma by computerized axial tomography. J Urol 120:349–351, 1978.
104. Harrison TS, Freier DT: Pitfalls in the technique and interpretation of regional venous sampling for localizing pheochromocytoma. Surg Clin North Am 54:339–347, 1974.
105. Baltaxe HA, Levin DC, Imperato JL: The angiographic demonstration of partially infarcted pheochromocytomas of the adrenal gland. AJR 119:793–795, 1973.
106. Sturman MF, Moses DC, Beierwaltes WH, Harrison TS, Ice RD, Dorr PR: Radiocholesterol adrenal images for the localization of pheochromo cytoma. Surg Gynecol Obstet 138:177–180, 1974.
107. Morales JO, Beierwaltes WH, Counsell RE: The concentration of radioactivity from labelled epinephrine and precursors in the dog adrenal medulla. J Nucl Med 8:800–809, 1967.
108. Wieland DM, Braun LE, Tobes ML: Imaging primate adrenal medullae with ^{123}I- and ^{131}I-meta-iodobenzylguanidine. J Nucl Med 22:353–364, 1981.
109. Gross MD, Frager M, Valk T, Sisson J, Kline R, Swanson D, Wieland D, Beierwaltes WH: Localization of pheochromocytomas with I-131-Iodobenzylguanidine (I-131-mIBG). Clin Res 29:292A, 1981.
110. Dunnick NR, Doppman JL, Geelhoed GW: Intravenous extension of endocrine tumors. AJR 135:471–476, 1980.
111. Gross MD, Thrall JH, Beierwaltes WH: The adrenal scan: A current status report on radiotracers, dosimetry and clinical utility. In Nuclear Medicine Annual 1980: LM Freeman, HS Weissman (eds) Raven Press, New York 1980, p 163.
112. Gyepes MT, Lindstrom R, Merten D, Goller D, Lachman R, Lippe B: Hormonally active adrenal adenomas and carcinomas in children. Am Radiol 20(1):123–131, 1976.
113. Fritzsche P, Andersen C, Cahill P: Vascular specificity in differentiating adrenal carcinoma from renal cell carcinoma. Radiology 125:113–117, 1977.
114. Behan M, Martin EC, Muecke EC, Kazam E: Myelolipoma of the adrenal: two cases with ultrasound and CT findings. AJR 129:993–996, 1977.
115. Fink DW, Wurtzebach LR: Symptomatic myelolipoma of the adrenal. Radiology 134:451–452, 1980.
116. Scheible W, Ellenbogen PH, Leopold GR, Siao NT: Lipomatous tumors of the kidney and adrenal: apparent echogenic specificity. Radiology 129:153–156, 1978.
117. Robbins SL: Pathologic basis of disease. Philadelphia, WB Saunders, 1974, p 1314.

118. Swischuk LE: Radiology of the newborn and young infant. Baltimore, Williams and Wilkins, 1973, p 393.
119. Mittelstaedt CA, Volberg FM, Merten DF, Brill PW: The sonographic diagnosis of neonatal adrenal hemorrhage. Radiology 131:453–457, 1979.
120. Gross MD, Freitas JE, Silver TM: Documentation of adrenal cyst by adrenal scanning techniques. J Nucl Med 19:1092, 1978.

8. The Surgical Management of Tumors of the Adrenal Gland

WILLIAM P. TUNELL

INTRODUCTION

Except for neuroblastoma, tumors of the adrenal gland are rare in childhood. Of necessity, adult experience must be transposed to children for maximum understanding of the surgical management of these adrenal neoplasms; nevertheless, children do present unique differences in adrenal pathology and endocrinology, in tumor localization, and in operative approach. These significant features are emphasized in this paper. The text is divided into two sections. The first considers general aspects of surgical management of tumors of the adrenal glands; anatomy, preoperative identification and localization of tumors, incision and exposure, and perioperative care. The second section considers specific tumors, emphasizing the unique features of their diagnosis and operative care. Pheochromocytoma is not discussed in this chapter.

1. GENERAL CONSIDERATIONS

The unifying feature of surgical procedures is the attempted safe and successful anatomic alteration of some structures of the body. Considerations of universal importance in surgical practice are anatomy, exposure, operative technique and perioperative patient management. These principles are germane to the surgical management of adrenal tumors and are discussed in this section.

The adrenal glands develop bilaterally as unitary and capsulated organs of distinct embryonic tissues, the cortex made up of mesoderm and the medulla of ectoderm. At birth, each lies medial to the upper pole of its respective kidney. In the perinatal period, the gland is relatively large and vascular. Hemorrhage into the gland, especially prevalent with difficult deliveries,

G. Bennett Humphrey et al. (eds), Adrenal and Endocrine Tumors in Children.

predisposes to subsequent calcifications and/or cyst formation. Either may ultimately require differentiation from an adrenal neoplasm.

The right adrenal is pyramidal in shape; the left more crescentric. They are indented by the adjacent superior medial curve of the kidney. Enveloping pseudocapsules are incomplete and consist of condensed surrounding fat and connective tissue [1]. The arterial supply is typically from an enveloping arcade, supplied by three adrenal arteries; they are the superior, a branch of the inferior phrenic, the middle from the aorta, and the inferior from the renal artery. Of greater importance to successful adrenal surgery, is the venous egress. Characteristically, a single adrenal vein arises from the inferior portion of the gland; the right vein is short and enters the vena cava, the left is somewhat longer and joins the left renal vein. The right adrenal gland lies posterior to the vena cava medially and to the duodenum laterally. It abuts the kidney inferiorly and the diaphragm and liver superiorly and posteriorly. The fusiform left gland adjoins the diaphragm and pleura posterior superiorly. Anteriorly lie the stomach, pancreas and spleen.

Anatomic variations are important in determining sensible treatment for specific adrenal lesions. Agenesis is uncommon and usually associated with ipsilateral renal agenesis. Fused kidneys may herald fused adrenal glands, but pelvic or ectopic kidneys and crossed renal ectopia typically have normally situated adrenal glands. Accessory adrenal glands are rare; more common is extra adrenal chromaffin (medullary) tissue along the sympathetic trunk of the thorax and especially the abdomen. Of greatest prevalence and importance is the chromaffin tissue (organ of Zuckerkandl) lying anterior along the abdominal aorta at the level of the inferior mesenteric artery. Extra adrenal cortical tissue, common in neonates, usually involutes and disappears but may persist in the area from normal gland caudally to the gonad.

Preoperative indication and evaluation of adrenal tumors are not the subject of this paper. It is enough to say adrenal scanning and especially abdominal computed tomography have provided enhanced localization of adrenal tumors and tissue which has been helpful to all surgeons [2]. Accurate localization of adrenal tumors permits unilateral flank or posterior exposure of the adrenal glands. Nevertheless, the transabdominal approach to the adrenal gland continues to predominate in childhood for two important reasons. In most children, pulmonary status, coexisting disease, and abdominal wall thickness are not likely to impede safe and adequate exposure transabdominally; and even with accurate preoperative localization the preponderance of childhood adrenal tumors mandates bilateral adrenal exploration and thorough intra-abdominal exploration. The abdomen may be entered through either an upper midline or transverse abdominal incision. The author prefers a flattened chevron transverse incision, exposing the left adrenal gland by mobilizing the spleen and pancreas anteriorly and medially. The colon is reflected inferiorly and medially and the duodenum is mobilized to the left (midline) to expose the right adrenal. In this instance the vena cava may need to be gently retracted medially with special care taken not to injure the right adrenal vein on its short course from inferior medial gland to vena cava. At dissection, meticulous attention is paid to controlling arterial and particularly venous blood supply of the adrenal gland. Adjacent major vessels are identified and protected; if injured, they are either anatomically repaired or ablated. Incomplete adrenal excision, to be avoided in most situations, is best prevented by initial mobilization of the superior aspect of the adrenal gland with dissection and excision preceeding caudally.

Most operations for adrenal tumors are on elective basis. In addition to specifying the preparation mandated by the particular tumor, certain general measures will be helpful in conducting a safe operation. The skin should be prepared by preoperative cleansing; the bowel should be emptied and decompressed prior to surgery, especially if a transabdominal exploration is planned.

Complications of adrenal surgery include hemorrhage, wound infection and poor healing. The two latter complications are less frequent in children than adults. Endocrinopathies may persist following adrenalectomy for Cushing's Disease. These will be discussed below.

1.1. Adrenal cortical tumors

Virilizing tumors. Most infants and children with virilization have congenital adrenal hyperplasia. The incidence of the rare virilizing tumors is uncertain. However, experience at a major children's hospital suggests that such a tumor ought to be considered and evaluated in the investigation of any infant or child with virilization [3]. The preferred treatment is removal if possible. Most tumors will be carcinomas with few cures and high disease mortality.

Cushing's syndrome. Unlike adults, most children with Cushing's Syndrome have an adrenal cortical tumor. Presenting symptoms resemble those of patients who have the syndrome on the basis of adrenal hyperplasia. Especially common are obesity, hirsutism, plethoric facies and acne. Accurate diagnosis is now invariably determined preoperatively by the endocrinologist. Biochemical analysis and manipulation is standardized and reliable. Abdominal computed tomography has been helpful in defining adrenal gland size and configuration and in localizing adrenal cortical tumors. Abdominal ultrasound can identify tumors of sufficient size and is particularly useful in establishing adrenal size and possible hypertrophy.

The surgical procedure, for reasons previously described, would utilize the abdominal approach in children. If an adenoma has been positively diagnosed and localized, the posterior approach or flank approach may be employed [4]. In uncertain cases, and with all suspected carcinomas, transabdominal exposure provides access to both adrenal glands and to the entire abdominal cavity. Pathologic confirmation of carcinoma while the operation is in progress is frequently not practical. Unfortunately, the best evidence of malignancy often is metastatic disease or extension of the tumor through the capsule and into adjacent organs. Adrenalectomy is the treatment of choice for tumor; in the event of carcinoma, excision of contiguous organs may also be required. Exogenous steroid is administered during the operative procedure [5]. This should be continued postoperatively and tapered as the patient's endocrinologic condition permits.

Recurrence of adrenal tumor following excision may be identified by hormone excretion assay. Recent techniques of adrenal scanning, particularly using ^{131}I-6-B-Iodomethyl-19-Norcholesterol have identified the site of recurrence with near anatomic accuracy [5]. This localization may enhance the possibility of re-exploration and excision if that is practical.

1.2. Cushing's Disease

The treatment of Cushing's Disease (pituitary tumor with excess ACTH production) is controversial at the present time. Historically, most children with Cushing's Disease have had bilateral adrenalectomy to provide prompt remission of their symptomatology. The high occurrence rate of postoperative pituitary tumors (Nelson's Syndrome) makes this treatment questionable [6]. Now alternate techniques including trans-sphenoidal microdissection, pituitary radiotherapy and chemotherapy are being investigated; and there are reports suggesting the efficacy of adrenal autotransplantation following removal for hyperplasia [7, 8].

1.3. Aldosteronism

An aldosterone producing adenoma of the adrenal cortex is one cause of hypersecretion of aldosterone. Such a functioning adenoma is the only cause for which surgical extirpation is clearly indicated. Diagnosis is dependent on the demonstration of high aldosterone excretion and of low plasma renin activity in a patient with hypertension and hypokalemia. Adenomas may be responsible for symptoms in up to 70% of patients with primary aldosteronism [9]. Girls predominate among those patients with adenomas, boys among those with hyperplasia. 60% of adenomas occur in the left adrenal gland. Localization of adrenal adenomas has been enhanced by adrenal vein sampling for aldosterone and by abdominal computed tomography.

Pediatric experience with aldosterone producing adenomas is scant but suggests that accurate localization can be accomplished preoperatively. In the event of such localization, a flank or posterior incision may be utilized for adrenalectomy. An anterior abdominal approach is indicated when bilateral adenomas are suspected or have been demonstrated. Spironolactone should be administered preoperatively in an attempt to render the patient normotensive and to normalize the patient's electrolytes. This effect of spironolactone enhances the safety of surgery and, in addition, identifies patients most likely to be cured by adrenalectomy. Excision of the adrenal gland containing the adenoma is the operative procedure of choice. Bilateral adenomas may require adrenalectomy and contralateral subtotal gland excision. In that event, postoperative steroid replacement may be necessary.

1.4. Non-functioning tumors, cysts and tumor-like lesions

Most adrenal tumors present with evidence of endocrinologic abnormality. Non-functioning tumors of the adrenal gland, either in the cortex or medulla, are rare. Presumably because of a lack of clinical signs, non-functioning tumors tend to be larger when diagnosis is made. Included in the possible cell types are adenoma and carcinoma of the cortex, ganglioneuroma of the medulla and hamartomas. None are common in children. If encountered, treatment is surgical removal.

Pseudocysts of the adrenal gland occuring in infancy and childhood have been reported [10]. An interesting presentation is that of an abdominal mass causing intestinal obstruction.

This has been reported in several infants and is presumed to be secondary to enteric displacement by the large cystic mass. These cysts may have crescentric calcification and are believed to be secondary to neonatal adrenal hemorrhage. Treatment is surgical removal, both for diagnosis and treatment. In some patients adrenal calcification clearly is secondary to adrenal hemorrhage. In most, the cause of a unilateral adrenal calcification is uncertain and the possibility of neuroblastoma a concern. Precise diagnosis requires gland removal. In most instances bilateral gland calcification may be presumed secondary to adrenal hemorrhage.

Tumor metastases to the adrenal gland are rare in children, presumably because the common offending cancers – breast, GI tract and lung – are infrequent in childhood. Metastases occasionally occur from a contralateral neuroblastoma.

REFERENCES

1. Hollinshead WH: Anatomy for surgeons, New York, Harper & Rowen 1971.
2. Dunnick NR, Schaner EG, Doppman JL, et al.: Computed tomography in adrenal tumors, AJR 132:43–46, 1979.

3. Burrington JD, Stephens CA: Virilizing tumors of the adrenal gland in childhood: Report of eight cases, J Pediatr Surg 4:291–302, 1969.
4. Scott HW, Foster JH, Rhamy RK, et al.: Surgical management of adrenocortical tumors with Cushing's Syndrome, Ann Surg 173:892–906, 1971.
5. Seabold JE, Haynie TP, DeAsis DN: Detection of metastatic adrenal carcinoma using ^{131}I-6-B-Iodomethyl-19-Norcholesterol total body scans, J Clin Endocrinol Metab 45:788–797, 1977.
6. McArthur RG, Hayles AB, Salassa RN: Childhood Cushing's Disease: Results of bilateral adrenalectomy. J Pediatr 95:214–219, 1979.
7. Kaplan NM, Shires GT: Apparent cure of Cushing's Disease by bilateral adrenalectomy and autotransplantation, Am J Med 53:377–380, 1972.
8. Hardy JD: Surgical management of Cushing's Syndrome with emphasis on adrenal autotransplantation, Ann Surg 188:290–307, 1978.
9. Audo SP, Brennan MF, Gill JR, Jr.: Evaluation of the surgical management of primary aldosteronism, Ann Surg 191:1–7, 1978.
10. VandeWater JM, Fonkalsrud EW: Adrenal cysts in infancy, Surgery 60:1267–1270, 1966.

9. Pathologic Features of Childhood Adrenocortical Tumors

R. PAUL WEATHERBY and J. AIDAN CARNEY

Excluding nonfunctioning adenomas, neoplasms of the adrenal cortex are rare. Although most commonly found in women between the ages of 20 and 50 years, the tumors may occur in both sexes and in patients of any age; but are particularly rare in children. In childhood, most of these neoplasms are hormone-secreting, as manifested by virilization, Cushing's syndrome, aldosteronism, or feminization (in decreasing order of frequency).

Because of the rarity of childhood adrenocortical tumors, experience with them is limited, even at large institutions. Recent reports on the neoplasms have not separated cases occurring in children from those in adults; in such reports, it is often not possible to determine whether the clinical behavior of the childhood tumors is similar to that of the adult group.

In this study, we will review the Mayo Clinic experience with 22 cases of adrenocortical tumors in children and discuss the pathologic features of these neoplasms as they relate to clinical manifestations and prognosis.

1. PATIENTS AND METHODS

Between 1907 and 1980, adrenocortical tumors were diagnosed in 28 Mayo Clinic patients who were age 16 years or younger. Some of these patients were included in previous reports [1, 2]. Two patients who died from their disease were excluded from this study because the adrenocortical carcinoma was diagnosed clinically. Two other patients were excluded because their adrenocortical tumors were a component of a multiple endocrine neoplasia syndrome. One patient who underwent operation elsewhere and in whom the diagnosis of adrenocortical carcinoma was confirmed histologically at the Mayo Clinic was excluded because the tissue was no longer available for our review; this patient also died from her tumor. Another patient, who initially had Cushing's syndrome, was excluded because review

G. Bennett Humphrey et al. (eds), Adrenal and Endocrine Tumors in Children.

of the case suggested that the tumor (initially interpreted as a carcinoma arising in an accessory adrenal gland) was probably a functioning islet-cell tumor originating in the tail of the pancreas. The remaining 22 patients with surgically proved adrenocortical tumors form the basis of this study. The clinical and pathologic findings in these cases were correlated with the clinical outcome and follow-up data.

1.1. Clinical material

Sex and age. Nineteen patients (86 %) were female and three were male. The age of patients at the time of detection of the tumor ranged from 1 3/12 to 16 years (mean, 7.1 years).

Symptoms and signs. Twenty patients (91 %) had symptoms related to adrenocortical hyperfunction, but 'pure' syndromes were relatively uncommon (Table 1). In 14 patients (64 %), the symptoms commenced before age 5 years; symptoms preceded the first birthday in 4 patients, but no patient was examined before the age of 1 year. The duration of symptoms before diagnosis ranged from 2 months to 10 years (mean, 18 months). In 10 patients, symptoms had been present for 6 months or less.

Table 1. Predominant clinical syndromes at time of diagnosis.

Syndrome	No. of patients	
Virilization		12
'Pure' virilization	4	
Virilization + Cushing's	2	
Virilization + feminization	5	
Virilization + feminization + Cushing's	1	
Cushing's syndrome		5
With hirsutism	5	
With hirsutism and other features of virilization	3	
Aldosteronism		2
Feminization (pure)		1
Hypoglycemia		1
Pain due to nonfunctioning metastases		1
Total		22

Virilization, usually manifested by the appearance of public hair and clitoral enlargement, was the outstanding clinical feature in 12 patients (55 %). Facial acne and generalized hirsutism were also frequently noted. Additionally, eight patients in this group had minor features suggestive of estrogen stimulation (breast development, isosexual precocious puberty), glucocorticoid excess (obesity, striae, cushingoid facies), or both.

The classic appearance of Cushing's syndrome was present in five patients (23%), all of whom exhibited some degree of virilism as well (public, axillary, facial, or generalized hirsitusm). Other signs of virilization (clitoral enlargement, deepened voice, male escutcheon) were present in three of these patients.

Symptoms due to severe hypertension led to the evaluation of the two patients with aldosteronomas. Hypertension was also present in two patients with Cushing's syndrome and in one patient whose initial symptoms were virilization and mild features of Cushing's syndrome.

Of the remaining three patients, at the time of initial examination one had feminization, one had hypoglycemia, and one had hip pain due to bony metastasis. An abdominal mass was palpable in only four patients (18%).

1.2. Laboratory and roentgenographic studies

Because the period of the study spanned over 70 years, the laboratory and roentgenographic studies used for detection of the neoplasms inevitably varied in number and sophistication. Among the laboratory results obtained were the following: twenty-four-hour urinary 17-ketosteroid levels were increased in 14 of 17 patients (82%); urinary 17-ketosteroid output was not suppressed after administration of dexamethasone sodium phosphate (in dosages equivalent to 8 mg/24 h in adults) in 9 of 10 patients (90%). Five patients studied more recently had plasma cortisol levels that lacked the normal diurnal rhythm, and two patients (one with aldosteronism and one with hypoglycemia) had normal levels of cortisol. A calcified mass was visible in plain abdominal roentgenograms in three patients. Results of excretory urography showed an adrenal mass in three patients and inferior displacement of the kidney in four patients; however, this test disclosed no abnormality in nine patients. Presently available techniques for evaluation of adrenocortical tumors in children will be discussed elsewhere in this volume [3].

1.3. Treatment

All patients underwent a surgical procedure at the Mayo Clinic. Twenty-one were treated by surgical excision of the tumor along with all or part of the involved adrenal gland; one patient had only biopsy of the tumor. Lesions that were thought by the surgeon to be malignant were removed by wide excision, and biopsy specimens were taken from adjacent lymph nodes. Nineteen patients were treated with corticosteroids preoperatively and postoperatively. No patient received either irradiation or chemotherapy.

2. PATHOLOGIC FINDINGS

Twelve of the tumors were located in the right and 10 in the left adrenal gland. Using the criteria of Heinbecker *et al.* [29], 13 were interpreted as adrenocortical adenomas and 9 as adrenocortical carcinomas. Small size, encapsulation, lack of necrosis, and paucity of mitoses were features of adenoma. Large size, gross lobulation, necrosis, local invasion, and frequent mitoses (including atypical ones) were features of carcinoma. In all tumors, the number of mitoses was determined by counting the number of division figures in at least 50 high-power (400 ×) fields (HPF) in the most mitotically active area of the tumor; the counts were expressed as the number of mitoses per 20 HPF.

2.1. Adenomas

Gross appearance. The 13 adenomas varied from 4.0 to 8.5 cm in greatest dimension (mean, 6.0 cm) and ranged in weight from 30 to 122 g (Table 2). All were encapsulated, ovoid or spherical, solitary tumors. They were usually uniform in color and appeared yellow-red, mahogany brown, or yellow. The cut surface of the tumor was generally smooth or finely nodular (Figure 1), but three tumors each exhibited a coarsely bosselated or lobulated appearance (Figure 2). Three adenomas contained gross calcium deposits, massive

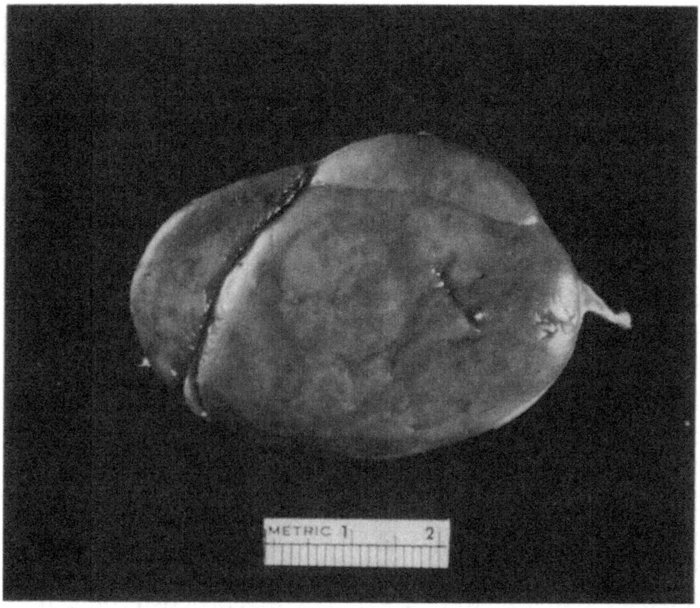

Figure 1. Encapsulated adrenocortical adenoma with smooth, relatively uniform cut surface. Extratumoral adrenal cortex to right of tumor is atrophic.

Table 2. Major pathologic features and clinical outcome in 22 childhood adrenocortical tumors.

Pt. No.	Sex	Age, yr.	Predominant clinical syndrome	Tumor weight, g	Necrosis	Capsular or vascular invasion	Nuclear pleo-morphism	Mitoses per 20 HPF*	Follow-up Status	Follow-up Years
Adenomas										
1	F	16	Virilization	80	–	–	–	Occ	Alive	12
2	F	3 6/12	Virilization	50	–	–	±	Occ	Alive	19
3	F	5 9/12	Virilization	61	–	–	–	0	Alive	7
4	M	1 3/12	Virilization	40	–	–	–	Occ	Alive	26
5	F	3 6/12	Virilization	36	–	–	–	Rare	Alive	24
6	F	1 6/12	Virilization	60	–	–	2+	Rare	Alive	1
7	F	1 11/12	Virilization	45	–	–	–	Occ	Alive	35
8	F	1 5/12	Cushing's	35	–	–	+	Rare	Alive	27
9	F	9 6/12	Cushing's	36	–	–	–	Rare	Alive	42
10	F	5 8/12	Cushing's	122	–	–	–	0	Alive	20
11	F	16	Aldosteronism	30	–	–	–	0	Alive	13
12	F	16	Aldosteronism	75	–	–	–	Occ	Alive	7
13	M	5 11/12	Feminization	30	+, old	–	–	0	Alive	5.5
Carcinomas										
14	F	6 4/12	Virilization	5	–	–	–	1.5 (A)	Alive	32
15	F	1 8/12	Virilization	40	+	–	2+	2 (A)	Alive	16
16	F	5	Virilization	12	–	–	+	1.5	Alive	5
17	F	2 9/12	Virilization	250	+	+	3+	4(A)	Alive	3
18	F	3 6/12	Virilization	460	+	+	2+	3 (A)	Died	5/12
19	F	16	Cushing's	250	+	+	–	7 (A)	Died	7/12
20	F	1 3/12	Cushing's	190	–	–	–	2	Alive	34
21	F	16	Hypoglycemia	1,700	+	+	–	8	Died	1
22	M	14	Nonfunctioning	80	+	+†	3+	10 (A)	Died	2/12

* HPF = high-power field; Occ = occasional; (A) = atypical mitotic figures present.
† = metastases present at diagnosis as well.

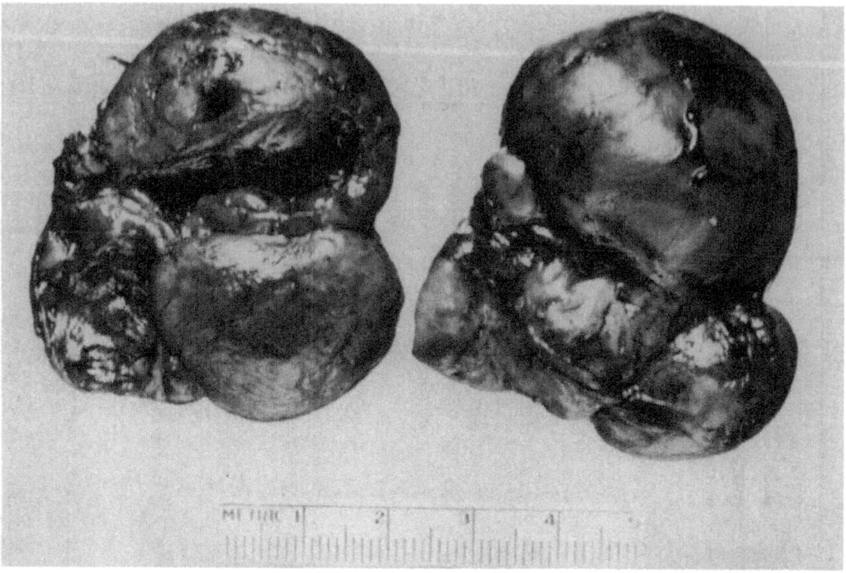

Figure 2. Adrenocortical adenoma (*left*, cut surface; *right*, external surface), showing gross lobulation.

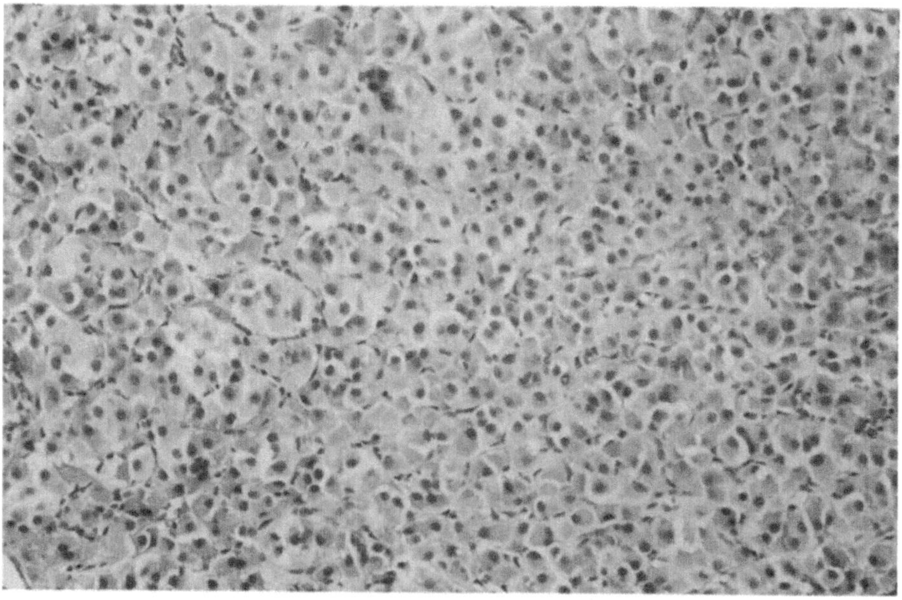

Figure 3. Virilizing adrenocortical adenoma, composed of cells with eosinophilic cytoplasm reminiscent of compact cells of normal zona reticularis. Note arrangement of cells in small alveolar clusters, variation in cell size, relatively uniform nuclei, and occasional multinucleated cells. (Hematoxylin and eosin; × 160.).

in one. Cystic areas were found in three tumors. Necrosis was not evident in any of the adenomas, but one had a hemorrhagic cut surface.

Microscopic appearance. Although all of the adenomas were composed of adrenocortical-like cells, they exhibited a variety of morphologic patterns. Typically, oval or polygonal cells with eosinophilic cytoplasm (resembling the compact cells of the normal zona reticularis) (Figure 3) and larger cells with clear or vacuolated cytoplasm (similar to the clear cells of the zona fasciculata) (Figure 4) were present. In 11 cases, however, compact cells

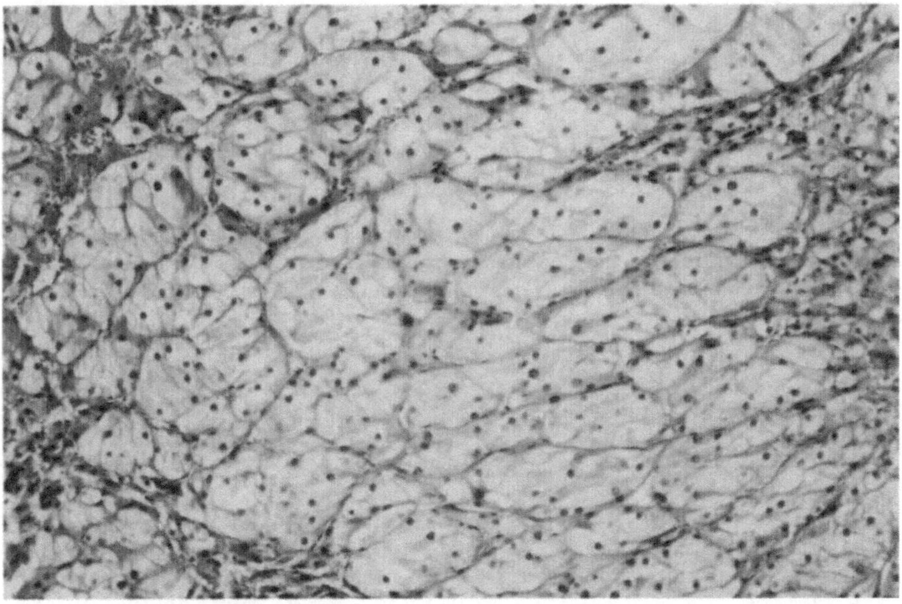

Figure 4. Adrenocortical adenoma showing small clusters and cords of cells with small uniform nuclei and abundant vacuolated cytoplasm, resembling clear cells of normal zona fasciculata. Other areas of tumor were similar to tumor shown in Figure 3. (Hematoxylin and eosin; ×100.)

were generally either the sole (six cases) or the predominant (five cases) cell type; in only two cases were clear cells the predominant component of the tumor. All tumors exhibited some variation in cell size, with a tendency toward cells that were larger than normal adrenocortical cells. One tumor was primarily composed of huge cells with eosinophilic cytoplasm and eccentric nuclei, which resembled ganglion cells (Figure 5), and two others exhibited cells that were smaller than normal adrenocortical cells. The cells were usually arranged in small or large alveolar clusters (Figure 3, 4, and 6), but three tumors exhibited a diffuse, sheet-like pattern of growth. Almost

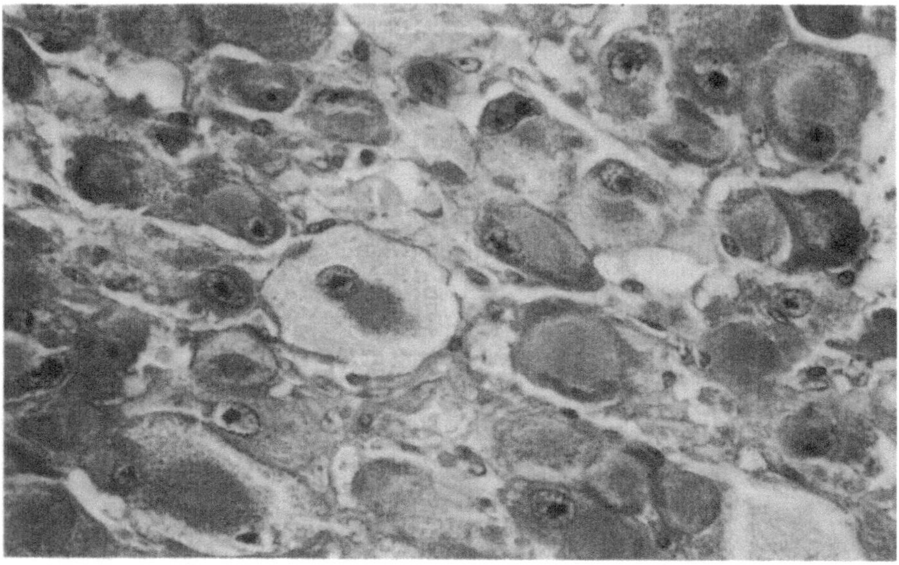

Figure 5. Huge cells with abundant granular, acidophilic cytoplasm and enlarged nuclei with prominent nucleoli from adrenocortical adenoma that caused Cushing's syndrome. Many cells superficially resemble ganglion cells. (Hematoxylin and eosin; ×400.)

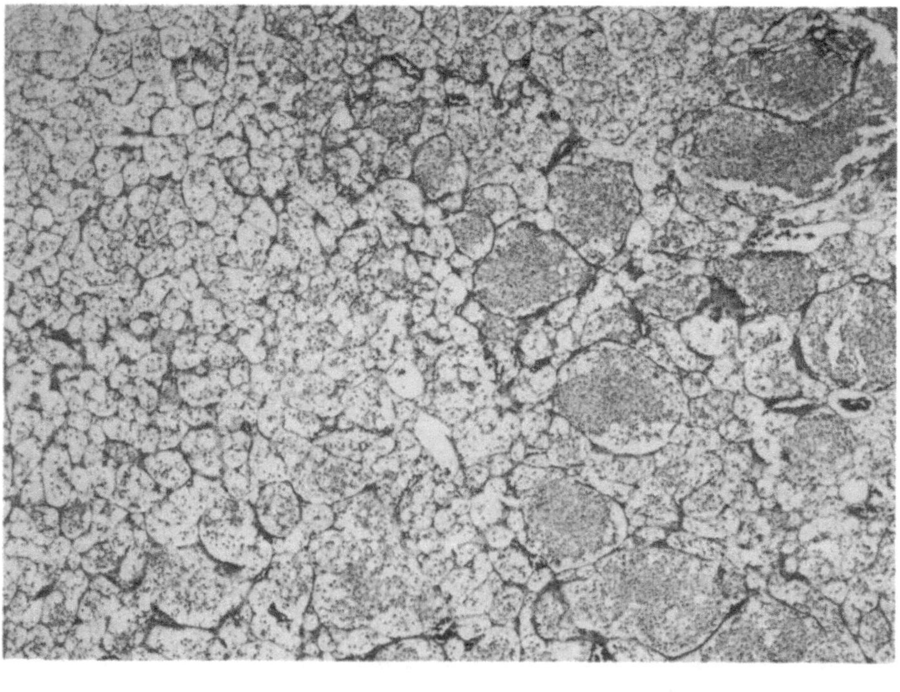

Figure 6. Adrenocortical adenoma that caused Cushing's syndrome. Large alveolar clusters of compact-type cells merge with smaller clusters of clear cells. (Hematoxylin and eosin; ×40.)

half of the tumors had focal areas in which the cells assumed a trabecular or ribbon-like arrangement; in two tumors, both in patients with aldosteronism, this was the predominant pattern. Clusters or sheets of tumor cells were frequently separated by thin-walled vascular sinusoids. In no adenoma was there microscopic evidence of vascular or capsular invasion.

The tumor nuclei were similar to or somewhat larger than normal adrenocortical cell nuclei; nucleoli were usually inconspicuous. The nuclear chromatin was typically smooth or finely stippled. Mitotic activity was minimal or absent in all of the adenomas. Two mitotic figures were seldom encountered in 50 contiguous HPF. Because the cells generally tended to be large, the ratio of nucleus to cytoplasm was low or intermediate. Several adenomas contained occasional enlarged nuclei, but only 3 of the 13 tumors exhibited substantial nuclear atypia (defined as the presence of cells with an abnormally high ratio of nucleus to cytoplasm or prominent variation in size and shape of hyperchromatic nuclei) [4]. Although nuclear pleomorphism was sometimes worrisome (Figure 7), in the absence of appreciable mitotic activity, necrosis, and invasion, we did not consider this feature sufficient to warrant a morphologic diagnosis of carcinoma. This particular nuclear atypicality is probably degenerative in origin. Occasional multinucleated tumor cells were found in more than half of the adenomas.

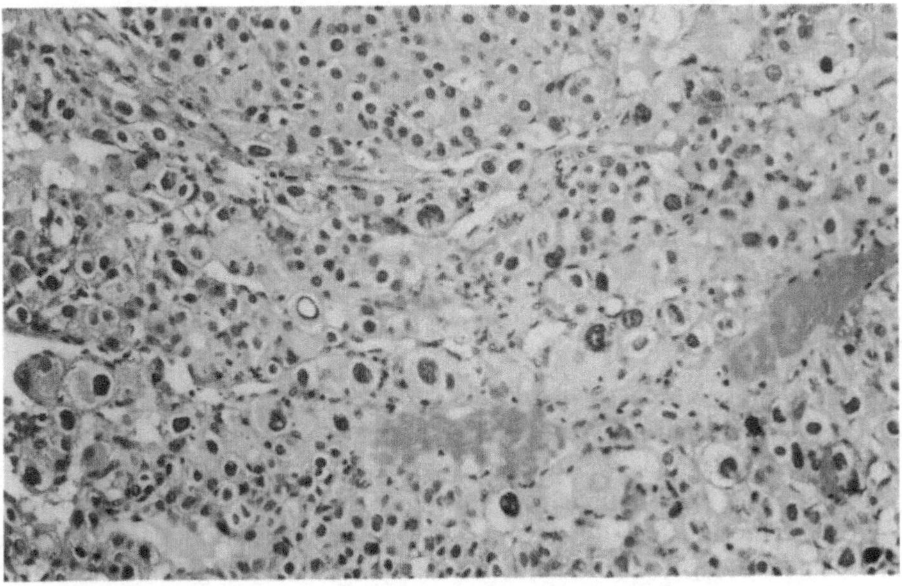

Figure 7. Nuclear pleomorphism in adrenocortical adenoma. In the absence of mitotic activity, this should not be considered as evidence of malignant lesion. Many degenerating nuclei are present. (Hematoxylin and eosin; × 160.)

Many of the tumors had a variety of secondary degenerative changes. Edema and hyalinization of the stroma were common; one case exhibited unusual stromal fibrosis that resulted in a small alveolar pattern. Calcification was noted in three tumors, two of which showed metaplastic bone formation; in these two tumors were many areas of 'psammomatous' calcification, apparently resulting from death of isolated individual cells. Focal lymphocytic infiltration was present in four of the tumors and prominent in one. Areas of fatty change were occasionally seen within the tumors; in one, myelolipomatous change (fat and hematopoietic elements) was observed (Figure 8). Foci of microcystic degeneration were present in three of the tumors. Isolated pyknotic and degenerating nuclei were observed in the majority of the adenomas.

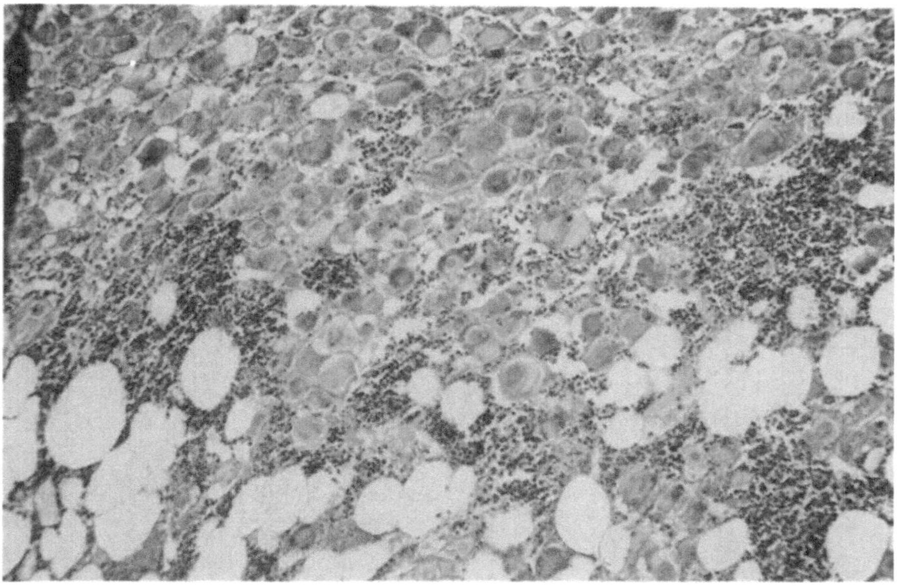

Figure 8. Myelolipomatous change in adrenocortical adenoma. Interspersed among tumor cells are fat cells and myeloid elements. (Hematoxylin and eosin; × 100.)

Extratumoral cortex was available for review in 12 of the cases. In nine, it was atrophic, including six of seven patients with virilization, the two patients with Cushing's syndrome (no uninvolved adrenocortical tissue was available in the third patient with this disorder), and the patient with feminization. The attached adrenal cortex was of normal thickness in three patients, including the two with aldosteronism and a girl whose initial symptoms were virilization and precocious breast development.

There was considerable overlap in the morphologic features of the tumors occurring in the patients with virilization and Cushing's syndrome as the predominant clinical manifestations and no microscopic features were found that would have enabled the pathologist to predict the predominant clinical features. In contrast, however, the tumors in the two patients with aldosteronism and the patient with feminization displayed distinctive morphologic features that merit separate description.

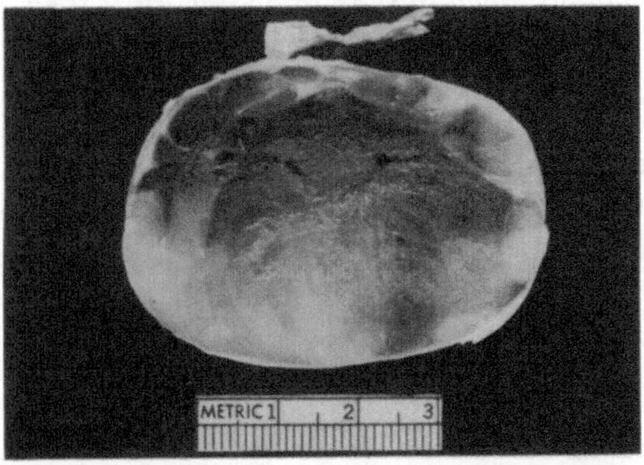

Figure 9. Gross appearance of encapsulated aldosterone-producing adenoma. Variations in color corresponded to variable amounts of stromal edema and hyalinization.

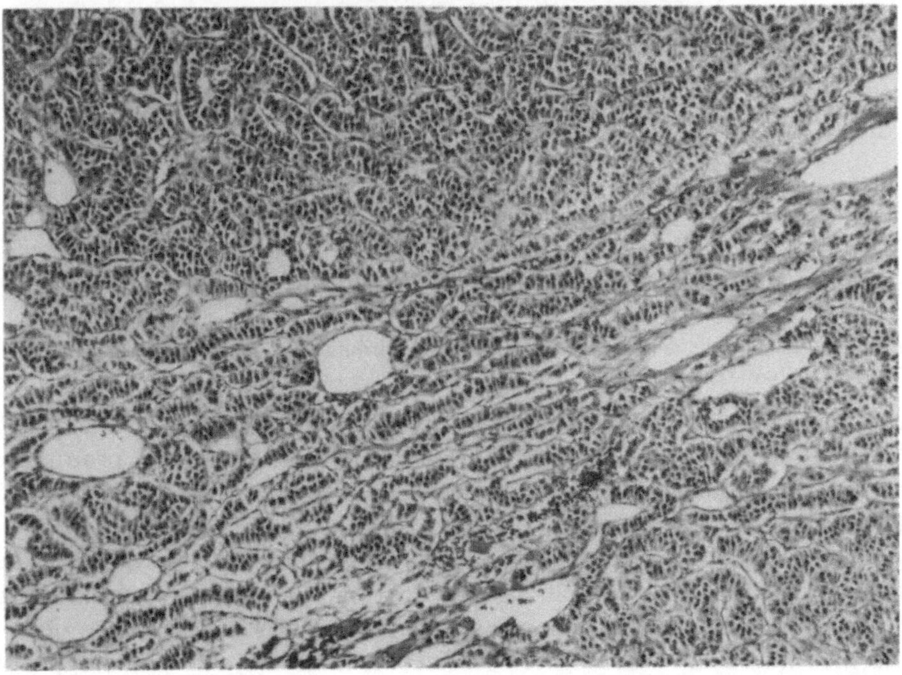

Figure 10. Trabecular arrangement of cells in aldosterone-producing adenoma. Similar areas were present focally in other nonaldosterone-producing adenomas. (Hematoxylin and eosin; ×100.)

The two tumors that caused aldosteronism weighed 30 and 75 g, respectively. The smaller tumor had a moist, relatively uniform, reddish yellow cut surface; the larger tumor had a more variegated cut surface, ranging in color from pale grayish tan to yellow-brown (Figure 9). Microscopically, the striking feature of both tumors was the pronounced ribbon-like arrangement of the cells throughout much of the tumor (Figure 10); elsewhere, an alveolar pattern was prominent. Both tumors were composed of medium-sized lipid-sparse cells with eosinophilic cytoplasm, relatively uniform nuclei, and few mitoses. Nuclear vesiculation was found in both tumors. Degenerative stromal changes - specifically, marked edema and hyalinization - were prominent (Figure 11). Microcyst formation was also conspicuous in both

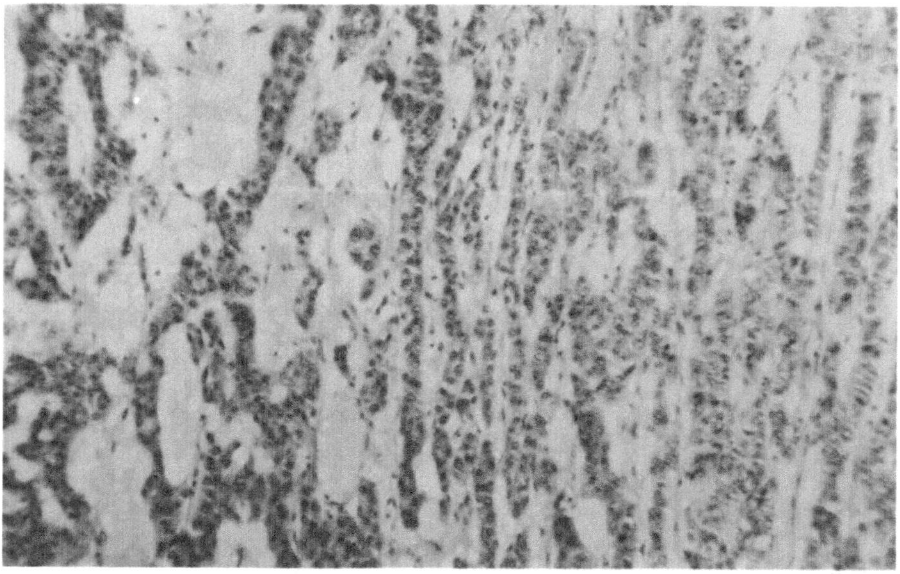

Figure 11. Ribbons of cells separated by edematous stroma in aldosterone producing adenoma. (Hematoxylin and eosin; × 160.)

tumors (Figure 12). The adjacent adrenal cortex was normal in thickness in both cases. In one gland the extratumoral cortex showed focal prominence of the zona glomerulosa and in the other this zone exhibited a striking diffuse thickening (Figure 13).

The patient whose major manifestation was feminization (Figure 14) had a heavily calcified tumor that was apparent on both plain abdominal roentgenograms and excretory urograms (Figure 15). The tumor was so densely calcified that a saw was required to bisect it in the surgical pathology laboratory. The coarsely bosselated tumor weighed 30 g and had a yellow-brown cut surface with massive central calcification (Figure 16). Microscopically, it was composed of a mixture of large vacuolated cells and smaller compact-

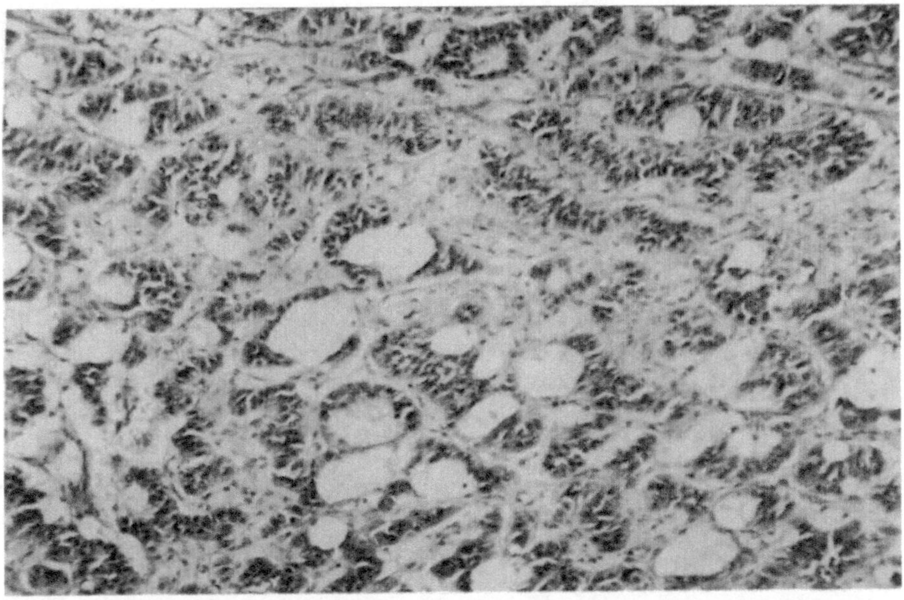

Figure 12. Early microcyst formation, apparently resulting from cystic degeneration within clusters of tumor cells. (Hematoxylin and eosin; ×100.)

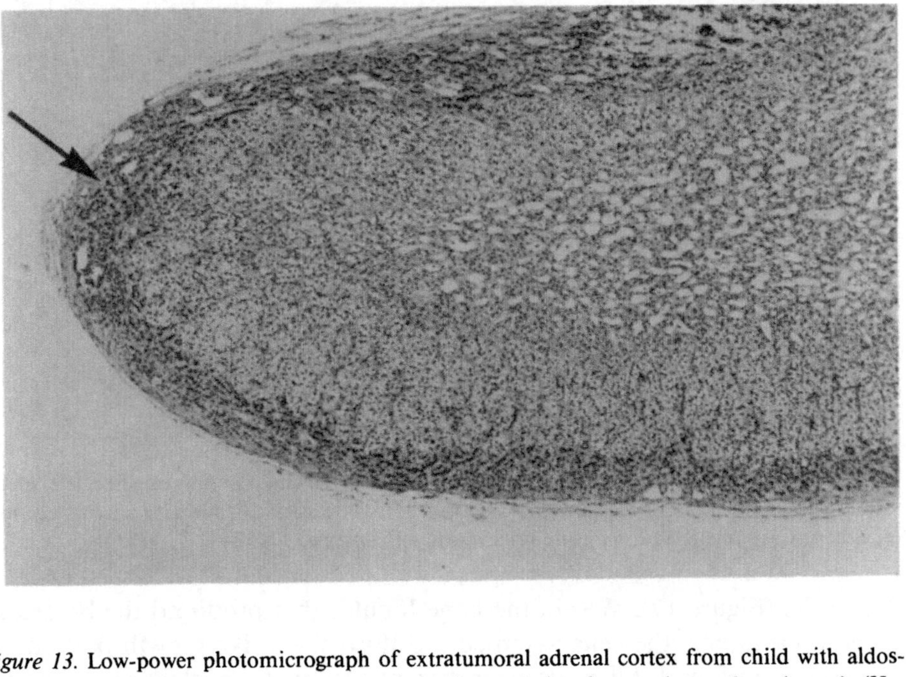

Figure 13. Low-power photomicrograph of extratumoral adrenal cortex from child with aldosterone-producing adenoma, showing prominent hyperplasia of zona glomerulosa (*arrow*). (Hematoxylin and eosin; ×40.)

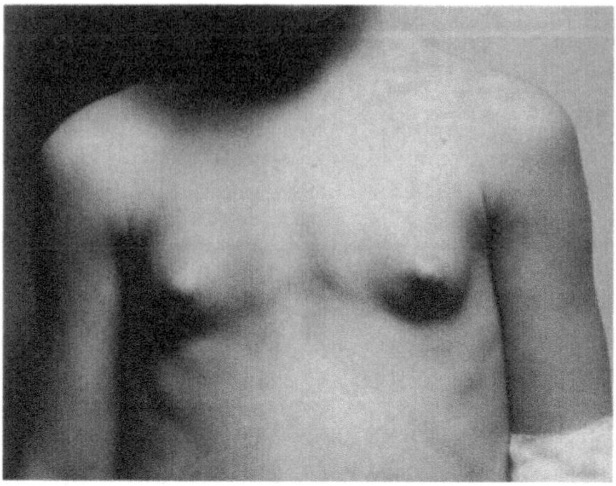

Figure 14. Bilateral breast enlargement in 5-year-old boy with feminizing adrenocortical adenoma. (Reproduced from Howard CP, Takahashi H, Hayles AB: Feminizing adrenal adenoma in a boy: case report and literature review. Mayo Clin Proc 52:354–357, 1977.)

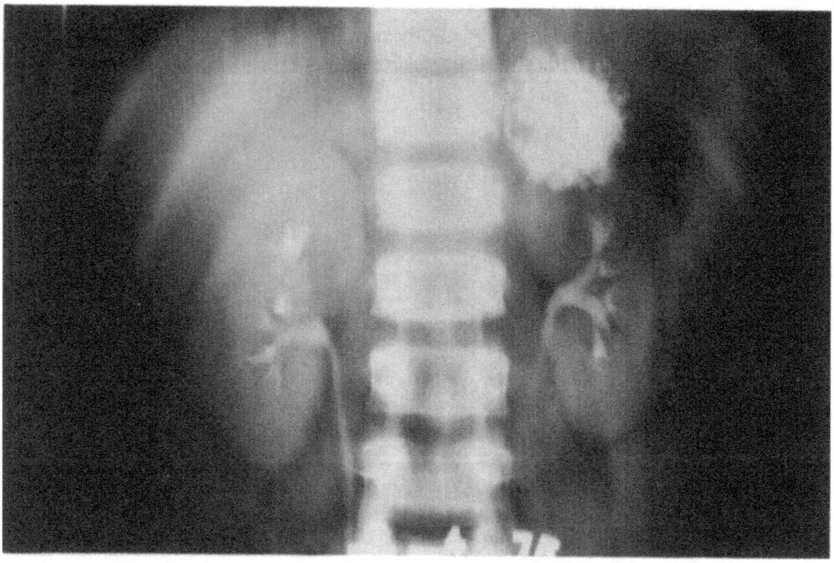

Figure 15. Excretory urogram of patient in Figure 14, showing densely calcified left adrenal tumor. (Reproduced from Howard CP, Takahashi H, Hayles AB: Feminizing adrenal adenoma in a boy: Case report and literature review. Mayo Clin Proc 52:354–357, 1977.)

type cells (Figure 17). Within the large lobules that produced the bosselated gross appearance, the cells assumed a diffuse sheet-like growth pattern. No mitoses were found. Many degenerating and pyknotic nuclei were seen, particularly in the compact-cell areas; these isolated degenerating cells fre-

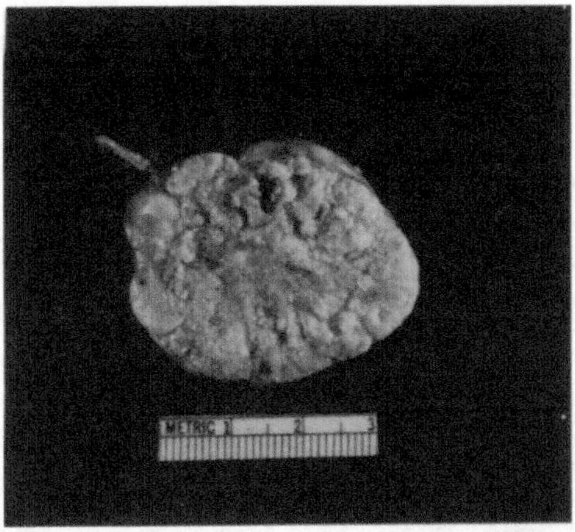

Figure 16. Gross appearance of feminizing adrenocortical adenoma, showing coarsely bosselated cut surface and massive central calcification. Extratumoral cortex (*upper left*) is atrophic.

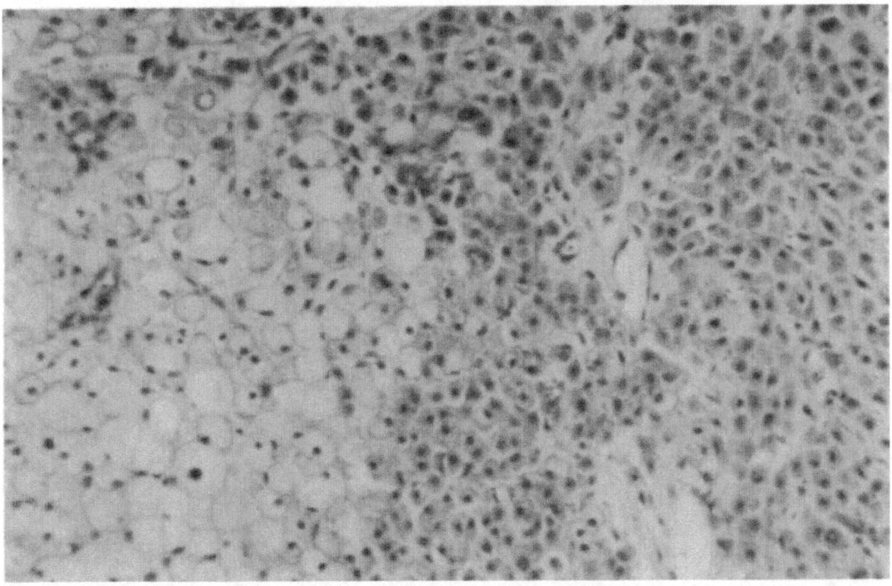

Figure 17. Mixture of compact-type and lipid-laden cells without tendency to form alveolar clusters, from tumor shown in Figure 16. (Hamatoxylin and eosin; × 100.)

quently became calcified and produced psammoma-like calcospherites (Figure 18). Coalescence of these bodies presumably led to massive areas of dense calcification and, ultimately, metaplastic bone formation within the tumor. Only in this tumor among all the adenomas was zonal necrosis observed (Figure 19), a process that, because of the cholesterol crystals present, possibly was a chronic degeneration and may have represented an

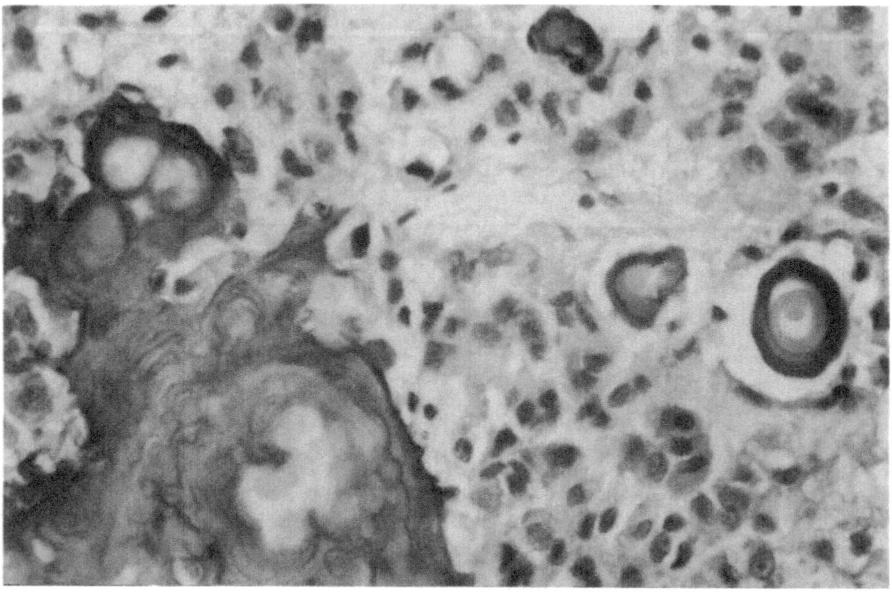

Figure 18. Psammomatous calcification in feminizing adrenocortical adenoma, resulting from degeneration of individual cells. Note coalescence of calcific bodies (at *left*), producing larger areas of calcification within tumor. (Hematoxylin and eosin; ×400.)

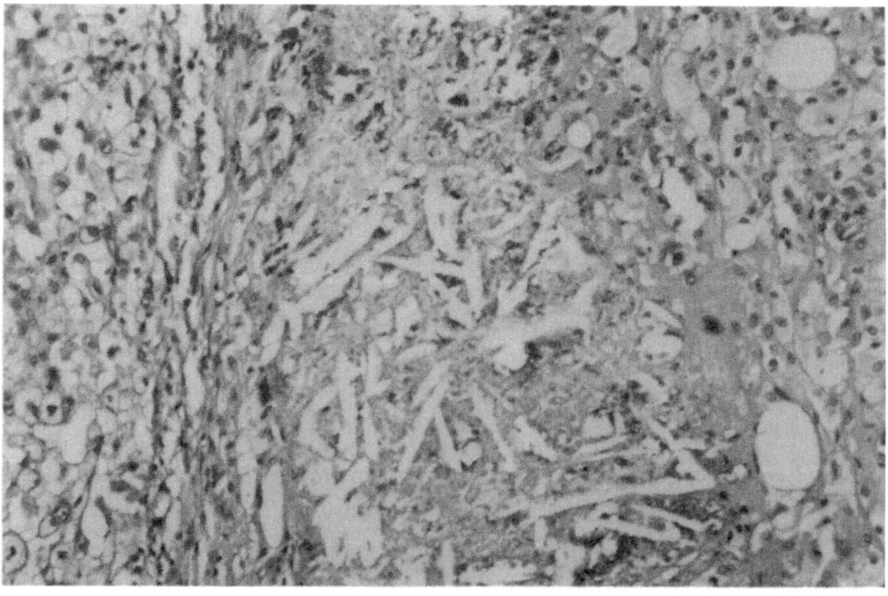

Figure 19. Necrotic focus of long duration in adrenocortical adenoma, composed of cellular debris, cholesterol crystals, and multinucleated phagocytes. (Hematoxylin and eosin; ×100.)

accentuation of the extensive single-cell necrosis that was present throughout the tumor.

2.2. Carcinomas

Gross appearance. The nine carcinomas varied in size from 2.5 to 20 cm in greatest dimension (mean, 9 cm). Tumor weight ranged from 5 to 1,700 g (mean, 332 g). Four of the carcinomas overlapped in size and weight with the adenomas. The tumor on which only biopsy had been performed was found at autopsy to weigh only 80 g. Most of the carcinomas appeared to be encapsulated, but gross invasion of adjacent tissues was present in three cases. The cut surface was grossly lobulated in six cases (Figure 20) and was

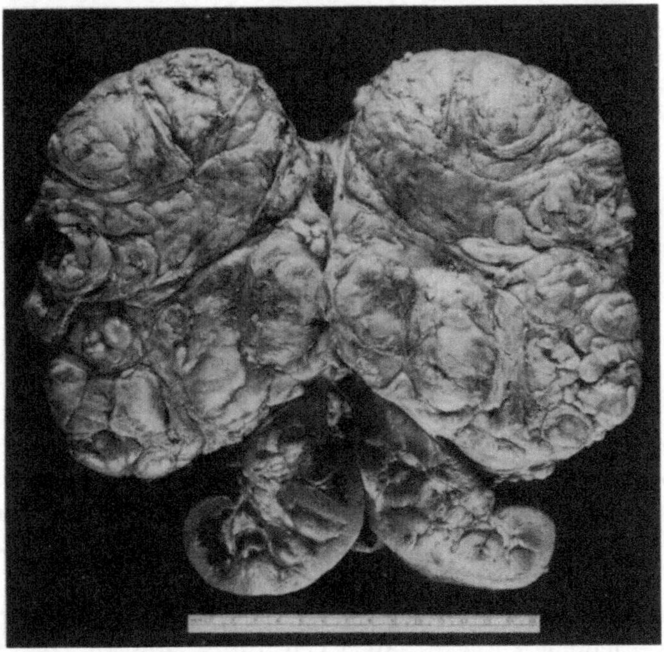

Figure 20. Gross appearance of huge (1,700-g) adrenocortical carcinoma, showing prominent lobulation and focal areas of necrosis.

usually variegated in color and consistency (Figure 21). Areas of necrosis were present in six tumors, and hemorrhage was observed in four. Cystic degeneration occurred in two of the tumors.

Microscopic appearance. Histologically, most of the carcinomas were composed of medium-sized or large cells with eosinophilic cytoplasm, and on low-power examination some of them closely resembled the adrenocortical adenomas. As a group, the features that distinguished them from the ade-

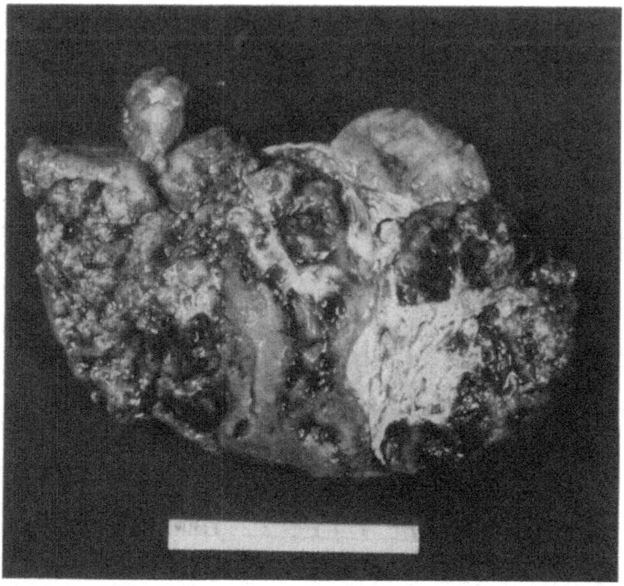

Figure 21. Variegated cut surface of 250-g adrenocortical carcinoma, with extensive necrosis and hemorrhage.

nomas were frequent mitoses (including atypical division figures), broad zones of necrosis, prominent pleomorphism, and invasion of blood vessels or tumor capsule.

Most of the carcinomas contained areas in which the cells were arranged in large or small alveolar clusters, and in five tumors this was the predominant pattern. In the other four cases, most of the tumor consisted of cells disposed in diffuse sheets. All of the carcinomas were composed predominantly of cells with eosinophilic cytoplasm; cells with clear or vacuolated cytoplasm were present only focally in a few of the tumors. Cells varied in size, with a tendency toward larger cell forms; however, two tumors were composed entirely of polygonal cells that were uniformly smaller than normal adrenocortical cells (Figure 22). Nuclei were usually enlarged, and the nuclear chromatin frequently was coarsely clumped or diffusely hyperchromatic, although in some cases the nuclear structure resembled that seen in adenomas. Nuclear vesiculation was frequently observed.

A feature common to all of the carcinomas was a mitotic rate in excess of that in the adenomas (Table 2). In the nine carcinomas, the mitotic rate ranged from 1.5 to 10 mitoses per 20 HPF; the count was less than two in two cases, from two to four in four cases, and greater than four in three cases. Abnormal mitotic figures (Figure 23) were found in five of the nine carcinomas.

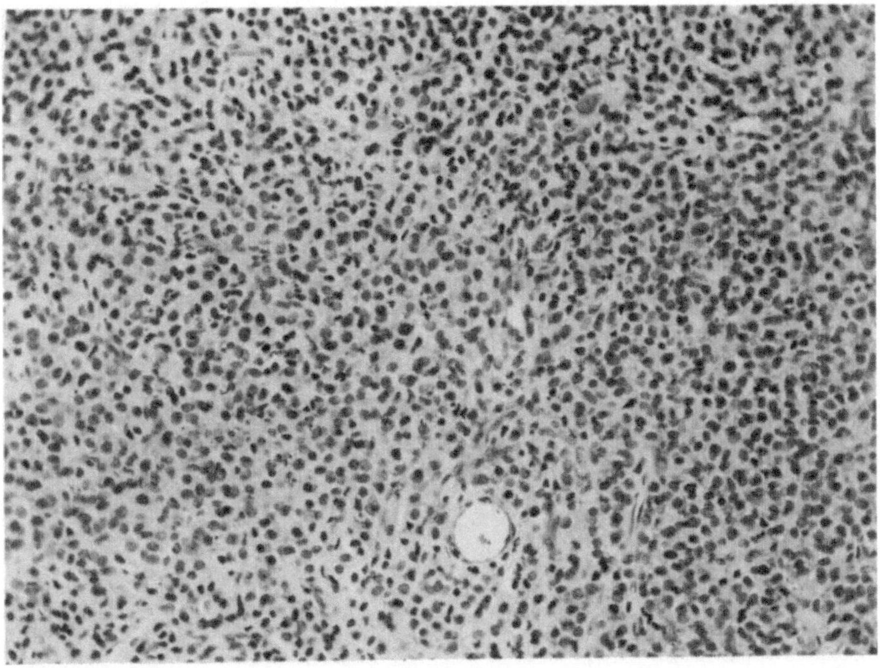

Figure 22. Adrenocortical carcinoma composed of diffuse sheet-like expanse of small cells with hyperchromatic nuclei. Numerous mitotic figures are present. (Hematoxylin and eosin; ×160.)

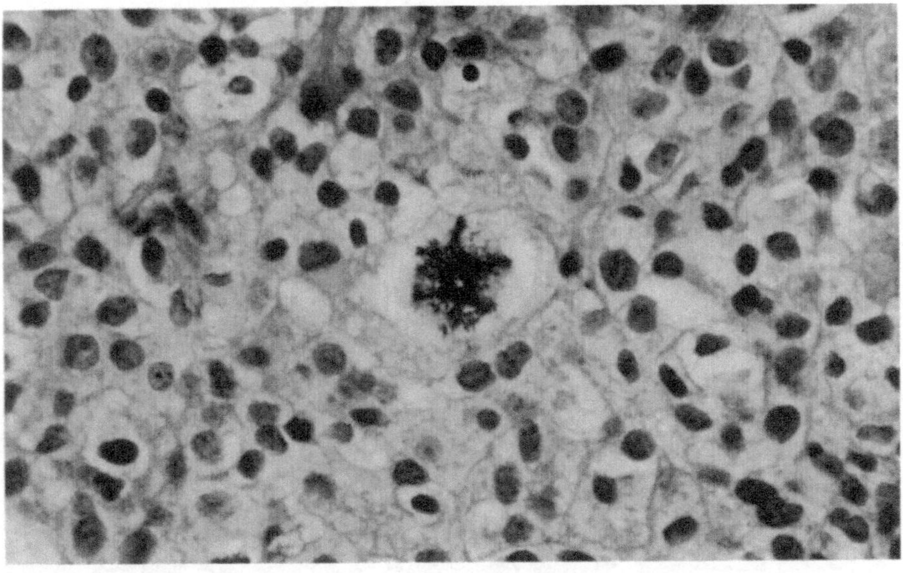

Figure 23. Abnormal multipolar mitotic figure in adrenocortical carcinoma. Other nuclei are enlarged, irregular, and hyperchromatic. (Hematoxylin and eosin; ×400.)

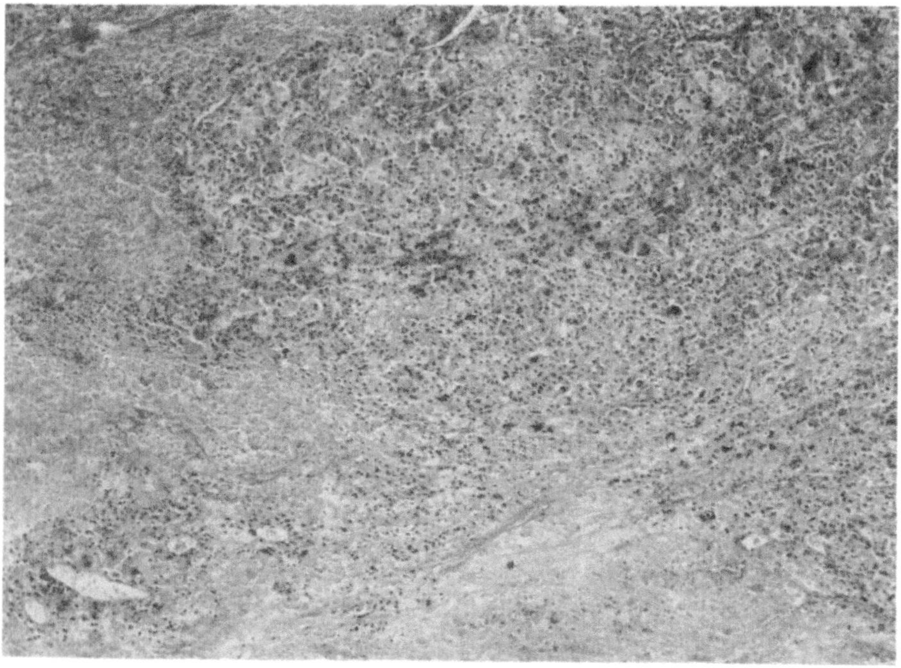

Figure 24. Broad zone of necrosis in 40-g adrenocortical carcinoma. Mitoses, including atypical forms, were readily found. Many multinucleated tumor cells are present in viable areas. (Hematoxylin and eosin; ×64.)

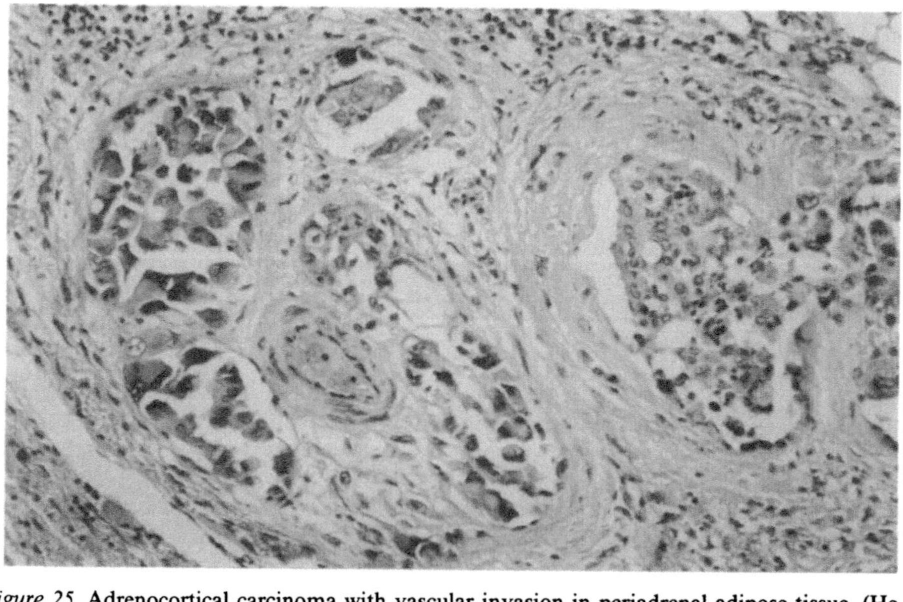

Figure 25. Adrenocortical carcinoma with vascular invasion in periadrenal adipose tissue. (Hematoxylin and eosin; ×160.)

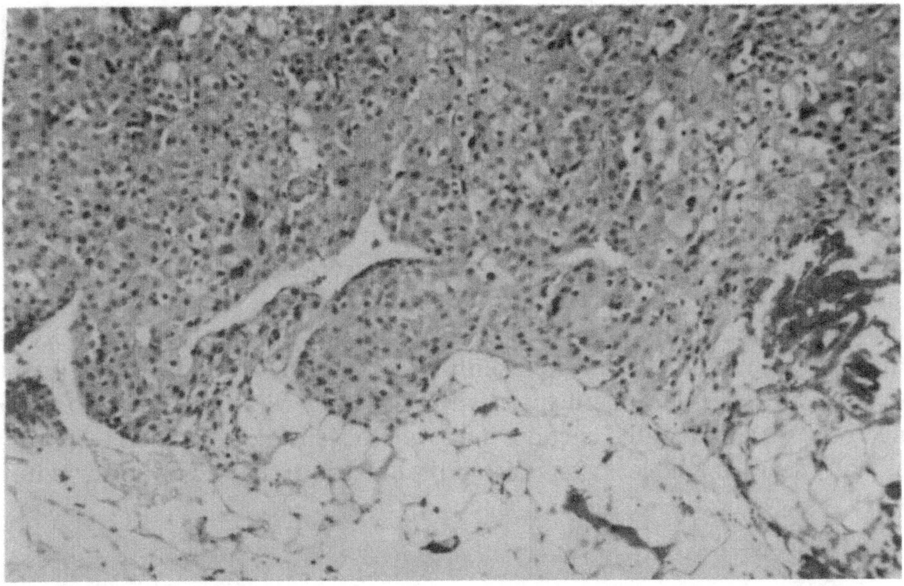

Figure 26. Adrenocortical carcinoma infiltrating periadrenal adipose tissue. (Hematoxylin and eosin; × 100.)

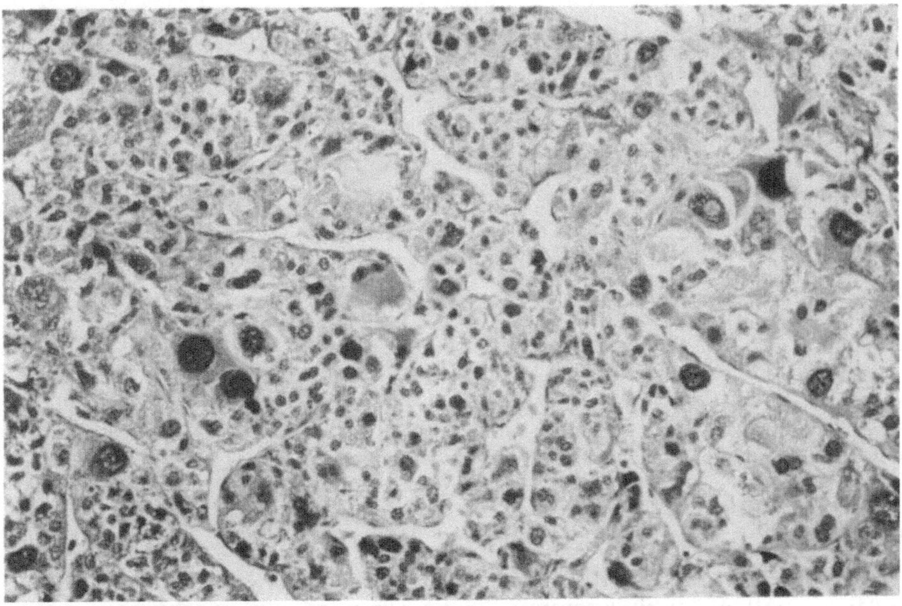

Figure 27. Prominent nuclear pleomorphism and sinusoidal vascular pattern in adrenocortical carcinoma. Numerous mitoses are present. (Hematoxylin and eosin; × 160.)

Broad zones of necrosis (Figure 24) were present in six carcinomas. Invasion of blood vessel walls (Figure 25), tumor capsule, or retroperitoneal fat (Figure 26) was interpreted as unequivocal evidence of a malignant lesion but was found in only five of the carcinomas. Nuclear pleomorphism (Figure 27) was prominent in five of the nine tumors but was notably absent or minimal in some of the tumors with very high mitotic rates.

The secondary degenerative changes, such as stromal edema and hyalinization, that were frequently observed in the adenomas were found in the smaller carcinomas only. Four carcinomas featured broad fibrous bands tranversing the tumors (Figure 28), and calcification was present in five of the tumors. In addition to the psammomatous type of calcification seen in three cases, irregular calcification within fibrous septa and about areas of necrosis was frequently encountered. Microcystic degeneration was occasionally seen; it tended to be more prominent in tumors with lower mitotic rates.

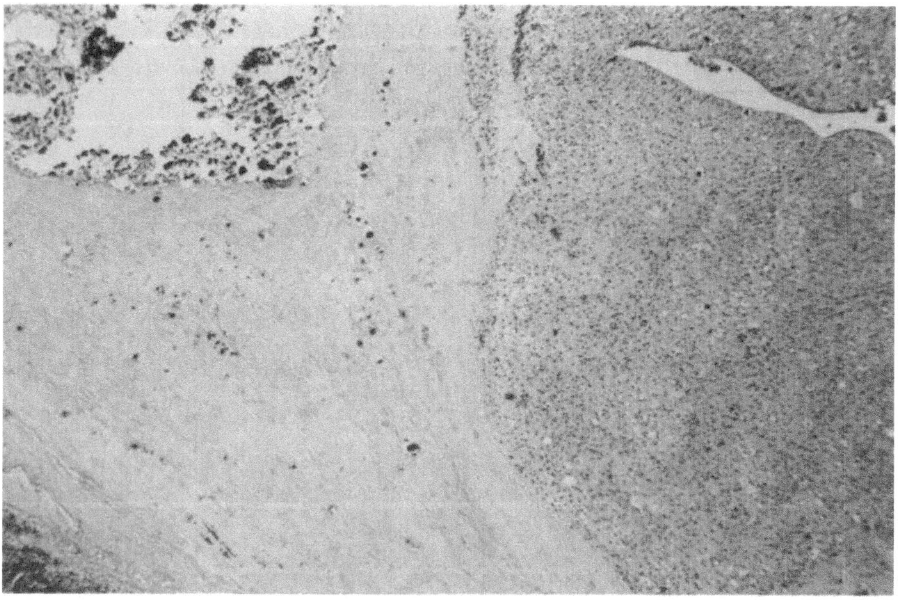

Figure 28. Broad collagenous band in adrenocortical carcinoma. Focal septal calcification is present (most prominent at *top left*). (Hematoxylin and eosin; $\times 40$.)

3. RESULTS OF TREATMENT

All 13 patients with adenomas have survived without recurrence. The duration of follow-up ranged from 1 to 42 years, all but one patient having been followed up for more than 5 years.

Four of the nine patients (44%) with carcinoma died with metastases within 1 year after operation; three of these patients were more than 10 years old. Autopsy, performed in two cases, disclosed metastases to the retroperitoneum, kidney, liver, and lung in one and disseminated visceral and nodal metastases in both the thorax and abdomen in the other. The two other patients who succumbed had clinical evidence of local recurrence and hepatic and pulmonary metastases at death. Five patients (56%) with carcinoma are alive without evidence of tumor recurrence from 3 to 34 years (mean, 18 years) postoperatively.

4. DISCUSSION

The 22 cases of adrenocortical tumors in this study represent 70 years' experience at a major referral center. Clinical features among these patients seem to be similar to those reported in the few other series available for comparison. Nineteen (86%) of the 22 patients were female, and 14 (64%) had symptoms before the fifth birthday. Among the 34 children studied by Benaily *et al.* [5], 65% were female; symptoms were noted in 80% before age 5 years and in 43% before age 2 years. Virilization was the most frequent manifestation of these childhood tumors; it was the predominant feature at the time of diagnosis in slightly more than 50% of Mayo Clinic patients and in 83% of the patients studied by Benaily and associates. In both series, 'mixed' virilizing syndromes (virilization associated with features of hypercortisolism, feminization, or both) were more common than virilization alone.

Although carcinomas outnumber adenomas among childhood adrenocortical tumors recorded in the literature, in the present study 13 of the 22 tumors were adenomas. The average age of patients with adenomas was not appreciably different from that of patients with carcinomas. The duration of symptoms before diagnosis was less than 6 months in the four patients with fatal carcinomas but also in five patients with adenomas and one with a nonfatal carcinoma. Biochemical tests of adrenocortical function, although extremely useful in distinguishing adrenocortical hyperplasia from tumors, were of less value in differentiating benign from malignant tumors, and there was considerable overlap in these test results between patients with adenomas and those with carcinomas.

4.1. *Functional-pathologic correlation*

Virilizing tumors. More than half of all virilizing adrenocortical tumors occur in children, and almost all male patients with virilization due to adrenal tumor have been children. Congenital adrenal hyperplasia, however, is a much more common cause of virilization in childhood than is tumor. Virilization as a predominant manifestation of an adrenocortical tumor is usually seen in young children; in this series, only 1 of 12 thus affected was initially examined after the age of 7 years, and in this patient the onset of symptoms had antedated the seventh birthday. In our experience, virilization associated with features of hypercortisolism or feminization occurred twice as frequently as 'pure' virilization. Although adrenal tumors that cause 'mixed' virilizing syndromes in adults are usually carcinomas, this was not true for children in our study; indeed, six of the eight patients with 'mixed' virilization had adenomas. Other investigators who have studied virilizing adrenocortical tumors in children have found that most were carcinomas, which usually proved to be fatal [6, 7]. In contrast, the prognosis for children with virilizing adrenocortical tumors in our series was very good: 7 of the 12 tumors were benign, and only one of five patients with virilizing carcinoma succumbed to the neoplasm.

The virilizing tumors in our material tended to be relatively small: 7 of the 12 tumors weighed 50 g or less, and only 2 weighed more than 100 g. The histologic pattern was similar in six of the seven virilizing adenomas, the tumors being composed of compact-type cells of varying size arranged in small nests, cords, and alveolar clusters separated by delicate fibrovascular septa. A similar histologic pattern was present in the three smallest carcinomas. These tumors overlapped in size with the adenomas but were interpreted as carcinomas because of frequent mitoses and other features associated with a malignant lesion. Neville and Mackay [8] have also noted considerable overlap in the size and weight of benign and malignant virilizing adrenocortical tumors. In the two large virilizing carcinomas in our study, the cells tended to aggregate in large alveolar clusters or solid sheets, and frequent and atypical mitoses, necrosis, invasion, and nuclear pleomorphism were prominent. A diffuse sheet-like arrangement was occasionally seen in the smaller tumors and was present in one of the adenomas in this group. Contrasting with the experience of Symington [9], who found the uninvolved ipsilateral or the contralateral adrenal cortex to be normal in most patients with virilizing tumors, varying degrees of cortical atrophy were found in 8 of 10 patients in this study (including 3 patients without clinical features of hypercortisolism).

Tumors that cause Cushing's syndrome. In adults, bilateral adrenocortical hyperplasia accounts for about 80% of cases of Cushing's syndrome [10]. In contradistinction, Neville and Symington [11] found that in children the underlying adrenal lesion was carcinoma, bilateral hyperplasia, and adenoma in 51%, 35%, and 14% of cases, respectively. At our institution, however, hyperplasia has been a much more common cause of Cushing's syndrome in children than has adrenocortical tumor. Survey of the records at the Mayo Clinic shows that only 5 patients of age 16 years or younger have undergone operation for adrenocortical tumors that have caused Cushing's syndrome, whereas 27 patients in the age group had surgically proved adrenocortical hyperplasia during the years 1947 through 1977 alone [12].

Adrenocortical adenomas that cause Cushing's syndrome are usually small, most weighing less than 40 g [9, 10, 13]; however, some extremely large adenomas have been reported in adults. In the current study, among the five tumors that caused Cushing's syndrome, the three adenomas weighed 35, 36, and 122 g, and the carcinomas weighed 190 and 250 g. Histologically, the tumors were virtually indistinguishable from their benign and malignant counterparts among the virilizing tumors. As would be expected, the attached uninvolved adrenal cortex was atrophic in all three cases in which it was available for review.

Feminizing tumors. Feminization is an extremely uncommon manifestation of adrenocortical tumors, particularly in children. In the most extensive review of feminizing adrenocortical tumors to date, Gabrilove *et al.* [14] found that most occurred in adults between 25 and 50 years of age. The tumors tended to be large; a palpable mass was present in more than half of the patients. Seventy-eight percent of the tumors were carcinomas, and in 30 of 41 patients with carcinomas, metastases developed subsequently. Feminizing adrenocortical tumors are indistinguishable pathologically from tumors that cause virilization or Cushing's syndrome. Occasionally, a feminizing tumor that subsequently metastasizes may have a deceptively benign histologic appearance. This has prompted some authors [8] to advocate treating all feminizing adrenocortical tumors as carcinomas.

Feminizing tumors in adolescents have been large carcinomas that have carried the same grim prognosis as those in adults. The outlook for prepubertal children with feminizing adrenocortical tumors is considerably better, however. The patient with feminization in this review was described in a 1977 report [2] as the seventh case of a feminizing adrenal tumor in a prepubertal male. In one of the previously reported cases, however, features of virilization predominated over those of feminization [15]. All six patients in whom feminization was the outstanding clinical feature had bilateral gynecomastia and advanced bone age; in addition, signs of virilization, such as axillary or pubic hair, enlarged penis, or acne, were present in four of the six. Four of the tumors were small, the largest measuring 5 by 3.5 by 3.5 cm and weighing 30 g. Three of these were interpreted as adenomas, and the fourth was diagnosed as a carcinoma because vascular invasion was present. All four patients were alive from 5 to 14 years after excision. The other two tumors were large, both weighing more than 200 g. One of these was interpreted as an adenoma on the basis of the histologic appearance, and the patient was alive 1 year after surgical excision. The importance of long-term follow-up in feminizing adrenocortical tumors is illustrated by the other case, reported by Bacon and Lowrey [16]. This patient had an encapsulated tumor that exhibited cells arranged in clusters and cords, vesicular nuclei with coarse nuclear chromatin, and occasional mitoses; a solitary nest of neoplastic cells was found within a dilated vein in the tumor mass. The lesion was interpreted as an adrenocortical adenoma with a neoplastic thrombus; the patient remained well for 7 years after excision, but metastases subsequently developed and he died within 1 year. Snaith [17] has reported a feminizing adenoma weighing 10.65 g in a 5½-year-old girl.

Tumors that cause primary aldosteronism. Primary aldosteronism is rare in children, but this syndrome accounts for up to 34% of cases of adrenocortical hyperfunction in adults [8]. In about two-thirds of cases in adults, the underlying adrenal lesion is a solitary adenoma, and most of the remaining cases are the result of adrenocortical hyperplasia; about 20 cases of aldosteronism due to malignant adrenocortical tumors have been described. In children and adolescents, primary aldosteronism is usually due to adrenocortical hyperplasia. Only five cases of pure primary aldosteronism due to adrenocortical tumor in children younger than 16 years of age have been reported [18–22].

The pathologic features of adrenocortical tumors that cause primary aldosteronism have been well studied [23]. Almost all are adenomas, and most are quite small; 60% weigh less than 6 g [9]. The typical small adenoma is a well-circumscribed, oval or round lesion with a distinctive golden-yellow or canary yellow cut surface. Microscopically, tumors with this gross appearance are composed of large lipid-laden clear cells with small vesicular nuclei, similar to those of the normal zona fasciculata, and arranged in small cords or alveolar clusters. On the basis of the pathologic descriptions of the five previously reported tumors in children, all apparently have had a morphologic pattern similar or identical to this. The largest of the five reported tumors weighed only 15 g.

The two aldosterone-producing tumors in our study weighed 30 and 75 g and differed in their gross and microscopic appearance from those that have been previously reported in children. The tumors, which were virtually identical histologically, were composed of medium-sized cells with acidophilic lipid-sparse cytoplasm, resembling cells of the zona glomerulosa or reticularis. The most striking features of these tumors were the areas of prominent trabecular arrangements of tumor cells and the formation of cords and acini separated by an edematous myxoid stroma. Neville and Symington [23] found this pattern in 2 of 18 aldosterone-producing tumors in adults. This pattern seems to be more common in larger aldosterone-producing adenomas.

Tumors that cause hypoglycemia. The clinical syndrome of hypoglycemia in association with extrapancreatic malignant tumors is well recognized. More than half of the reported cases have been associated with malignant mesenchymal tumors of the abdomen and thorax; hepatocellular carcinoma accounts for another 20% of cases. About 20 cases of hypoglycemia due to adrenocortical carinoma have been reported. These tumors are invariably quite large, most weighing more than 1,000 g; they may cause other endocrine syndromes, such as virilization or Cushing's syndrome, in addition to hypoglycemia. Broster and Patterson [24] have reported such a case in a 14-year-old girl in whom virilization had been evident for 18 months before the onset of hypoglycemic attacks. The mechanism of hypoglycemia due to adrenocortical carcinoma remains unclear and may involve consumption of glucose by the tumor, impaired gluconeogenesis due to substantially increased production of anabolic steroids [25], or production by the tumor of substances with nonsuppressible insulin-like activity [26].

'Nonfunctioning' tumors. About 5% of childhood adrenocortical tumors produce no clinical evidence of endocrine dysfunction. This does not mean that they are incapable of steroidogenesis (many are capable of forming precursor steroids such as pregnenolone [27]) but only that they do not produce an excess of active hormones. Because they do not produce symptoms due to hormonal excess, these tumors are usually extremely large at the time of diagnosis – many weigh more than 1,000 g; a palpable abdominal mass is present in about half of the patients. They are usually composed predominantly of compact-type cells and are histologically indistinguishable from functioning adrenocortical carcinomas [28]. The prognosis for these patients is extremely poor, 70% dying within 1 year. The 'nonfunctioning' carcinoma in our series is unusual because of its relatively small size (80 g); most adrenal carcinomas attain a relatively large size before dissemination becomes clinically apparent.

4.2. Diagnosis of a malignant process in adrenocortical tumors

Accurate prognostication of the behavior of all adrenocortical tumors on the basis of pathologic findings still remains an elusive goal. Gross pathologic findings such as necrosis, hemorrhage, penetration into periadrenal fat, and extension of tumor into adrenal or renal veins are obvious indications of a malignant lesion. In other cases, adenoma or carcinoma can be diagnosed on the basis of the histopathologic findings, supplemented by clinical and operative data and the tumor weight.

In assessing the 22 childhood adrenocortical tumors in the current study, we have used histologic criteria similar to those proposed by Heinbecker, O'Neal, and Ackerman [29] in their review of 16 tumors, which included 7 tumors in children. The regarded frequent mitoses, venous invasion, and capsular invasion as definite criteria of a malignant lesion and necrosis, hemorrhage, calicification, pleomorphism, and nuclear atypia as helpful supportive findings. Other investigators [4, 13, 30–34] have found similar criteria to be useful. Broad zones of necrosis, characteristic of carcinomas, must be distinguished from single-cell necrosis, a common finding in adenomas. Nuclear pleomorphism in the absence of mitotic activity or other features of a malignant process is insufficient to render a diagnosis of carcinoma. We did not find microscopic calcification to be a helpful criterion in distinguishing adenomas from carcinomas; it was found in three tumors that were classified as adenomas and five of the carcinomas, including three in patients who survived. Other criteria, such as broad collagenous bands traversing the tumor [4, 9], a diffuse sheet-like pattern of growth [4, 9], and enlarged vesicular nuclei [8, 9], have also been suggested as helpful in distinguishing adenomas from carcinomas. Nevertheless, we would hesitate to diagnose adrenocortical carcinoma solely on the basis of one or more of these features; they are merely findings suggestive of or consistent with this diagnosis.

In practice, the classification of most adrenal tumors as adenoma or carcinoma by applying the criteria described is relatively easy. Encapsulated tumors weighing less than 100 g with minimal or no mitotic activity and no necrosis, capsular invasion, or vascular invasion are classified as adenomas, even if nuclear pleomorphism is present. Likewise, large tumors with necrosis, abundant mitoses, and invasion of veins or tumor capsule are readily classified as carcinomas; a high percentage will recur locally or metastasize and lead to the death of the patient. Two groups of adrenocortical tumors may pose problems in distinguishing adenomas from carcinomas: (1) small encapsulated tumors with increased mitotic activity and nuclear pleomorphism and (2) large tumors with apparently benign histologic features.

Most patients with small (less than 50 g) adrenocortical tumors are cured by excision of the tumor and the attached adrenal gland, regardless of the histologic characteristics of the tumor. This by no means justifies considering all small adrenocortical tumors to be adenomas. On the basis of the assumption that adrenocortical carcinomas are malignant from their inception and do not arise in preexisting adenomas, we consider a tumor with histologic features of a malignant process to be a carcinoma regardless of its size. In this series, carcinoma was diagnosed on the basis of histologic evidence in three virilizing tumors that weighed less than 50 g; two of these weighed less than the smallest adenoma. All three tumors had increased mitotic activity; in addition, one tumor contained abnormal mitotic forms (including tripolar mitoses), another displayed prominent nuclear pleomorphism, and the third contained broad zones of necrosis, prominent pleomorphism, and abnormal mitoses. No capsular or vascular invasion was identified in any of these three tumors, and the patients are alive without recurrence, 5, 16, and 32 years postoperatively.

Tang and Gray [32], in a study of 39 adrenocortical tumors, encountered 3 tumors that weighed 30 g or less which were characterized by histologic features indistinguishable from those in 12 of 13 fatal carcinomas, including architectural disarray, prominent pleomorphism, aboundant mitotic figures, and vascular invasion. All three patients were apparently cured by surgical excision, and two of them were children 18 months and 3 years of age. It should be noted, however, that metastasizing tumors that weigh less than 50 g have been reported [4, 5]. Thus, although the risk of subsequent metastasis from a small but histologically malignant adrenocortical tumor is low, the potential for recurrence or metastasis must be recognized, and these patients should be under close surveillance.

Tumors that weigh more than 100 g with equivocal histologic findings pose perhaps the most difficult diagnostic problem for the pathologist. Although some extremely large adrenocortical adenomas have been reported, they are far outnumbered by large benign-appearing tumors that have subsequently metastasized. Any large tumor should arouse suspicion of a malignant process, regardless of its histologic appearance. Benaily *et al.* [5] found that all children with tumors that weighed more than 250 g died with metastasis. If mitotic activity is increased in a large tumor, or if any other histologic features suggestive of a malignant lesion are found, the tumor must be considered a carcinoma. We have seen large adrenocortical tumors with benign histologic features which have subsequently metastasized in adults, but we have not encountered similar examples in children.

In this series, six tumors weighed more than 100 g. Four had obvious histologic features of a malignant lesion, and three metastasized. Another tumor, which caused Cushing's syndrome in a 15-month-old girl, weighed 190 g and was interpreted as carcinoma on the basis of increased mitotic activity (2 mitoses/20 HPF), although there was no evidence of necrosis, capsular invasion, or vascular invasion; the patient is alive 34 years after surgical excision. A tumor that weighed 122 g (and also produced Cushing's syndrome) was diagnosed as an adenoma. The tumor was encapsulated; thorough sampling of the lesion revealed no evidence of mitotic activity, vascular or capsular invasion, necrosis, or nuclear atypia. The patient is alive 20 years postoperatively.

4.3. Prognosis

In the Mayo Clinic series, the outlook for children with adrenocortical tumors was relatively good. All 13 patients with adenomas are alive from 1 to 42 years postoperatively, and 5 (56%) of 9 patients with carcinomas have survived without recurrence for 3 years or more after surgical excision. Benaily and associates [5] did not distinguish adenomas from carcinomas in their study of 34 children with adrenocortical tumors, but found that 52% of their patients were well from 4 to 17 years postoperatively. Of note in their series is the relatively large size of the tumors; 19 of 29 patients for whom actual or estimated tumor weights were available had tumors that weighed 80 g or more. Three of four children with adrenocortical carcinoma studied by Stewart and associates [35] were alive without recurrence from 1 to 6 years after surgical excision and postoperative radiotherapy.

The prognosis for children with adrenocortical carcinoma seems considerably better than that for adults. Most larger series of adrenocortical carcinoma in the recent literature have included children together with adults, children constituting from 0 to 25% of the total; in these series, the overall 5-year survival rates have ranged from 10 to 35% [30, 31, 34, 36]. How much these rates have been affected by the inclusion of children in the series is difficult to estimate. Sullivan and associates [37] found that adrenocortical carcinomas in children were more frequently confined in the adrenal gland at the time of diagnosis, and thus more amenable to successful surgical excision, than those in adults.

In our experience, the prognosis for prepubertal children with adrenocortical carcinomas was much better than that for adolescents; only one of six patients younger than 10 years old died, whereas all three patients whose symptoms began after an ostensibly normal puberty died with metastases.

Our experience with childhood adrenocortical tumors indicates that the application of standard pathologic criteria is useful in predicting the clinical outcome in these patients. Of the 13 tumors classified as adenomas on the basis of the criteria outlined in this chapter, none has subsequently recurred or metastasized. The histologic criteria of increased and abnormal mitoses, capsular invasion, vascular invasion, and broad zones of necrosis and hemorrhage were useful in distinguishing carcinomas from adenomas. The presence of either capsular or vascular invasion was associated with a high frequency of subsequent metastasis. Five carcinomas in this series exhibited infiltration beyond the tumor capsule, and intratumoral vascular invasion was found in four of these. Four of the five patients died with metastases, and the other (whose tumor displayed both capsular and vascular invasion) is alive without recurrence 3 years postoperatively. Alternatively, a tumor that weighs less than 100 g and shows no invasion of vessels or tumor capsule is unlikely to metastasize.

REFERENCES

1. Hayles AB, Hahn HB, Sprague RG, Bahn RC, Priestley JT: Hormone secreting tumors of the adrenal cortex in children. Pediatrics 37:19–25, 1966.
2. Howard CP, Takahashi H, Hayles AB: Feminizing adrenal adenoma in a boy: Case report and literature review. Mayo Clin Proc 52:354–357, 1977.
3. Gross MD, Bowerman RA, Mori KW, Cho KJ: The role of ultrasonography, computed tomography, scintigraphy and angiography in the localization of adrenal disease. In: This volume.
4. Hough AJ, Hollifield JW, Page DL, Hartmann HW: Prognostic factors in adrenal cortical tumors: a mathematical analysis of clinical and morphological data. Am J Clin Pathol 72:390–399, 1979.
5. Benaily M, Schweisguth O, Job J-C: Les tumeurs cortico-surrenales de l'enfant. Arch Franc Ped 32:441–454, 1975.
6. Kenny FM, Hashida Y, Askair HA, Siber WH, Fetterman GH: Virilizing tumors of the adrenal cortex. Am J Dis Child 115:445–458, 1968.
7. Burrington JD, Stephens CA. Virilizing tumors of the adrenal gland in childhood: Report of eight cases. J Pediatr Surg 4:291–302, 1969.
8. Neville AM, Mackay AM: The structure of the human adrenal cortex in health and disease. Clinics in Endocrinol Metabol 1:361–395, 1972.
9. Symington T: Functional Pathology of the Human Adrenal Gland. Edinburgh and London, E & S Livingstone, 1969.
10. Neville AM, Symington T: The pathology of the adrenal gland in Cushing's syndrome. J Pathol Bacteriol 93:19–35, 1967.
11. Neville AM, Symington T: Bilateral adrenocortical hyperplasia in children with Cushing's syndrome. J Pathol 107:95–106, 1972.
12. McArthur RG, Hayles AB, Salassa RM: Childhood Cushing disease: results of bilateral adrenalectomy. J Pediatr 95:214–219, 1979.
13. Schteingart DE, Oberman HA, Friedman BA, Conn JW: Adrenal cortical neoplasms producing Cushing's syndrome: a clinicopathologic study. Cancer 22:1005–1013, 1968.
14. Gabrilove JL, Sharma DC, Wotiz HH, Dorfman RI: Feminizing adrenocortical tumors in the male: a review of 52 cases, including a case report. Medicine 44:37–79, 1965.
15. Castleman B, Scully RE, McNeely RU: Case records of the Massachusetts General Hospital (case 46-1972). N Engl J Med 287:1033–140, 1972.
16. Bacon GE, Lowrey GH: Feminizing adrenal tumor in a six-year-old boy. J Clin Endocrinol Metab 25:1403–1406, 1965.
17. Snaith AH: A case of feminizing adrenal tumor in a girl. J Clin Endocrinol Metab 18:318–322, 1958.
18. Orndahl G, Hökfelt B, Ljunggren E et al.: Two cases of primary aldosteronism: comments on differential diagnosis and difficulties in screening. Acta Med Scand 165:445–452, 1959.
19. Crane MG, Holloway JE, Winsor WG: Aldosterone-secreting adenoma: report of a case in a juvenile. Ann Intern Med 54:280–291, 1961.
20. Canell B, Sandegard E, Hökfelt B: Primary aldosteronism due to an adrenal adenoma in a three-year-old child. Acta Pediatr Scand 53:205–212, 1964.
21. Kelch RP, Connors MH, Kaplan SI et al.: A calcified aldosterone producing tumor in a hypertensive, normokalemic, prepubertal girl. J Pediatr 83:432–437, 1973.
22. Kafrouni G, Oakes MD, Lurvey AN, DeQuattro V: Aldosteronoma in a child with localization by adrenal vein aldosterone: collective review of the literature. J Pediatr Surg 10:917–924, 1975.

23. Neville AM, Symington T: Pathology of primary aldosteronism. Cancer 19:1854–1868, 1966.
24. Broster LR, Patterson J: Unusual case of adrenal carcinoma with a note on the application of a new colour test. Br Med J 1:781–782, 1948.
25. Eymontt MJ, Gwinup G, Kruger FA, Maynard DE, Hamwi GJ: Cushing's syndrome with hypoglycemia caused by adrenocortical carcinoma. J Clin Endocrinol Metab 25:46–52, 1965.
26. Hyodo T, Megyesi K, Kahn CR, McLean JP, Friesen HG: Adrenocortical carcinoma and hypoglycemia: Evidence for production of nonsuppressible insulin-like activity by the tumor. J Clin Endocrinol Metab 44:1175–1184, 1977.
27. Fukushima DK, Gallagher TF: Steroid Production in 'nonfunctioning' adrenal cortical tumor. J Clin Endocrinol Metab 23:923–927, 1963.
28. Lewinsky BS, Grigor KM, Symington T, Neville AM: The clinical and pathologic features of 'nonhormonal' adrenocortical tumors. Cancer 33:778–79, 1974.
29. Heinbecker P, O'Neal LW, Ackerman LV: Functioning and nonfunctioning adrenal cortical tumors. Surg Gynecol Obstet 105:21–33, 1957.
30. Huvos AG, Hajdu SI, Brasfield RD, Foote FW: Adrenal cortical carcinoma: clinicopathologic study of 34 cases. Cancer 25:354–361, 1970.
31. Ibanez ML: The pathology of adrenal cortical carcinoma: study of 22 cases. Endocrine and Non-endocrine Hormone-Producing Tumors. Chicago, Yearbook Medical Publishers, 1971, 231–239.
32. Tang CK, Gray GF: Adrenocortical neoplasms: prognosis and morphology. Urology 5:691–695, 1975.
33. Kay S: Hyperplasia and neoplasia of the adrenal gland. Pathol Ann 11:103–139, 1976.
34. King DR, Lack EE: Adrenal cortical carcinoma: a clinical and pathologic study of 49 cases. Cancer 44:239–244, 1979.
35. Stewart DR, Jones PHM, Jolleys A: Carcinoma of the adrenal gland in children. J Pediatr Surg 9:59–67, 1974.
36. Hajjar RA, Hickey RC, Samaan NA: Adrenal cortical carcinoma: a study of 32 patients. Cancer 35:549–554, 1975.
37. Sullivan M, Boileau M, Hodges CV: Adrenocortical carcinoma. J Urol 120:660–665, 1978.

10. The Multiple Endocrine Neoplasia Syndromes

R. NEIL SCHIMKE

1. THE MULTIPLE ENDOCRINE NEOPLASIA SYNDROMES

There are at least three distinct syndromes that feature hyper- or neoplasia of the endocrine glands, termed appropriately enough, multiple endocrine neoplasia (MEN), types I-III [1]. The former designation of multiple endocrine adenoma syndrome is also used, but it implies that the conditions are inherently benign, which is clearly not true, and for this reason, substitution of neoplasia for adenoma is more accurate. Since types II and III have certain features in common, some prefer a IIa and IIb designation. However, as will be shown, the two conditions differ from one another substantially enough that the former enumeration seems more appropriate. There are also 'overlap' patients whose clinical characteristics may be shared by more than one of the MEN syndromes. Usually these are isolated instances that prove or disprove nothing in regard to the relationship between the established MEN syndromes, either from a genetic or an etiologic point of view. A few of these endocrine tumor associations can be explained on the basis of a common embryologic origin of the tissues in question or a common exposure to a given environmental insult. In other instances, the reason for the assocation is not at all apparent. Some may actually be due to chance, while others may result from as yet poorly defined gene defects; i.e., it is quite possible and even likely that additional MEN syndromes exist.

1.1. MEN, Type I

Erdheim was one of the first to record a combination of endocrine tumors when he described an acromegalic who also had parathyroid hyperplasia at autopsy [2]. The first description of an affected family and the association with peptic ulcer appeared 36 years later [3]. Wermer [4] and, independently, Moldawar *et al.* [5] summarized the available information and, with

G. Bennett Humphrey et al. (eds), Adrenal and Endocrine Tumors in Children.

their own case material, clearly established MEN I as a heritable entity. The condition, also called the Wermer syndrome, comprises adenomas or hyperplasia of the parathyroids, pancreatic islet cells, pituitary, adrenal cortex and thyroid follicular cells in decreasing order of frequency. Carcinoid tumors and, curiously, lipomas also occur. More than 60% of patients have adenomas or carcinomas in at least two glands and about 20% eventually have three or more different glands involved [6]. More than 90% present with hypercalcemia and/or its various complications: peptic ulcer, hypoglycemia, diarrhea, or symptoms referable to a pituitary mass lesion such as headache or visual field defects [7]. The remaining patients may appear with other endocrine disorders like acromegaly, Cushing's syndrome or more commonly in recent years, amenorrhea-galactorrhea in females and decreased libido in males, the latter complications induced by excessive prolactin secretion [8]. Less commonly, patients may exhibit flushing due to carcinoid syndrome or inanition because of far-advanced metastatic disease. Ectopic hormone production by the various tumors does occur and should be considered before any surgical approach is contemplated.

The parathyroid glands are involved in more than 90% of patients, many of whom may be quite asymptomatic, the disease having been discovered after systematic family screening studies [9]. Hyperparathyroidism in MEN I behaves no differently than the nonfamilial disease [10]. Diffuse hyperplasia of all glands is quite common; in fact, when such is detected, the patient should be considered a MEN I suspect. In one series of patients with primary hyperparathyroidism 17.5% had evidence of another endocrine gland tumor [11]. In another the incidence was 16% [12]. A Mayo Clinic review of 475 patients with hyperparathyroidism showed 53 (11.2%) with hyperplasia, and of these, nearly 23% had evidence of MEN [13].

Tumors of the pancreatic islet cells can produce numerous symptoms, the most common of which is the Zollinger-Ellison syndrome. The pathologic lesion may be either a single adenoma or more commonly multiple adenomas or diffuse hyperplasia of the pancreatic islet cells. About 15% of the time the tumor is in the duodenum [14]. At least 25% of patients with the true Z-E syndrome; i.e., islet cell tumors or hyperplasia and not antral gastrinosis or ectopic hypergastrinemia, actually have MEN I. Insulinomas, glucagonomas, somatostatinomas and mixed tumors develop with an often confusing array of symptoms [15]. The pancreatic islet cells are particularly prone to produce ectopic hormones such as ACTH, ADH and even calcitonin [16]. Serum levels of pancreatic polypeptide are often elevated in patients with MEN I [17], and one personally observed case has been noted in which the pancreatic tumor produced only this substance. Diarrhea may be related to excessive gastrin-induced secretion of high volumes of low pH gastric juice. Other secretogogues have also been implicated in the etiology of the diarrhea, termed the pancreatic cholera syndrome in recognition of its secretory characteristics, including vasoactive intestinal polypeptide (VIP), gastric inhibitory polypeptide (GIP), pancreatic polypeptide or even prostaglandins [18]. The islet cell lesions frequently have the histological characteristics of carcinoid tumors and they may elaborate more than one hormone [16, 19]. True carcinoid tumors in MEN I are almost invariably of foregut origin with other common locations being in the bronchi or thymus. In a recent series of 74 cases of thymic carcinoid, 13 had a family history consistent with MEN [20]. Carcinoid tumors in MEN I also regularly elaborate ectopic polypeptides, especially ACTH.

Adrenal cortical hyperfunction may be due to a pituitary tumor, single or multiple adrenal adenomas or ectopic ACTH. Both Cushing's syndrome and hyperaldosteronism have been described, the latter rather infrequently [21]. Any of the pituitary hormones theoretically could be hyper-secreted but excess gonadotropins or TSH have not been convincingly demonstrated. Thyroid lesions in MEN I have been reported, but the pathology is not specific – goiter, adenoma, non-medullary carcinoma, Graves' disease and thyroiditis all having been described. In view of the commonality of these lesions in the general population, one wonders whether the thyroid involvement is truly part of the basic gene defect.

Individuals with MEN I may develop symptoms at any age but the condition is rare in childhood and uncommonly presents initially over the age of 60. For the most part, affected children are ascertained not by symptoms but by family screening studies. As expected, hypercalcemia is the most common finding [22]. In one study of 43 children with hyperparathyroidism, another common clue to the diagnosis was radiographic evidence of osteoporosis [23]. More than half had nonspecific presenting symptoms such as fatigue, weakness, anorexia and vomiting. Interestingly, about one-third had hypertension. In this series 7/43 were noted to have diffuse hyperplasia, a finding again that would suggest the possibility of MEN I, but unfortunately, no family studies were reported in these patients. The Zollinger-Ellison syndrome is not at all common in childhood. In one review of 15 cases, ages 8–15 years, the father of one child also had the syndrome documented [24]. Since there is such a wide variation in age of onset of symptoms in MEN I, it is possible that adult members of these families harbored the mutant gene but were asymptomatic. No detailed family studies have been performed in this setting, but it would seem likely that a proportion of children with Zollinger-Ellison syndrome might actually have MEN I, especially those in whom the operative findings are of diffuse islet cell hyperplasia or multiple pancreatic adenomas.

Insulinomas are likewise rare in children [25], although they have been reported as a cause of neonatal hypoglycemia [26]. Almost invariably they are single adenomas and their removal results in cure. There is no evidence at present to warrant any more detailed endocrine evaluation on these children or their families, since MEN I has not been reported in this setting. Diffuse hyperplasia of the islet cells with hyperinsulinemia (nesidioblastosis) has been described in sibs and appears to be an autosomal recessive defect independent of MEN I. Other islet cell tumors have not been reported in children. Likewise, adrenal adenomas or carcinomas do not seem to be part of the MEN I spectrum in children; however, it is important to emphasize that very little attention has generally been paid to the family history in reported cases.

Pituitary tumors in children are usually craniopharyngiomas and are not secretory, although hyperprolactinemia has been recorded. This tumor type is not part of MEN I. Carcinoid tumors virtually never occur in children.

MEN I is an autosomal dominant disorder with a high degree of penetrance. Effective therapy depends on which gland is involved and is mostly surgical. Controversy surrounds the treatment of the Zollinger-Ellison syndrome, some preferring surgical exploration and total gastrectomy and others favoring a medical approach with control of symptoms using the H_2-blocker cimetadine with or without subtotal gastrectomy [27, 28]. It makes good sense to at least explore, since the tumor may be single and resectable, thereby reserving cimetadine for more extensive disease, although it is true that 60% or more of the tumors are indeed malignant when discovered [29]. Moreover, in the small series of 15 children with the Z-E syndrome alluded to earlier, seven children treated with total gastrectomy survived for months to years despite the fact that four of the seven had documented metastatic disease at the time of surgery. Gastrin levels remained elevated in some, but surprisingly, dropped to normal in others even after having been above normal for up to six years. One further case subjected to total gastrectomy at age 15 for Z-E syndrome with multiple metastases was found to be disease free at age 34 [30]. What this means is not clear, but one possibility is that the Z-E syndrome in children is a different disease. Whether the Z-E syndrome in children when it occurs as part of MEN I is more or less benign thatn the sporadic non-heritable disease is totally unknown. Streptozotocin therapy may be useful in the management of non-resectable islet cell lesions of any secretory type. A promising new approach advocates the use of long-acting somatostatin analogue that suppresses pancreatic endocrine tumor secretion for up to twenty-four hours [31]. There is no evidence that any of the component tumors of MEN I, whether in children or adults, differ histologically from their sporadically occurring counterparts.

1.2. MEN, type II

In 1961, Sipple collated a number of patients with both pheochromocytoma and thyroid carcinoma [32]. Later workers, notably Schimke and Hartman in the United States [33] and Williams in Wales [34], pointed out that the thyroid carcinoma was invariably a medullary carcinoma, that hyperparathyroidism was an associated endocrinopathy, and the entire complex was inherited.

The thyroid tumor is always malignant, and as is the case with most familial tumors, tends to develop at an earlier average age and be multifocal within the thyroid gland. Calculations of age of onset are likely somewhat biased by inclusion of families studied because the proband was recognized as having the complete syndrome. Medullary thyroid carcinoma (MTC) is remarkably variable from patient to patient even within the same family. The most common presentation is of a thyroid mass which may contain radiographically visible calcification [35]. It is not at all uncommon to find family members who have tumors in the absence of a palpable mass or in the presence of a normal radionuclide scan. This latter group is detected by the measurement of serum calcitonin levels which are characteristically elevated with frank MTC. At operation, cervical lymph nodes are involved in more than 60% of patients and more distant spread to lungs, liver and adrenals will eventually occur [36]. A few patients may actually present with metastatic disease without an obvious thyroid source. While stromal amyloid is a characteristic histologic feature, it is not invariably present, and the tumor cells may be quite pleomorphic. The pathology of the lesion has been described in detail [37]. Peculiarly, the tumor has a quite variable clinical course, some individuals dying shortly after the primary is discovered, whereas others may live for many years even with obvious metastatic disease [38]. The reason for this is obscure but immunologic mechanisms may be involved [39]. Rarely the tumor may herald its presence because of seemingly unrelated symptoms. Diarrhea is not uncommon and has been related to excessive tumor production of calcitonin, VIP, serotonin, or prostaglandins [40]. The MTC in from 2–5% of patients secretes excessive ACTH and the patients may initially present with Cushing's syndrome [41]. This feature is not prognostically favorable, since one compilation of 23 such patients noted that 18 were dead within five months of the diagnosis [42].

It is now reasonably certain that MTC is derived from the parafollicular or C-cell of the thyroid. There is also good evidence that C-cell hyperplasia precedes actual tumor formation for quite literally years [43]. The hyperplastic C-cells are capable of secreting excess calcitonin, but only with pharmacologic provocation with calcium or pentagastrin or, perhaps better, a combination of the two [44]. Such provocative tests are extremely useful in family screening since they will identify the individual with subclinical, or at least non-invasive disease.

Pheochromocytomas are found in about 50% of patients with MEN II [9]. They are bilateral and/or multifocal about 70% of the time, and even when unilateral, the opposite adrenal may show diffuse medullary hyperplasia or nodularity [45]. Bilateral hyperplasia may also occur and these changes have been likened in a predictive sense to C-cell hyperplasia of the thyroid. As is true with other familial endocrine tumors, the two adrenals need not be synchronously involved. Oddly enough, the pheochromocytomas are often asymptomatic, and may not even respond to the usual provocative tests. The reason for this is not entirely clear, although vasodilatory substances elaborated by the MTC have been implicated [1], since MTC almost invariably preceeds development of the adrenal tumors. Alternatively, it is possible the pheochromocytoma in MEN II is at least biochemically different, since it tends to produce more epinephrine, in contrast to the sporadic tumor where norepinephrine predominates [46]. The incidence of malignant degeneration of the pheochromocytomas in MEN II is also somewhat higher than in the isolated tumors, but this may be related to the longer duration of asymptomatic disease and hence potential for tumor growth and dedifferentiation with the familial lesion.

The initial observations suggested that parathyroid hyperplasia might have been a compensatory effect of prolonged hypercalcitoninemia. This possibility no longer seems tenable. About 25% of patients with MEN II eventually show evidence of hyperparathyroidism, either on clinical or biochemical grounds [9].

The various facets of MEN II rarely appear before the age of 20. Most workers feel that everyone with the syndrome will develop MTC. Since C-cell hyperplasia is the precursor lesion, and as this state can be detected by provocative testing, it seems feasible to offer early surgery for those individuals who have a positive response to calcium/pentagastrin, even when no palpable nodules exist or radioimaging is nondiagnostic. One large family has been regularly examined by this technique and small foci of frank MTC have been detected in the second decade, with children as young as 8 having had prophylactic total thyroidectomy on the basis of calcitonin hyperresponsiveness [41].

No documented case of a pheochromocytoma has been described in a child with MEN II. Certainly, pheochromocytomas do develop in children and they are frequently multifocal, the latter finding not inconsistent with the operation of genetic factors, even in the absence of a positive family history [48]. There is evidence, however, that familial pheochromocytoma do exist outside the genetic confines of MEN II or III. It seems unlikely that children with multifocal or bilateral pheochromocytomas have MEN II, but again, appropriate testing has not been carried out. It is important to remember in this context that a moderate rise in calcitonin secretion may be seen in patients with pheochromocytoma [49], as well as in those with a host of other tumors such as oat cell carcinoma, hepatoma and breast carcinoma [50] and this fact should be taken into consideration when the results of the provocative tests are evaluated, especially in adults. A moderate response to calcium/pentagastrin infusion in a child who has had a previous pheochromocytoma may indicate the presence of another pheochromocytoma rather than MTC.

Parathyroid tumors or hyperplasia have not been described in children with MEN II.

The syndrome is an autosomal dominant with full penetrance probably by the age of 30 if C-cell hyperplasia is considered as a minimal diagnostic criterion. Many patients do not develop MTC until later life, however, and as mentioned previously, prolonged survival has been reported. There is no sex predilection and the syndrome has been described in the United States, in Europe and in Japan.

Treatment for all the tumors is surgical. Total thyroidectomy is vital and limited node dissection may be of value, especially if baseline calcitonin levels are elevated. Measurement of plasma calcitonin has been used to assess adequacy of resection, but on a few occasions, elevated levels did not decline to normal for 6 months or more [51]. There is no good evidence that radioiodine or the currently available chemotherapeutic agents are of significant value in the patient with more extensive disease. The pheochromocytoma, if not resectable, may be treated with a combination of alpha and beta blockers or with alpha-methyl tyrosine, a competitive analogue of tyrosine that interferes with the rate-limiting conversion of tyrosine to DOPA and hence catecholamines [52].

1.3. MEN III

MEN III also includes MTC and pheochromocytoma but there are some additional major findings that clearly differentiate this syndrome from MEN II. First of all, there is a striking physical difference. Patients with MEN II are outwardly normal, whereas those with MEN III have a very unusual habitus: peculiar facies with mucosal neuromas, megacolon, musculoskeletal abnormalities, and pigmentary alterations such as diffuse lentigines or cafe-au-lait spots, and on occasion findings similar to those of patients with neurofibromatosis [53, 54]. Secondly, hyperparathyroidism is a rare occurrence in MEN III. Most descriptions of parathyroid hyperplasia probably represent anatomic variation and should not necessarily be equated with hyperfunction [55]. Third, the MTC behaves in a much more aggressive fashion [56], the average age of death being in the third decade with MEN III and in the sixth to seventh decade in MEN II [57]. The pheochromocytoma behaves in similar fashion in the two disorders, although there is some suggestive evidence that it may develop on the average a few years earlier in MEN III [45]. Thus the tendency to 'lump' MEN II and III under the collective rubric of the Sipple syndrome would hardly seem justifiable.

By the same token, to consider MEN III as a forme fruste of von Recklinghausen's disease on the basis of a few cutaneous similarities and the occasional pheochromocytoma in neurofibromatosis is also not appropriate. Patients with MEN III have discrete mucosal neuromas throughout the gastrointestinal tract, a finding that is rare in von Recklinghausen's disease. Virtually all the MEN III patients have some involvement of the autonomic, sensory or motor neurons largely attributed to the presence of neuromas [58]. Their physical features are quite literally pathognomonic, whereas the diagnosis of generalized neurofibromatosis is often difficult to make clinically. Then, too, MTC is not a regular feature of von Recklinghausen's disease. The few patients in which this association was described could have easily have had MEN III with an unusual number of peripheral neuromas or neurofibromas [59, 60].

Unlike MEN II, MEN III can be diagnosed in childhood largely on the basis of the physical findings, the features of which have been referred to as the phenotype of malignancy, since they appear to always indicate at least C-cell hyperplasia and often frank MTC [61]. In accord with the early average of death of MEN III patients when compared to MEN II, MTC has been found to be fully developed in children even prior to the age of 2 [62, 63]. The treatment of MEN III, like MEN II, is surgical with the caveat that within reason the earlier the total thyroidectomy, the better [64]. Survival data from a Mayo Clinic series of patients with MEN III (IIb in their terminology) suggested that cure in the literal sense of the word could only be accomplished if thyroidectomy were performed prior to age 12 [65]. It would appear feasible to operate as soon as possible when the characteristic physiognomy is recognized.

MEN III is also an autosomal dominant condition. Penetrance appears high in affected families but many cases are sporadic. Whether this indicates overall reduced penetrance, a high spontaneous mutation rate, or underdiganosis in less severely affected relatives; i.e., variable expressivity, is not knwon. Treatment of the non-endocrine facets of the condition is not readily available, and surgical intervention, even on cosmetic grounds, may be less than satisfactory due to the diffuse nature of the disease process. Megacolon which is due to autonomic neurinomatosis, may require surgery but again, partial colectomy may not be curative because of generalized autonomic dysfunction.

1.4. Possible additional MEN syndrome

There are a number of reports in the literature describing patients with two or more endocrine tumors. Virtually all of these have been isolated cases and the tumors are generally single. In some instances the association can be at least potentially explained on the basis of a common environmental insult, as for example with parathyroid adenoma and thyroid carcinoma after external irradiation in childhood. Other times, there might be an underlying, perhaps unrecognized disorder, that predisposes to more than one endocrine tumor, simply on the basis of a common developmental defect, as with the combination of pheochromocytoma and carcinoid tumor [66]. More puzzling are the reports of parathyroid hyperplasia with carcinoid tumors, unless these patients have MEN I [61]. One such patient had a positive family history of hyperparathyroidism, a setting that would strongly favor a diagnosis of MEN I in the minds of many [68]. Oddly enough, there does seem to be a strong association, not recognizably genetic, of gastrointestinal carcinoids with a host of tumors: e.g., thyroid, breast, ovary and cervix, implying a more generalized tendency to malignancy in patients with carcinoid tumors [69].

If patients harbor two or more tumors, each of which appears as a facet of one of the MEN syndromes, it will obviously prompt speculation that the MEN syndromes are not distinct. Since the entire endocrine system, save for the gonads, is represented in the MEN syndromes, such overlap is inevitable and actually provides no evidence one way or another about the possibility of one inclusive syndrome or many. For example, a patient with MEN II had the Z-E syndrome with hypergastrinemia [70]. Yet, the source of the excessive gastrin was not determined and the pancreas was not examined. Gastrin-stimulating activity has been described with MTC [71], and ectopic gastrin production by MTC is certainly possible, given the array of peptides the MTC has been shown to produce [72]. Similarly, the discovery of an incidental microscopic pituitary adenoma in a patient with MEN II is not sufficient evidence to combine MEN I and II [73], any more than the presence of cafe-au-lait spots in Gaucher's disease, tuberous sclerosis, neurofibromatosis and McCune-Albright syndrome indicates that they are all in reality a single entity. In other words, overlapping features do not invariably imply fundamental identity.

It is quite possible, and even probable, that additional MEN syndromes exist. A respectable candidate is the combination of pheochromocytomas with islet cell tumors of the pancreas [74]. Each of these tumors is a part of a different MEN syndrome; however, there are certain differences indicating that the association is unique. The pheochromocytomas tend to be multiple, as in MEN II, but appear on the average a decade or more earlier. The islet cell lesion, which runs the gamut from hyperplasia through adenoma to carcinoma is generally nonfunctional as determined either by lack of hormone secretion or by the absence of other usual or unusual intracellular peptides as detected by immunoperoxidase staining techniques. These findings are in contrast to those in MEN I where the bulk of islet cell neoplasms are hormonally active. In one family, the proband had multiple islet cell lesions and multicentric pheochromocytoma, her daughter had a unilateral pheochromocytoma, and her mother had bilateral pheochromocytomas and a pituitary tumor [75]. The findings in this family may well support the existence of yet another MEN syndrome.

At the present time, however, there are reasons why this addition may not be appropriate. More than half the reported patients with pheochromocytoma and islet cell tumors either had the von Hippel-Lindau syndrome or had relatives with the disorder [76]. Even in the three generation family just described, the proband had bilateral renal adenomas, a finding common in the von Hioppel-Lindau syndrome. A recent compilation of data on von Hippel-Lindau syndrome noted that of 29 autopsy records, 21 contained references to pancreatic cysts and two others recorded pancreatic adenomas, cell type unknown [77]. One other patient not in the autopsy series had a non-beta-islet cell tumor of the pancreas. It is therefore conceivable that patients with pheochromocytoma and islet cell and pituitary tumors actually have the von Hippel-Lindau syndrome, which in any case is a quite variable condition. Perhaps the findings are more indicative of heterogeneity within the von Hippel-Lindau syndrome, one type having the classical variety with hemangioblastomas of the retina and cerebellum, the other expanded to include certain endocrine tumors. Obviously, this question needs to be answered, not only for nosologic reasons, but for improved patient care. As a corollary, it is important to continue to record endocrine tumor associations of all types in order to develop a better understanding of the interrelationships among the various glands and provide insight into the molecular mechanism underlying gene influenced endocrine tumor formation.

1.5. Molecular basis of the MEN syndromes

A number of theories have been proposed to account for the MEN syndromes. Wermer initially proposed that MEN I was the embodiment of what he called mosaic pleiotropism. This term is in reality only descriptive and could actually be considered tautological, since pleiotropism by definition indicates that a single gene effects different tissues, or in the case of the endocrine system, different glands [4]. Vance *et al.* postulated nesidioblastosis, by that meaning that the various secretory cells of the pancreas could secondarily influence other glands with the eventual development in those glands of hyperplasia and/or tumors; e.g., insulin-induced hypoglycemia, if prolonged, could lead to compensatory HGH secretion and perhaps a pituitary tumor [78]. The term nesidioblastosis currently has a bit different meaning (see later), and in any case there is no evidence at all that the pancreas is responsible for the various tumors comprising MEN I.

In 1968 Azzopardi and Williams, in a discussion of tumors producing ectopic hormones, hypothesized that all cells capable of producing peptide hormones might be derived from a common ancestral cell [79]. Pearse subsequently established that such cells shared certain cytochemical and ultrastructural properties presumably indicative of functional similarities [80]. He offered the acronym APUD (*A*mine *P*recursor *U*ptake and *D*ecarboxylation) to emphasize the ability of these cells to synthesize and secrete bioactive amines and peptides. Elegant embryologic mapping techniques established that some of these cells were of neural crest origin and, moreover, they seemed to be the progenitors of at least part of the classic endocrine system. In a scientific world perhaps grasping for simple solutions, the terms APUD (or its tumorous extension, apudoma), neural crest and endocrine tumor became practically synonymous [81]. The MEN syndromes were thus considered to represent abnormalities in differentiation of neural crest tissue and hence be collectively classified as neurocristopathies [82].

There is indeed good evidence that the adrenal medulla and the thyroid C-cell are derived from neural crest [83], although the source of the latter still is disputed [84]. The data favoring a neural crest origin of the remaining components of the endocrine system is less compelling; indeed, there is strong evidence against this hypothesis. A variety of transplant studies using quail embryos or quail-chick embryonic allografts seem to clearly indicate that the APUD cells of the gut and pancreas are not derived from neural crest [85–87]. The parathyroid glands have similarly not been shown in any studies to be anything other than from epithelial anlage. The adrenal cortex is clearly a mesodermal derivative. Pearse, in an attempt to rationalize these discrepancies, suggested that the endocrine cells in the primitive gut endothelium were programmed by neuroendocrine tissue during their development from the embryonic epiblast [88]. At present this is an unproved hypothesis. It is now clear, however, that the possession of APUD characteristics and the ability to produce hormones does not necessarily imply a neural crest origin of the cell in question [89]. In fact, the ability to synthesize peptides may be a nearly universal concomitant of neoplasia [90]. Thus, the attractive neurocristopathy concept is no longer tenable, at least insofar as the MEN syndromes are concerned, although it does remain useful as a starting point for future investigation [91].

At the present time, the molecular lesions giving rise to the MEN syndromes remain enigmatic. In view of the fact that months or years can elapse between involvement of one endocrine tissue and another, it is sensible to postulate that the environment might play a precipitating role. Baylin *et al.*, using tumor cells from a patient with MEN II who was also heterozygous for the X-linked trait, glucose-6-phosphate dehydroxygenase (G6PD) deficiency, found that each tumor expressed either type A or the B phenotype and hence each was derived from a single clone [92]. These findings are compatible with the Knudson hypothesis in that the original germinal mutation could be considered as having given rise to multiple susceptible cells, the development of a frank tumor being then dependent on a second mutational event. The exact nature of this second mutational event is conjectural, but the temporally disparate tumor development supports the idea of some environmental insult. The initial findings need to be confirmed in other patients and also extended to the other MEN syndromes. Perhaps studies of this type would also help establish whether or not a given patient with two endocrine tumors has a heritable basis for his disease; i.e., are the two (or more) tumors derived from one or a number of clones. Clearly, more readily available polymorphic markers are needed since G6PD differences have only limited applicability.

REFERENCES

1. Schimke RN: Multiple endocrine adenomatosis syndromes. Adv Intern Med 21:249–65, 1976.
2. Erdheim J: Zur normalen und pathologischen Histologie der Glandula Thyreoides, Parathyreoidea, und Hypophysis. Beitr Path Anat 33:158–236, 1903.
3. Rossier PH, Dressler M: Familiare Erkrankung innerskretorischer Drusen kombiniert mit Ulcuskrankheit. Schweiz Med Wschr 69:985–990, 1939.
4. Werner P: Genetic aspects of adenomatosis of endocrine glands. Am J Med 16:363–371, 1954.
5. Moldawer PM, Nardi GL, Raker JW: Concomitance of multiple adenomas of the parathyroids and pancreatic islets with tumor of the pituitary: a syndrome with familial incidence. Am J Med Sci 228:190–206, 1954.
6. Schimke RN: Disorders affecting multiple endocrine systems. In: Harrison's Textbook of Internal Medicine, Isselbacher K, Adams R, Braunwald E, Petersdorf R, Wilson J (eds), New York, McGraw-Hill, 1980, Ed 9, p 1820–1824.
7. Rimoin DL, Schimke RN: Genetic disorders of the endocrine glands. New York, Plenum Press, Ed 2 (in press).
8. Veldhuis JD, Green JE III, Kovacs E, Worgul TJ, Murray FT, Hammond JM: Prolactin-secreting pituitary adenomas. Association with multiple endocrine neoplasm, Type I. Am J Med 67:830–7, 1979.
9. Baylin SB: The multiple endocrine neoplasm syndromes: implications for the study of inherited tumors. Semin Oncol 5:35–45, 1978.
10. Lamers CB, Froeling PG: Clinical significance of hyperparathyroidism in familial multiple endocrine adenomatosis Type I. (MEAI) Am J Med 66:422–4, 1979.
11. Boey JH, Cooke TJC, Gilbert JM, Sweeney EC, Taylor S: Occurrence of other endocrine tumours in primary hyperparathyroidism. Lancet 2 pt. 2:781–784, 1975.
12. Mallette LE, Bilezikian JP, Heath DA, Aurbach GD: Primary hyperparathyroidism: clinical and biochemical features. Medicine 53:127–146, 1974.

13. Scholz DA, Purnell DC, Edis AJ, Van Heerden JA, Woolner LB: Primary hyperparathyroidism with multiple parathyroid gland enlargement: review of 53 cases. Mayo Clinic Proc 53:792–97, 1978.
14. Evans WE, Armstrong RG, Schulte W, Garancis JC: Ulcerogenic tumor of the duodenum. Am J Surg 124:596–599, 1972.
15. Schimke RN: Syndromes with multiple endocrine gland involvement. Prog Med Genet (NS) 3:143–175, 1979.
16. Yamaguchi K, Kameya T, Abe K: Multiple endocrine neoplasia Type I. Clin Endocrinol Metab 9:261–84, 1980.
17. Lamers CB, Diemel J, Roeffen W: Serum levels of pancreatic polypeptide in Zollinger-Ellison Syndrome and hyperparathyroidism from families with multiple endocrine adenomatosis type I. Digestion 18:297–302, 1978.
18. Larsson L-I, Schwartz T, Lundqvist G, et al.: Occurrence of human pancreatic polypeptide in pancreatic endocrine tumors: possible implication in the watery diarrhea syndrome. Am J Pathol 85:675–684, 1976.
19. Boden G, Owen OE, Rezvani I, Elfenbein BL, Quickel KE. An islet cell carcinoma containing glucagon and insulin. Diabetes 26:128–37, 1977.
20. Wick MR, Scott RE, Li CY, Carney JA: Carcinoid tumor of the thymus: A clinico-pathologic report of seven cases with a review of the literature. Mayo Clin Proc 55:246–54, 1980.
21. Ballard HS, Frame B, Hartsock PJ: Familial multiple endocrine adenoma peptic ulcer complex. Medicine 43:481–516, 1964.
22. Betts JB, O'Malley BP, Rosenthal FD: Hyperparathyroidism: a prerequisite for Zollinger-Ellison syndrome in multiple endocrine adenomatosis Type I—report of a further family and review of the literature. Q J Med 49(193):69–76, 1980.
23. Bjernulf A, Hall K, Sjogren I, Werner I: Primary hyperparathyroidism in children. Acta Paediatr Scand 59:249–258, 1970.
24. Wilson SD, Schulte WJ, Meade RC: Longevity studies following total gastrectomy in children with the Zollinger-Ellison syndrome. Arch Surg 103:108–115, 1971.
25. Rickham PP: Islet cell tumors in childhood. J Pediatr Surg 10:83–86, 1975.
26. Baerentsen H: Neonatal hypoglycemia due to islet cell adenoma. Acta Paediatr Scand 62:207–210, 1973.
27. McCarthy DM: The place of surgery in the Zollinger- Ellison syndrome. N Engl J Med 302(24):1344–7, 1980.
28. Drake DP, Maciver AG, Atwell JD: Zollinger-Ellison syndrome in a child: medical treatment with cimetidine. Arch Dis Child 55:226–8, 1980.
29. Schein PS, DeLellis RA, Kahn CR, Gorden P, Kraft AR: Islet cell tumours; current concepts and management. Ann Intern Med 79:239–257, 1973.
30. Davis CE Jr, Vansant JH: Zollinger-Ellison syndrome. Spontaneous regression of advanced intra-abdominal metastases with 20 year survival. Ann Surg 189:620–6, 1979.
31. Long RG, Barnes AJ, Adrian TE, et al.: Suppression of pancreatic endocrine tumour secretion by long-acting somatostatin analogue. Lancet 2(8146):764–7, 1979.
32. Sipple JH: The association of pheochromocytoma with carcinoma of the thyroid gland. Am J Med 31:163–166, 1961.
33. Schimke RN, Hartmann WH: Familial amyloid-producing medullary thyroid carcinoma and pheochromocytoma: A distinct genetic entity. Ann Intern Med 63:1027–39, 1965.
34. Williams ED: A review of 17 cases of carcinoma of the thyroid and pheochromocytoma. J Clin Pathol 18:288–292, 1965.
35. Pearson KD, Wells SA, Keiser HR: Familial medullary carcinoma of the thyroid, adrenal pheochromocytoma and parathyroid hyperplasia. Radiology 107:249–256, 1973.

36. Williams ED, Brown CL, Doniach I: Pathologic and clinical findings in a review of 67 cases of medullary carcinoma of the thyroid. J Clin Pathol 19:103–113, 1966.
37. Williams ED: Medullary carcinoma of the thyroid. In: Endocrinology, Vol. 2, Martin L, Potts JT Jr, Nelson DH, Steinberger E, Winegrad AI (eds), New York, Grune and Stratton, 1979, p 777–792.
38. Ljunberg O: On medullary carcinoma of the thyroid. Acta Pathol Microbiol Scand (Supp) 231:1–57, 1972.
39. Rocklin RE, Gagel R, Feldman Z, Tashjian AH Jr: Cellular immune responses in familial medullary thyroid carcinoma. N Engl J Med 296 pt. 2:835–838, 1977.
40. Steinfeld CM, Moertel CG, Woolner LB: Diarrhea and medullary carcinoma of the thyroid. Cancer 31:1237–1239, 1973.
41. Goltzman D, Huang SN, Browne C, Solomon S: Adrenocorticotropin and calcitonin in medullary thyroid carcinoma: frequency of occurrence and localization in the same cell type by immunocytochemistry. J Clin Endocrinol Metab 49:364–9, 1979.
42. Keusch G, Binswanger U, Damubacher MA, Fischer JA: Ectopic ACTH syndrome and medullary thyroid carcinoma. Acta Endocrinol 86:306–316, 1979.
43. Wolfe HJ, Melvin KE, Cervi-Skinner SJ, et al.: C-cell hyperplasia preceding medullary thyroid carcinoma. N Engl J Med 289 pt. 1:437–441, 1973.
44. Wells SA Jr., Baylin SB, Linshaw WM, Farrell RE, Cox EB, Cooper CW: Provocative agents and the diagnosis of medullary carcinoma of the thyroid gland. Ann Surg 188:139–141, 1978.
45. Webb TA, Sheps SG, Carney JA: Differences between sporadic pheochromocytoma and pheochromocytoma in multiple endocrine neoplasm, Type 2. Am J Surg Pathol 4:121-6, 1980.
46. Hamilton BP, Landsberg L, Levine RJ: Measurement of urinary epinephrine in screening for pheochromocytomas in multiple endocrine neoplasm, Type II. Am J Med 65:1027–1032, 1978.
47. Graze K, Spiler IJ, Tashjian AH Jr: Natural history of familial medullary thyroid carcinoma. N Engl J Med 299:980–985, 1978.
48. Stackpole RH, Melicow MM, Uson AC: Pheochromocytoma in children. J Pediatr 63:315–330, 1963.
49. Raue F, Bayer JM, Rahn KH et al.: Hypercalcitoninemia in patients with pheochromocytoma. Klin Wochenschr 56:697–701, 1978.
50. Schwartz KE, Wolfsen AR, Forster B, Odell WD: Calcitonin in non-thyroid cancer. J Clin Endocrinol Metab 49:438–44, 1979.
51. Stepanas AV, Samaan NA, Hill CS, Hickey RC: Medullary thyroid carcinoma importance of serial serum calcitonin measurement. Cancer 43:825–37, 1979.
52. Jones NF, Walker G, Ruthven CR, Sandler M: α-methyl-p-tyrosine in the management of phaeochromocytoma. Lancet 2:1105–1112, 1968.
53. Williams ED, Pollock DJ: Multiple mucosal neuromata with endocrine tumours; a syndrome allied to von Recklinghausen's disease. J Path Bact 91:71–80, 1966.
54. Schimke RN, Hartmann WH, Prout TE, Rimoin DL: The syndrome of bilateral pheochromocytoma, medullary thyroid carcinoma and multiple neuromas. N Engl J Med 279:1–7, 1968.
55. Carney JA, Roth SI, Heath H III, Sizemore GW, Hayles AB: The parathyroid glands in multiple endocrine neoplasm, type 2b. Am J Pathol 99:397–400, 1980.
56. Norton JA, Froome LC, Farrell RE, Wells SR Jr: Multiple endocrine neoplasia Type IIb: the most aggressive form of medullary thyroid carcinoma. Surg Clin North Am 59(1):109–18, 1979.
57. Williams ED: Thyroidectomy for genetically determined medullary carcinoma. (Letter)

Lancet 1(8025):1309–10, 1977.
58. Dyck PJ, Carney JA, Sizemore GW, Okazaki H, Brimijoin WS, Lambert EH: Multiple endocrine neoplasia, type 2b: phenotype recognition; neurologic features and twin pathological basis. Ann Neurol 6:302–14, 1979.
59. Pages A, Marty CH, Baldet P, Peraldi R: Le syndrome neurofibromatose carcinome medullaire thyroidien-pheochromocytome. Arch Anat Pathol 18:137–142, 1970.
60. Hansen OP, Hansen M, Hansen HH, Rose B: Multiple endocrine adenomatosis of mixed type. Acta Med Scand 200:327–331, 1976.
61. Schimke RN: Phenotype of malignancy: the mucosal neuroma syndrome. Pediatrics 52:283–4, 1973.
62. Moyes CD, Alexander FW: Mucosal neuroma syndroma presenting a neonate. Dev Med Clin Neurol 19:518–34, 1977.
63. Stjernholm MR, Freudenbourg JC, Mooney HS, Kinney FJ, Deftos LJ: Medullary carcinoma of the thyroid before age 2 years. J Clin Endocrinol Metab 51:252–3, 1980.
64. Leape LL, Miller HH, Graz K, Feldman ZT, Gagel RF, Wolfe HJ, DeLellis RA, Tashjian AHJ, Reichlin S: Total Thyroidectomy for occult medullary carcinoma of the thyroid in children. J Pediatr Surg 11:831-7, 1976.
65. Carney JA, Sizemore GW, Hayles AV: C-cell disease of the thyroid gland in multiple endocrine neoplasia, Type 2b. Cancer 44:2173–83, 1979.
66. Warner RR, Blaustein AS: Coexistence of pheochromocytoma and carcinoid syndrome produced by metastatic carcinoid of the ileum. Mt Sinai J Med 37:536–48, 1970.
67. Samaan NA, Hickey RC, Bedner TD, Ibanez ML: Hyperparathyroidism and carcinoid tumor. Ann Intern Med 82:205–207, 1975.
68. Lokich JJ, Li F: Carcinoid of the thymus with hereditary hyperparathyroidism. Ann Intern Med 89:364–5, 1978.
69. Godwin JG II: Carcinoid tumors. Cancer 36:560-9, 1975.
70. Cameron D, Spiro HM, Landsberg L: Zollinger-Ellison syndrome with multiple endocrine adenomatosis Type II. N Engl J Med 299:152–3, 1978.
71. Friesen SR, Schimke RN, Pearse AG: Genetic aspects of the Zollinger-Ellison syndrome. Ann Surg 176:370–83, 1972.
72. Iwanaga T, Koyama H, Uchiyama S, Takahashi Y, Nakono S, Itoh T, Horai T, Wada A, Tateishi R: Production of several substances by medullary carcinoma of the thyroid. Cancer 41:1106–12, 1978.
73. Wolf LM, Duduisson M, Schrub JC, Metayer J, Laumonier R: Syndrome la Sipple associé à des adenômes hypophysaires et parathyroidiens. Ann Endocrinol 33:455–63, 1972.
74. Carney JA, Go VL, Gorden H, Northcutt RC, Pearse AG, Sheps SG: Familial pheochromocytoma and islet cell tumor of the pancreas. Am J Med 68:515–21, 1980.
75. Janson KL, Roberts JA, Varela M: Multiple endocrine adenomatosis: in support of the common origin theories. J Urol 119:161–5, 1978.
76. Hull MT, Warfel KA, Muller J, Higgins JT. Familial islet cell tumors in von Hippel-Lindau's disease. Cancer 44:1523–26, 1979.
77. Horton WA, Wong V, Eldridge R: Von Hippel-Lindau disease. Arch Intern Med 136:769–77, 1976.
78. Vance JE, Stoll RW, Kitabchi AE, Buchanan KO, Hollander D, Williams RH: Familial nesidioblastosis as the predominant manifestation of multiple endocrine adenomatosis. Am J Med 52:211–27, 1972.
79. Azzopardi JG, Williams ED: Pathology of non-endocrine tumors associated with Cushing's syndrome. Cancer 22:274–86, 1968.
80. Pearse AGE: The cytochemistry and ultrastructure of polypeptide hormone-producing cells of the APUD series and the embryologic, physiologic and pathologic implications of the

concept. J Histochem Cytochem 17:303–13, 1969.
81. Weichert RF: The neural ectodermal origin of the peptide-secreting endocrine glands. Am J Med 49:232–41, 1970.
82. Bolande RP: The neurocristopathies. Hum Pathol 5:409–429, 1974.
83. Pearse AG, Polak JM: Cytochemical evidence for the neural crest origin of mammalian ultimobranchel C cells. Histochemistry 27:96–102, 1971.
84. Kameda Y, Ikeda A: Immunochemical and immunohistochemical studies on the 27S iodoprotein of dog thyroid with reference to thyroglobulin-like reaction of the parafollicular cells. Biochim Biophys Acta 577:241–47, 1979.
85. Andrew A: An experimental investigation into the possible neural crest origin of pancreatic APUD (islet) cells. J Embryol Exp Morphol 35:577–93, 1976.
86. Fontaine J, LeDouarin NM: Analysis of endoderm formation in the avian blastoderm by the use of quail-chick chimeras: problem of the neuro-ectodermal origin of the cells of the APUD series. J Embryol Exp Morphol 41:209–22, 1977.
87. Pictet RL, Rall LB, Phelps P, Rutter WJ: The neural crest and the origin of the insulin-producing and other gastrointestinal hormone producing cells. Science 191:191–2, 1976.
88. Pearse AG, Takor TT: Embryology of the diffuse neuroendocrine system and its relationship to the common peptides. Fed Proc 38:2238–94, 1979.
89. Baylin SB, Mendelson G: Ectopic (inappropriate) hormone production by tumors: mechanisms involved and the biological and chemical implications. Endo Rev 1:45–77, 1980.
90. Odell WD, Wolfsen AR: Humoral syndromes associated with cancer. Annu Rev Med 29:379–406, 1978.
91. Schimke RN: The neurocristopathy concept: fact or fiction. In: Advances in Neuroblastoma Research, Evans AE (ed), New York, Raven Press, 1980, p 13–24.
92. Baylin SB, Hsu HS, Gann DS, Smallbridge RC, Wells SA Jr: Inherited medullary thyroid carcinoma: a final monoclonal mutation in one of multiple clones of susceptible cells. Science 199:429–31, 1978.

11. Adrenal Cortical Carcinoma in Children: 42 Patients Treated from 1958 to 1980 at Villejuif

M. LEFEVRE, R. GERARD-MARCHANT, J.P. GUBLER, J.L. CHAUSSAIN and J. LEMERLE

INTRODUCTION

Adrenal cortical carcinoma in children is rare, but when present is a special challenge to the pathologist as well as other members of the pediatric oncology team. We report here our experience with 42 children seen between 1958 and 1980. We have correlated both traditional histopathology and tumor size to outcome.

Table 1a. Initial clinical features. 42 patients.

No.	Age		Sex	Virilization	Cushing's syndrome	Abdominal mass	Gyneco-mastia.
1	6 y	5 m	F	+	+	−	−
2	3 y	11 m	F	+	−	−	−
3	2 y	4 m	M	+	+	−	−
4	6 y		F	+	+	−	−
5	12 y	9 m	M	+	−	+	+
6	10 y	2 m	F	+	+	+	+
7	5 y	10 m	F	+	+	−	−
8	2 y	5 m	F	+	+	−	−
9	13 y	2 m	F	+	−	−	−
10	1 y		F	+	−	+	−
11	17 y		F	+	−	−	−
12	1 y	5 m	M	+	−	+	−
13	4 y	4 m	M	+	−	+	−
14	1 y	6 m	F	+	−	+	−
15	4 y	8 m	F	+	+	−	−
16	4 y	5 m	M	+	+	−	−
17	4 y	6 m	M	+	−	+	−
18	5 y	8 m	F	+	−	+	−

G. Bennett Humphrey et al. (eds), Adrenal and Endocrine Tumors in Children.

Table 1a. Initial clinical features. 42 patients (*continued*).

No.	Age		Sex	Virilization	Cushing's syndrome	Abdominal mass	Gyneco-mastia.
19	1 y	11 m	F	+	–	–	–
20	3 y	7 m	F	+	+	–	–
21	3 y	8 m	F	+	–	–	–
22	1 y	10 m	F	+	+	–	–
23	4 y	6 m	M	+	–	+	–
24	1 y	1 m	M	?	?	+	–
25	1 y	3 m	F	+	+	–	–
26	5 y	5 m	F	+	+	–	–
27	4 y	2 m	F	+	+	+	–
28	1 y	5 m	M	?	–	+	–
29		7 m	F	+	+	–	–
30	2 y	9 m	M	+	–	–	–
31	14 y		M	+	–	–	–
32	11 y		F	–	–	+	–
33		6 m	M	+	+	–	–
34	1 y	3 m	M	+	–	+	–
35		6 m	M	+	–	+	–
36	4 y		F	+	–	+	–
37	2 y	5 m	F	+	–	+	–
38	5 y	2 m	F	+	–	–	–
39	5 y	1 m	M	+	–	+	–
40	1 y	10 m	F	+	–	–	–
41		18 m	M	+	+	+	–
42	6 y	10 m	F	+	–	–	–

Table 1b. Initial clinical features. 42 patients.

Age at diagnosis:	median age = 3 years 11 months mean age = 4 years 7 months under 1 year = 3 patients/42 (7%) under 2 years = 14/42 (33%) under 5 years = 28/42 (66%)	
Sex ratio:	Female 26 (= 62%)	Male 16 (= 38%)
Symptoms at presentation:		
Virilization 39/42 93%	Cushing's syndrome 16/42 38%	Abdominal mass 19/42 45%
17 KS > Normal values = 25/31 80%		
17 OH > Normal values = 7/28 25%		

Table 2. Endocrinologic findings.

No.	24 hour urinary levels for 17 OH (mg/24 h, N2.2–7.3)	17 KS (mg/24 h, N1.5–5)	DHA (mg/24 h)	Basal plasma levels for Cortisol (μg/100 ml, N 12±1)	Testosterone (ng/100 ml)
1	10	5.5	1.3	36	
2	0.6	3			
3	7	3.8	1	27	
4	2.5	49		16	10
5	18.5	23.5	4	5.3	55
6	11.9	8.7	1.3	21	27
8	1.95	77	70	17.8	
9	8	420	325	8.1	28
10					
11	7.6	9.7		40	
12		320	310	29.3	1170
13	4.5	115	81	26	
14	4.2	14.6	9.5		
15					
16	2.5	12.5	5	13.2	840
17		1600			
18	9	280	296		5
19		48.5	33		
20	8.5	140	130	40	44
21	1.6	8	1.7		
22	1.2	1.2		35	76
23	5.6	124	114	12.8	57
24					
25		14			
26	14.5	14	1	22.1	
27	14.2	402	340		
28					
29					
30	0.7	245	233	24.5	
31					
32					
33					
34	0.7		3,8 mg/ml*	98	
35					
36					
37					
38	4.9	75.2	30	16.2	5.5
39	0.9	192	134		Normal
40	2	25	32,3 mg/ml*	Normal	0.35
41	1.5	81		43	10
42	Normal	250			

* This is a basal plasma level: normal values for DHA = 1 à 5 ng/ml.

PATIENTS

This tumor is seen mainly in young children and girls (Table 1a and 1b). Virilization syndrome is consistently found (93% of the cases). Other frequent symptoms are: abdominal mass (45%) and Cushing's syndrome (38%). The 24 h urinary 17-ketosteroid levels are elevated in 80% of the cases and in 25% for the 17 OH (Table 2 and 1b).

PROGNOSTIC FACTORS

Pathologic features do not seem to be reliable to establish the diagnosis of malignancy when surgery has been possible. The weight of the tumor seems to be the best indicator of a malignant tumor when there is no metastasis. Cytologic and architectural features are often misleading, making pathologic features less reliable indicators [1]. Of the 35 surgically resected tumors, the weight of which was known, 16/17 of the patients who had a tumor of less than 150 g are alive. The patient who died (No. 16) had a very small tumor, 22 g, and histologic diagnosis was malignant. 14/18 of the patients bearing a tumor over 150 g are dead (Table 3a and 3b). The five patients who had only biopsy are dead. Five patients among the 22 still alive had a tumor of more than 150 g.

TREATMENT

(1) *Surgery.* Prognosis is best when the tumor is resected totally and easily (Table 4a, 4b).

When surgery was not thought possible, two treatments were tried before surgery: mitotane (OP'DDD) and/or radiotherapy.

(2) *Radiotherapy* was used in 11 cases. In only one case were we able to observe a measurable action of radiotherapy in a patient who is still alive. This patient received radiotherapy before surgery on an unresectable tumor. Surgery became possible after XRT.

No patient has been cured by radiotherapy alone.

(3) *Mitotane (= OP'DDD)* was used in 21 cases. Efficacy is measurable only in 13 cases.

OP'DDD before surgery: objective effect in 2 cases out of 4 – these 2 patients are alive. Of the 2 others, one is alive although there was no objective effect of the OP'DDD and one is dead.

OP'DDD after surgery for incomplete resection: 4 cases – an objective

Table 3a. Pathologic findings after surgery.

No.	Pathologic diagnosis (M = Malignant, D = Doubtful, B = Benign)	Tumor's weight	Last known status (D = Dead, A = Alive)
1	B	50 gr	A
2	M	750	D
3	D	50	A
4	D	135	A
5	M	1400	D
6	D	1200	D
7	D	1170	D
8	D	110	A
9	B	120	A
10	M	Biopsy	D
11	B	30	A
12	?	200	A
13	M	740	D
14	No surgery	No surgery	D
15	M	820	D
16	M	22	D
17	M	Biopsy	D
18	M	>1000 gr	A
19	M	50	A
20	M	180	D
21	D	20	A
22	M	30	A
23	?	Biopsy	D
24	M	300	A
25	B	80	A
26	M	180	D
27	M	Biopsy	D
28	M	295	D
29	D	50	A
30	D	300	A
31	M	?	D
32	M	300	D
33	M	320	D
34	M	150	A
35	M	235	D
36	?	?	A
37	M	700	D
38	B	20	A
39	D	70	A
40	B	55	A
41	M	500	A
42	B	88	A

Table 3b. Prognostic factors.

Tumor weight	Total	Dead	Alive
<150 gr	17	1	16
>150 gr	18	14	4
No data	2	1	1
No surgery	1	1	0
Exploratory laparotomy (no resection)	4	4	0

Table 4a. Treatment.

		OP'DDD			Radiotherapy			
No.	Surgery	Before surgery	After surgery	For recurrence or metastas.	Before surgery	After surgery	For recurrence or metastas.	Survival (A = Alive, D = Dead)
1	Easy-complete	+	+					A
2	Difficult-complete			+				D
3	Difficult		+					A
4	Easy							A
5	Difficult		+			+		D
6	Difficult		+					D
7	Difficult			+				D
8	Easy							A
9	Easy							A
10	Exploratory lapar.							D
11	Easy							A
12	Partial	+	+			+		A
13	Difficult							D
14	No surgery							D
15	Partial							D
16	Easy		+					D
17	Explo.					+		D
18	Partial		+	+				A
19	Difficult							A
20	Partial	+						D
21	Easy							A
22	Easy							A
23	Explo.		+					D
24	Difficult							A
25	Easy				+			A
26	Easy			+			+	D
27	Explo.				+			D

Table 4a. Treatment.

No.	Surgery	OP'DDD Before surgery	OP'DDD After surgery	OP'DDD For recurrence or metastas.	Radiotherapy Before surgery	Radiotherapy After surgery	Radiotherapy For recurrence or metastas.	Survival (A = Alive, D = Dead)
28	Difficult			+	+			D
29	Easy							A
30	Easy							A
31	Partial		+			+		D
32	Difficult			+				D
33	Difficult		+			+		D
34	Easy	+	+			+		A
35	Easy		+					D
36	?			+				A
37	Difficult		+			+		D
38	Easy							A
39	Easy							A
40	Easy							A
41	Easy		+					A
42	Easy							A

Easy = easy and complete. Difficult = difficult but complete. Partial = incomplete. Explo. = exploratory laparotomy without resection.

Table 4b. Treatment.

	Total	Dead	Alive
Surgery			
Complete and easy resection	19	3	16
Complete but difficult resection	12	9	3
Incomplete resection	5	3	2
No resection at all	4	4	0
No data	1	0	1
Radiotherapy			
Before surgery	3	2	1
After surgery, systematically	7	5	2
On abdominal mass when surgery was impossible	1	1	0
On metastasis (lung)	1	1	0
OP'DDD			
Before surgery	4	1	3
After incomplete resection	4	2	2
For recurrence or metastasis	7	5	2

Table 5. Follow up.

No.	Status	Duration of survival from diagnosis to death or last time the patient was seen	Reason for death		
			Local recurrence	Metastasis	Other
1	Alive	6 y			
2	Dead	2 y 8 m	+	Skin	
3	Alive	11 y 8 m			
4	Alive	6 y			
5	Dead	1 y 6 m	+	Liver	
6	Dead	9 m	+	Liver	
7	Dead	1 y 8 m	+	Lung	
8	Alive	6 y 7 m			
9	Alive	7 y 9 m			
10	Dead	6 m			
11	Alive	7 y			
12	Alive	9 y 6 m			
13	Dead	1 y 9 m	+	Liver	
14	Dead	3 y		Lung	Died suddenly
15	Dead	6 m			
16	Dead	1 y	+	Liver + lung	
17	Dead	4 y		Brain	
18	Alive	11 y	+ *	Liver + lung	
19	Alive	15 y			
20	Dead	1 y	+		
21	Alive	8 y			
22	Alive	6 y 8 m			
23	Dead	2 y 6 m		Liver + lung	
24	Alive	9 y			
25	Alive	19 y			
26	Dead	2 y 8 m	+	Liver	
27	Dead	9 m		Liver + lung	
28	Dead	9 y		Brain + lung	
29	Alive	10 y			
30	Alive	9 y			
31	Dead	1 y 4 m	+	Lung	
32	Dead	1 y 1 m		Liver + lung	
33	Dead	9 m	+	Liver	
34	Alive	4 y 1 m			
35	Dead	6 m			Died suddenly at 6 m
36	Alive	1 y 3 m	+ *	Lung	
37	Dead	10 m	+	Liver	
38	Alive	3 m	+	Liver	
39	Alive	3 y 10 m			
40	Alive	1 y 4 m			
41	Alive	4 y 7 m			
42	Alive	7 m			

* These two patients are alive = their metastasis were cured by OP'DDD.

effect was observed in 1 case – (one of those who also received OP′DDD before surgery and is alive).

OP′DDD for recurrence and/or metastasis: 7 cases – an objective and definitive effect was noted in 2 cases who are cured and a temporary effect in one case.

An objective effect was noted in 5 cases out of 13 patients who received OP′DDD. No patient has been cured by OP′DDD alone.

FOLLOW UP: TABLE 5

Of the 42 patients treated here at Villejuif 22 are alive and 20 are dead, including 3 unexplained deaths. Eleven of the 17 whose death was due to this tumor had local recurrence; all 17 had metastases. The metastatic sites were: liver in 11 cases, lung in 8 cases, brain in 2 cases and skin in one case.

The mean duration of survival from date of diagnosis to death is one year 11 months (from 6 months to 9 years) (see Table 6 and Figure 1).

Some of the patients treated with mitotane had iatrogenic complications (Table 7). The most frequent complications were neurological and psychological. Some acute adrenal failures were observed. We did not find any correlation between dose of OP′DDD and complication. No patient died because of OP′DDD.

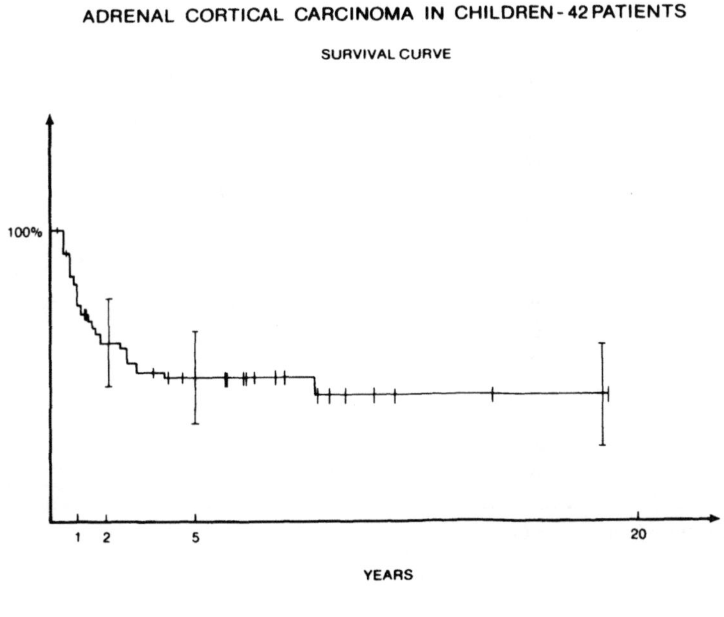

Figure 1.

Table 6. Survival duration between diagnosis and first metastase and/or 1st recurrence.

No.	Alive or Dead	Time
1	A	×
2	D	3 Months
3	A	×
4	A	×
5	D	1 Year
6	D	Primary tumor and metastase were simultaneous
7	D	4 m
8	A	×
9	A	×
10	D	?
11	A	×
12	A	×
13	D	5 m
14	D	Simultaneous
15	D	?
16	D	8 m
17	D	×
18	A	2 m
19	A	×
20	D	?
21	A	×
22	A	×
23	D	3 m
24	A	×
25	A	×
26	D	8 m
27	D	5 m
28	D	7 y 6 m
29	A	×
30	A	×
31	D	1 y 4 m
32	D	7 m
33	D	6 m
34	A	×
35	D	?
36	A	1 y
37	D	9 m
38	A	×
39	A	×
40	A	×
41	A	×
42	A	×

× : Nor metastase, neither recurrence.

Table 7. OP'DDD side effects.

No.	Dose/m² in gr/m²/day	Duration of treatment	Acute adrenal failure	Neuro-toxicity	Psycho-logical troubles	Growth impair-ment	Rickets	Gyne-comastia
3	6	3 y 6 m	–	–	+	+	–	+
26	6	1 y 6 m	–	–	+	–	–	–
5	6	13 m	–	–	+	–	–	+
12	6.5	2 y 6 m	+	+	+	+	+	+
16	6	11 m	–	–	–	–	–	–
31	5.5	15 m	+	–	–	–	–	+
32	10	6 m	–	–	–	–	–	–
33	12	6 m	–	–	+	–	–	–
34	11	1 y 6 m	–	+	+	–	–	–
35	?	3 m	?	?	?	?	?	?
28	10	3 m	–	?	?	?	?	?
2	3	8 m	–	?	?	?	?	?
36	10	1 y 6 m	–	–	+	+	–	+
18	2	5 y	–	–	+	–	–	–
41	5	3 y 6 m	+	–	–	–	–	+
1	3	At least 1 m	–	–	–	+	–	–
6	6	2 m	–	–	–	–	–	–
7	5	2 weeks	–	–	–	–	–	–
20	3	2 days	–	–	–	–	–	–
23	6	2 m	–	–	–	–	–	–
37	6	10 m	–	–	–	–	–	–

DISCUSSION

In our experience, tumor size is the most important prognostic determinant. Sixteen out of seventeen children with small tumors are alive while only four out of eighteen with large tumors are alive. Complete resection at surgery is also important as none of the five patients who were only biopsied are alive. While very subjective, the ease of surgical resection suggest a good prognosis (Table 4a).

Our data is limited but suggest that in cases where complete resection is not thought to be possible, preoperative chemotherapy with OP'DDD should be considered. Recurrent or metastatic tumor should be treated with OP'DDD. Finally, a prognosis should be guarded for at least the first two years after diagnosis. Rare deaths may occur five years after diagnosis.

REFERENCES

Benaily M, Schweisguth O, Job JC: Les tumeurs cortico-surrenales de l'enfant. Etude rétrospective de 34 cas observés de 1954 à 1973. Arch Fr Pédiatr 32(5):441–453, 1975.

12. Functioning Adrenocortical Tumors in Childhood

JOHN H. HOLCOMBE, THEODORE J. PYSHER and REBECCA T. KIRKLAND

INTRODUCTION

Neoplasms of the adrenal cortex are rare during childhood [1]. Their presentation is often a dramatic example of the effects of steroid over-production. The diagnosis is usually suspected in a child who manifests signs of adrenocortical hyperfunction, such as virilization, sexual precocity or Cushing's syndrome.

The frequency of adrenocortical carcinoma is estimated to be 0.2% of all childhood malignancies [2]. This tumor represented between 1–3% of all solid childhood tumors seen at a Brazilian hospital [3]. The rarity of this disease has precluded an accumulation of a large number of cases in a single series. Hayles, *et al.* [4] found 222 cases reported prior to 1962, and discussed 12 of their own patients which had been collected since 1933. In a more recent review, Zaitoon, *et al.* [5] described an additional 7 patients. The sex ratio favors females 2:1, regardless of age. Adrenocortical tumors have been described in all age groups, including the newborn period [6] and in siblings [7]. The well described association between these tumors, hemihypertrophy and central nervous system tumors [8] will not be discussed in this review.

VIRILIZING TUMORS

The majority of adrenal tumors in children present with signs of androgen excess [4], with the remainder presenting with Cushing's syndrome. However, most children with Cushing's syndrome also have some degree of virilization. These virilizing features include acne, deepening of the voice, muscular appearance, pubic hair, rapid statural growth, and enlarged penis or clitoris. The differential diagnosis in a virilized male is quite limited. Con-

G. Bennett Humphrey et al. (eds), Adrenal and Endocrine Tumors in Children.

ditions which must be excluded are late onset congenital adrenal hyperplasia, Leydig cell tumor of the testicle, and true isosexual precocity. The physical examination permits narrowing of the diagnostic possibilities. Both testicles remain small in cases of extra-testicular virilization, such as adrenal hyperplasia, while both testes are enlarged in true sexual precocity. A single enlarged testicle indicates the presence of an intratesticular tumor. An adrenal tumor in a prepubertal female must be differentiated from mild congenital adrenal hyperplasia and the rare ovarian arrhenoblastoma.

The clinical presentation of adrenal tumors is best understood in terms of the steroids produced. Virilization is due to tumor production of various androgens. These steroids include dehydroepiandrosterone (DHA), androstenedione, and testosterone [9–12]. The predominant urinary steroid metabolite in most cases is DHA and its sulfate. These compounds may contribute more than 50 percent of the total 17-ketosteroids [11], and it is not uncommon to find 17-ketosteroid excretion in excess of 100 mg/24 hours. Other androgen metabolites often found in the urine are etiocholanolone and androsterone [13]. Urinary 17-ketosteroids are usually markedly elevated in cases of malignancy. Benign tumors may produce sufficient testosterone to cause virilization, but the 17-ketosteroids may remain normal. The explanation for this is the observation that testosterone metabolites contribute only a small portion of the total 17-ketosteroids. Therefore, an increased testosterone production may not be reflected as an elevated ketosteroid [14]. Adrenal adenomas tend to secrete a limited number of steroids, such as testosterone and cortisol, whereas malignant tumors tend to produce a wide range of hormones [9, 10, 15]. The availability of steroid radioimmunoassays has made it relatively easy to complement urinary steroid studies with plasma androgen concentrations.

In spite of exaggerated hormone production, tumors may show a relative deficiency of the enzymes required for normal steroid biosynthesis. High urinary concentrations of tetrahydro-substance S in many patients with tumors indicates partial 11-hydroxylase deficiency with decreased conversion of 11-deoxycortisol to cortisol [15]. This enzyme block may also contribute to excess deoxycorticosterone production resulting in hypertension. Other enzymes that may show partial blocks are the 21-hydroxylase, the 17 α-hydroxylase, and the 3 β-hydroxysteroid dehydrogenase [15].

CUSHING'S SYNDROME

Endogenous Cushing's syndrome in children less than 10 years of age is usually due to an adrenal tumor [16], whereas in older children adrenal hyperplasia may exceed tumors in frequency [17]. Cushing's syndrome without virilization is rarely observed. The classical features of Cushing's syndrome include obesity, muscle wasting, plethora, round facies, striae, and short stature. Linear growth may be normal in the child that has associated virilization. Truncal obesity may be observed in older children, but infants tend to demonstrate generalized obesity. Hypertension is commonly found in Cushing's syndrome.

Cortisol production is increased in children with Cushing's syndrome and is usually reflected in elevated plasma cortisol concentrations and loss of the diurnal pattern of cortisol secretion. Adrenal malignancies tend to give rise to far greater cortisol levels than does adrenal hyperplasia. Although urinary excretion of 17-hydroxycorticosteroids is markedly increased in adrenal malignancy, especially when expressed as mg/gram creatinine/24 hours, the measurement of urinary free-cortisol is perhaps the most sensitive indicator of cortisol excess [18].

FEMINIZING TUMORS

Pure feminizing tumors are rarely encountered in pediatrics. Only seven cases of feminizing adenomas in males have been recorded [19]. However, it is not unusual to find adrenal malignancies which cause feminizing features in addition to virilization and Cushing's syndrome. The urinary 17-ketosteroids are usually elevated, and the predominant androgen is dehydroepiandrosterone. Production of estrogen, particularly estradiol, is increased in these tumors.

DIAGNOSIS

The evaluation of an adrenal tumor centers around documentation of both the type and amount of steroids being produced by the tumor. Baseline urine collections for 17-ketosteroids and 17-hydroxycorticoids should be obtained. Also, plasma cortisol and serum androgens (testosterone, DHA, androstenedione) should be measured.

ACTH stimulation and dexamethasone suppression tests have been used to assist in the differentiation between adrenal tumors and adrenocortical hyperplasia. Patients with hyperplasia hyper-respond to ACTH, whereas there is usually no change in cortisol levels in the patient with an autonomously functioning tumor [14]. Dexamethasone in high doses should suppress the cortisol secretion in patients with hyperplasia [20]. However, there are exceptions to these findings, and an occasional tumor may show apparent ACTH dependency or dexamethasone suppression [21, 22]. Steroid induced electrolyte abnormalities include hypokalemia and metabolic alkalosis [23].

Bone x-rays may show osteoporosis and bone age retardation, but in the case of virilizing tumors an advanced bone maturation can be seen with minimal osteoporosis. Plain films of the abdomen may rarely demonstrate calcification in a tumor. Recently, CT scanning of the abdomen has aided in tumor localization in children [24]. Abdominal ultrasound evaluation may be beneficial, especially in the delineation of right sided lesions. Arteriography and venography should be reserved for cases in which the suspected tumor cannot be visualized by any other means.

Adrenal scintigraphy utilizing various labelled cholesterol analogues can localize some adrenal tumors [25, 26, 27, 28]. Adrenocortical malignancies are capable of concentrating radiocholesterol, but to a lesser degree than does normal adrenal tissue [25]. This differential uptake makes it possible in most cases to distinguish between adrenal hyperplasia, adenoma, and carcinoma. Bilateral visualization of the adrenal area indicates hyperplasia, whereas an adenoma is suspected in the area of unilateral uptake. Through its steroid secretion an adenoma suppresses the contralateral adrenal and the suppressed gland will show no uptake of labelled cholesterol. Carcinomas concentrate the agent so poorly that the scan usually shows bilateral nonvisualization [29]. The experience with these compounds, particularly ^{131}I-6-β-iodomethyl-19-nor-cholesterol, remains limited in children, but their expanded use may antiquate the more laborious and time consuming suppression and stimulation testing.

TREATMENT

The primary treatment of adrenal tumors remains that of surgical excision. An anterior transverse approach is preferred in order that both adrenal glands may be examined since adrenal malignancy is bilateral in as many as 10% of cases [30]. The contralateral gland is often atrophic as a result of chronic suppression of ACTH by the steroid producing tumor, and exogenous steroid coverage should be provided before, during, and following the procedure even in the absence of clinical evidence of cortisol excess. Prolonged steroid maintenance (3 to 4 months) and gradual tapering is necessary when the remaining adrenal is atrophic.

The use of adrenolytic agents, such as o,p,,DDD (1,1-dichloro-2-(o-chlorophenyl)-2-(p-chlorophenyl)-ethane) and enzyme inhibitors, such as aminoglutethimide, has been advocated for the treatment of recurrent disease [31, 32]. Their use in children has been limited because of the infrequency of this disease. Decreased steroid synthesis by the tumor can occasionally be demonstrated, but either drug's effect on increasing survival time remains unproven [33].

Adrenal tumors and their metastases are usually radioresistant in adults, but palliative responses have been recorded [34]. Although the role of tumor bed radiation following surgery has not been well defined in children, its use in some instances has been encouraging [1]. Tumor recurrence may or may not be heralded by clinical evidence of steroid secretion. When recurrence is found, the only treatment currently available for palliation is o,p,DDD.

Adrenal tumors at Texas Children's Hospital and Oklahoma Children's Memorial Hospital

The combined experience with adrenal tumors of Texas Children's Hospital (1956-1980) and Oklahoma Children's Memorial Hospital (OCMH) (1971-1981) is shown in Table 1. The overall sex ratio favored females, 9:4. The mean age at diagnosis was 2.1 years, with a range of 0.25 to 9.2 years. Virilization was the predominant presenting sign in 6 of the cases, while 5 demonstrated predominantly Cushing's syndrome. Patient 12 presented with a palpable abdominal mass and underwent tumor removal before a complete endocrine evaluation was completed. He had very mild virilization, consisting of scrotal thinning and acneform lesions on the forehead, but the excretion of 17-ketosteroids preoperatively was marked (117 mg/24 h).

All OCMH patients except patient 12 received endocrine evaluation preoperatively. The minimum work-up consisted of urinary 17-ketosteroids, 17-hydroxycorticoids, and plasma cortisols. Plasma androgens were elevated in the three OCMH patients in whom they were measured. A dexamethasone suppression test was done in four OCMH patients, and the results were consistent with tumor in each case. In addition, an I.V. ACTH stimulation test showed no response in patient 13.

All of the OCMH patients had some degree of virilization and elevated 17-ketosteroids, and all but one had increased urinary 17-hydroxy corticosteroids. The 17-ketosteroid excretion in the fatal case at OCMH was 164 mg/24 hrs (normal for age <2.0 mg/24 hrs). Fractionation of androgen metabolites was not done in this case.

Patient 13 underwent adrenal scintigraphy using ^{131}I-6-β-iodomethyl-19-nor-cholesterol after an abdominal CT scan failed to reveal an adrenal tumor. The radioisotope study showed unilateral uptake in the region of the right adrenal. At surgery, the tumor was found in the right adrenal gland.

There have been two deaths in our combined series. The tumors of patients who died weighed 1200 gms and 344 gms. Tang and Gray [35] suggested that tumor size best correlated with histologic behavior, and that a

Table 1. Clinical and quantitative morphologic features of adrenocortical tumors.

	Sex	Age of presentation (years)	Predominant symptom	Diagnosis	Affected adrenal location	Weight of tumor (grams)	Size (cm)	Follow-up (years after surgery)
1.	M	1.3	Virilization	CA	Left	389	14 × 7.5 × 5	Alive and well 5 years post op. then lost to follow-up
2.	F	3.5	Cushings	A	Right	24	3.4 × 3.5 × 2.5	18
3.	F	0.5	Cushings	CA	?	24	4.0 × 3.0 × 2.8	25
4.	F	0.25	Cushings	CA	Bilateral w/liver metastasis	4.5 (R) 2.0 (L) 4.5 liver	4.2 × 2 × 1.5 3.5 × 1 × 2 4.5 cm	21
5.	F	1.8	Virilization	CA	Right	41	4.5 × 3.9 × 4.1	2.5
6.	F	1.0	Virilization	Tumor	Right	46	6.2 × 4 × 3.1	3.5
7.	F	0.75	Cushings	Tumor	Right	-	3.5	2.1
8.	M	9.2	Feminization (Gynecomastia)	Tumor	Left	1200	-	Expired with widespread metastasis 5 months after tumor removal
9.	F	1.1	Cushings	A	Right	28.5	5 × 4.5 × 3.5	11
10.	F	4.3	Virilization	CA	Right	344	9 × 11.5 × 7	Died 7 months after tumor removal
11.	M	1.2	Virilization	CA	Left	-	6.5 × 3.5 × 4	3.6
12.	M	0.75	Abdominal mass	CA	Left	470	13.5 × 9.5 × 7	1.5
13.	F	2.2	Virilization	Tumor	Right	8	2.8 × 2.2 × 0.6	-

CA = carcinoma, A = adenoma.

tumor weighing more than 95 gms should be considered malignant. However, two other patients (1 & 2) with tumors weighing 389 gms and 470 gms have had no recurrence at least 1.5 years after surgery.

Tumor size was also expressed as a percentage of total body weight. Hayles, *et al.* [4] reported a lower rate of metastasis in children whose tumor weight was below the arbitrary figure of 0.7 gm/100 gm body weight. This value in 7 of our patients ranged from .23 to 4.90 gm/100 gm body weight. Patient 12 had the highest value (4.90), but he has remained tumor free 19 months postoperatively. Both older patients who died of their disease had high relative tumor weights of 2.98 and 1.17 gm/100 gm body weight.

Both patients that died received o,p,DDD. In addition, patient 8 received 5-Fluorouracil. There was no measurable tumor response in either case as assessed by tumor size or steroid production in spite of a maximal dose of o,p,DDD of 16 gms per day (patient 8).

Patient 4 had bilateral adrenal tumors with a large liver metastasis. Without any treatment other than adrenalectomy and removal of the metastasis, the patient was alive and well 21 years postoperatively.

PATHOLOGY

Since 1978 at Texas Children's Hospital and most recently at OCMH adrenocortical neoplasms have been labelled 'tumor' unless distant metastases were present at the time of surgery. Table 2 lists the morphologic features of the five tumors resected at OCMH. There was considerable overlap at the gross, microscopic, and ultrastructural levels among tumors displaying divergent biologic behavior.

Table 2. Morphologic features of adrenocortical tumors.

Gross features				Histologic features			
Case	Hemorrhage	Necrosis	Calcification	Architecture	Cell type	Nuclear pleomorphism	Capsular or vascular invasion
9	–	–	+	Organoid	Small compact	1+	–
10	+	+	–	Organoid	Granular dimorphic	3+	+
11	–	–	–	Cords	Vacuolated	3+	–
12	+	+	–	Cords	Granular	1+	+
13	–	–	–	Cords	Granular	2+	–

+ – present, – absent, 1+ – 3+ – minimal, moderate, and severe pleomorphism.

All five of the tumors resected at OCMH manifested a firm but spongy consistency, and ranged from tan-yellow to tan-red in color. Gross hemorrhage and necrosis were noted only in the two largest tumors, and calcification was appreciated by gross examination in only one tumor (case 9).

Microscopically, these tumors were characterized by broad cords of large, polygonal cells with distinct cell boundaries separated by sinusoidal capillary networks or thin fibrovascular trabebeculae (Figure 1). One case (case 9), however, was composed of compact cells in an organoid arrangement (Figure 1A), and the lone fatal tumor (case 10) manifested a mixture of large and small cells (Figure 1B). Small foci of hemorrhage and individual cell necrosis were present in all tumors, and three (cases 9, 10, and 12) showed microscopic calcification. A very sparse and patchy mononuclear cell infiltrate was noted in a single tumor (case 11).

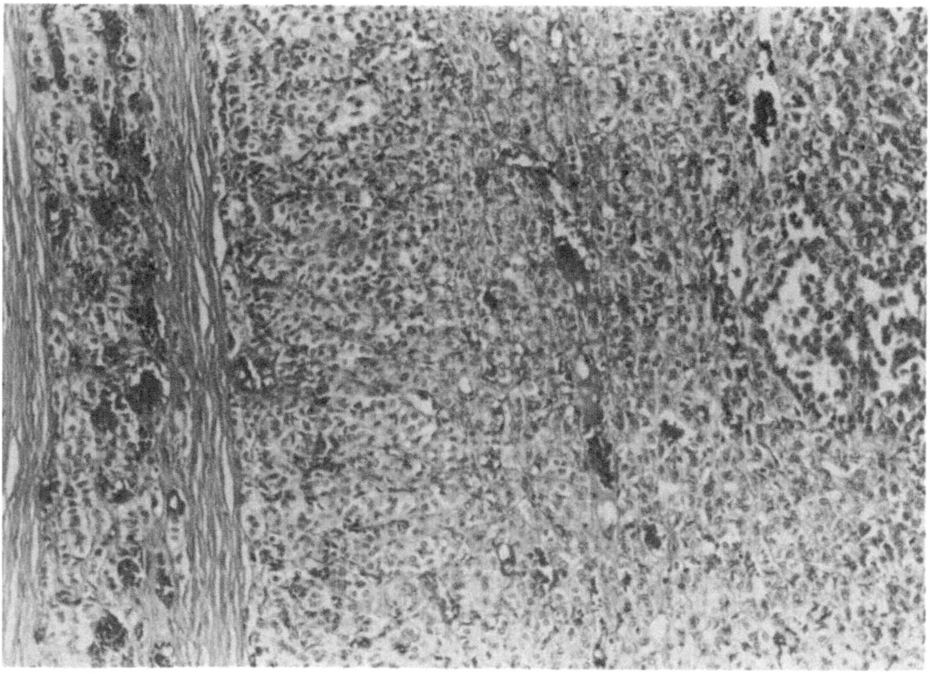

Figure 1. Histologic appearance of adrenocortical tumors. A. Case 9, compressed normal gland and organoid arrangement of small compact cells. B. Case 10, mixed, diffuse pattern with marked cytoplasmic and nuclear pleomorphism and nucleoli in some of the larger nuclei. C. Case 11, broad cords with marked pleomorphism and numerous vesicular nuclei containing large nucleoli. D. Case 12, broad cords of vacuolated cells with less cytoplasmic and nuclear pleomorphism than B or C, and no large nucleoli. Hemotoxylin and eosin. Original magnification 40×.

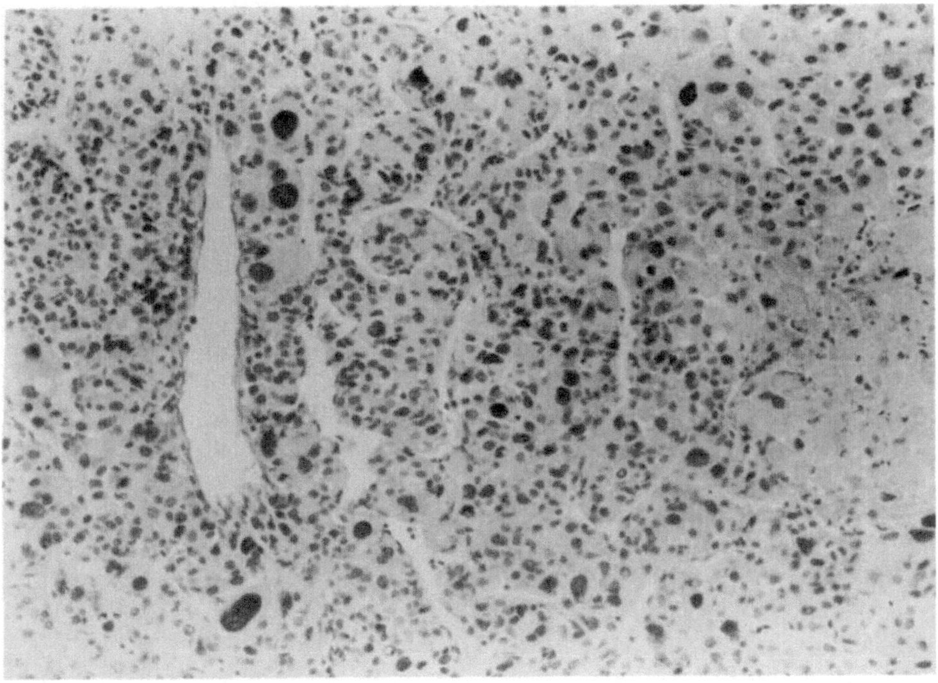

Figure 1B.

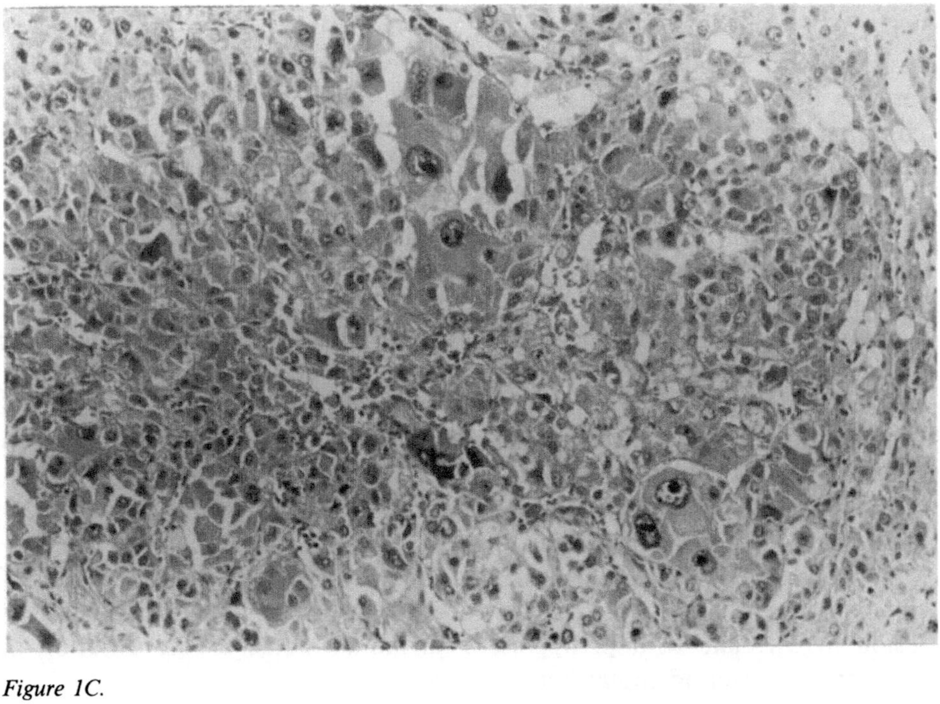

Figure 1C.

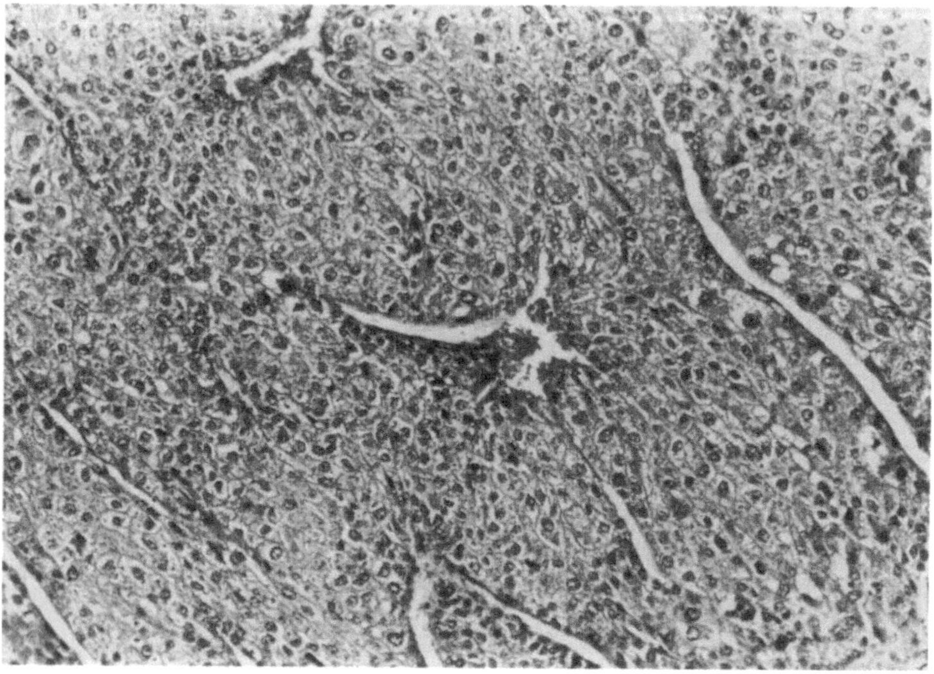

Figure 1D.

There was considerable variation in the size, shape and staining characteristics of nuclei among these tumors. Multinucleate forms were not uncommon, but mitotic figures were extremely rare. There was no relationship between nuclear atypia and other criteria of malignancy. Small tumors without evidence of local invasion (Figures 1A and 1C) showed nearly as much nuclear pleomorphism as the 344 gram tumor with extensive, eventually fatal, metastases (Figure 1B) and more than the 470 gram tumor with local invasion (Figure 1D).

Cytoplasmic contents ranged from fine granules to coarse vacuoles, but ultrastructural study of two tumors (cases 12 and 13), both associated with markedly elevated levels of urinary 17-ketosteroids, showed essentially the same features (Figure 2). Organelles included variable amounts of smooth endoplasmic reticulum (more abundant in the adenoma) and mitochondria with tubulo-vesicular cristae, indicative of steroid synthesis, as well as occasional lipid droplets and profiles of rough endoplasmic reticulum.

Portions of the ipsilateral adrenal gland were available for study in four of the five cases. There were varying degrees of atrophy, but no consistent lesion to correlate with preoperative hormonal status or the duration of postoperative steroid replacement.

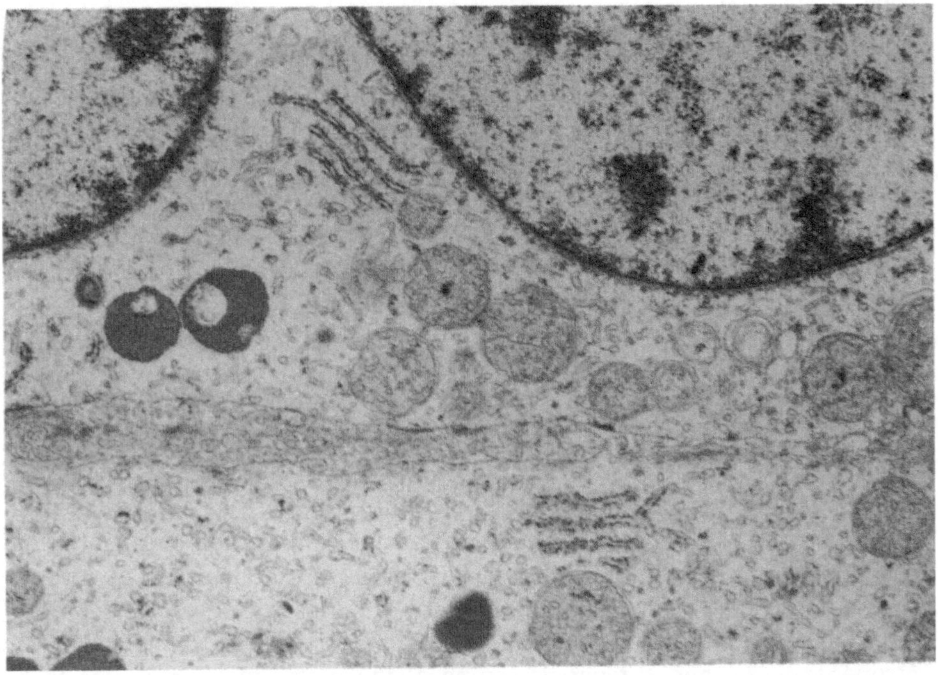

Figure 2. Ultrastructure of an adrenocortical tumor. Case 12. Note evidence of steroid synthesis (abundant smooth endoplasmic reticulum and tubular cristae in mitochondria) and rare profiles of rough endoplasmic reticulum. Uranyl acetate and lead citrate. 10,500×.

Autopsy of the patient who died of metastatic disease showed a large tumor in the retroperitoneum with extension to the vena cava, and metastases to both lungs and the liver.

Beyond actual demonstration of extracapsular extension or vascular invasion, no pathologic features, alone or in combination, consistently separate those tumors that will eventually metastasize from those that do not [36]. As stated above, Tang and Gray [35] concluded that tumor size was the best predictor of biologic behavior. Hough, *et al.* [37] studied 41 tumors in patients aged 9 months to 71 years and noted a number of features, including tumor mass, weight loss, broad fibrous bands, vascular invasion and a diffuse growth pattern to be associated with subsequent metastases. However, it was necessary to group several of these features in order to obtain reliable separation of benign and malignant behaving tumors. Contrariwise, no patient in their series with local recurrence escaped subsequent metastasis. In a series dealing only with carcinoma, defined by the presence of capsular or vascular invasion or distant metastases, Hogan, *et al.* [38] studied 21 patients, 16 to 67 years of age, and found that survival was predicted by the degree of nuclear pleomorphism. Large, pleomorphic nuclei were present in greater than 50% of cells in seven cases and all of those patients died of metastatic disease within nine months of diagnosis. By contrast, only two of the remaining 14 patients died within 19 months, and both deaths were related to chemotherapy rather than metastatic tumor. Patients in the group with nuclear pleomorphism tended to be males (57%) with no clinical or laboratory evidence of hormone production, features previously associated with a poor prognosis [39]. King and Lack [40] reported 49 cases of adrenal cortical carcinoma (ages 5 months to 77 years) and could find no statistically significant difference in survival based upon size of tumor, duration of symptoms prior to diagnosis, endocrine function of the tumor, or sex. In fact, the only criterion that correlated with survival was the completeness of resection.

Application of this confusing data to the present series is further complicated by the paucity of reports of adrenal cortical carcinoma in childhood [1, 9] and the long latent period which may elapse before metastases become apparent [37]. Nevertheless, it would appear that adrenal cortical tumors in children behave in a more indolent fashion than similar tumors in adults, and that long survival, even in the face of metastases, is the rule. Deaths do occur, however, and the pattern of metastatic spread observed in our fatal cases, direct extension to the inferior vena cava, local spread in the retroperitoneum, and extensive seeding of the lung and liver, seems to be characteristic.

A small, well encapsulated tumor seems to portend a good prognosis, but, as described in this series, tumors with all the characteristics of malignancy, including metastasis, may also be compatible with long survival.

SUMMARY

Thirteen children with functioning adrenocortical tumors are presented. All patients had evidence of steroid excess, the most common manifestation of which was virilization. Laboratory studies confirmed elevated steroid levels and autonomous tumor function. The patients were treated by surgical excision of the tumor, but recurrence in two patients was treated unsuccessfully with o,p,DDD. Tumor size seemed inversely related to prognosis, but no single gross or histologic feature consistently predicted eventual outcome.

REFERENCES

1. Stewart DR, Morris-Jones PH, Jolleys A: Carcinoma of the adrenal gland in children. J Pediatr Surg 9:59–67, 1974.
2. Young JL, Miller RW: Incidence of malignant tumors in U.S. children. J Pediatr 86:254–258, 1975.

3. Marigo C, Muller H, Davies JNP: Survey of cancer in children admitted to a Brazilian charity hospital. J Nat Cancer Inst 43:1231–1240, 1969.
4. Hayles AB, Hahn HB, Sprague RG, Bahn RC, Priestley JT: Hormone-secreting tumors of the adrenal cortex in children. Pediatrics 37:19–25, 1966.
5. Zaitoon MM, Mackie GG: Adrenal cortical tumors in children. Urology 12:645–649, 1978.
6. Kenny FM, Hashida Y, Askari A, Sieber WH, Fetterman GH: Virilizing tumors of the adrenal cortex. Am J Dis Child 115:445–458, 1968.
7. Mahloudji M, Ronaghy H, Dutz W: Virilizing adrenal carcinoma in 2 siblings. J Med Genet 8:160–163, 1971.
8. Fraumeni JF, Miller RW: Adrenal cortical neoplasms and hemihypertrophy, brain tumors and other disorders. J Pediatr 70:129–138, 1967.
9. Burr IM, Graham T, Sullivan J, Hartman WH, O'Neill J: A testosterone-secreting tumor of the adrenal producing virilization in a female infant. Lancet 2:643–644, 1973.
10. Schteingart DE, Woodbury MC, Tsao HS, McKenzie AK: Virilizing syndrome associated with an adrenal cortical adenoma secreting predominantly testosterone. Am J Med 67:140–146, 1979.
11. Saez JM, Rivarola MA, Migeon CJ: Studies of androgens in patients with adrenocortical tumors. J Clin Endocr 27:615–623, 1967.
12. Baulieu E-E: Studies of conjugated 17-ketosteroids in a case of adrenal tumor. J Clin Endocr 22:501–510, 1962.
13. Gallagher TF: On alterations in adrenal function, especially with adrenocortical carcinoma. Cancer Res 17:520–529, 1957.
14. Lipsett MB, Hertz R, Ross GT: Clinical and pathophysiologic aspects of adrenocortical carcinoma. Am J Med 35:374–383, 1963.
15. Lipsett MB, Wilson H: Adrenocortical cancer: Steroid biosynthesis and metabolism evaluated by urinary metabolites. J Clin Endocr Metab 22:906–915, 1962.
16. Guin GH, Gilbert EF: Cushing's syndrome in children associated with adrenal cortical carcinoma: A case report with review of the literature. Am J Dis Child 92:297–307, 1956.
17. McArthur RG, Cloutier MD, Hayles AB, Sprague RG: Cushing's disease in children: Findings in 13 cases. Mayo Clin proc 47:318–326, 1972.
18. Eddy RL, Jones AL, Gilliland PF, Ibarra JD, Thompson JQ, McMurray JF: Cushing's syndrome: A prospective study of diagnostic methods. Am J Med 55:621–630, 1973.
19. Sultan C, Descomps B, Garandeau P, Bressot N, Jean R: Pubertal gynecomastia due to an estrogen-producing adrenal adenoma. J Pediatr 95:744–746, 1979.
20. Liddle GW: Tests of pituitary-adrenal suppressibility, the diagnosis of Cushing's syndrome. J Clin Endocr Metab 20:1539-1560, 1960.
21. Kendall JW, Sloop PR: Dexamethasone suppressible adrenocortical tumor. N Eng J Med 279:532–535, 1968.
22. Rayfield EJ, Rose LI, Cain JP, Dluhy RG, Williams GH: ACTH-responsive, dexamethasone-suppressible adrenocortical carcinoma. N Engl J Med 284:591–592, 1971.
23. Bagshawe KD: Hypokalemia, carcinoma and Cushing's syndrome. Lancet 2:284–287, 1960.
24. Boldt DW, Reilly BJ: Computed tomography of abdominal mass lesions in children. Radiology 124:371–378, 1977.
25. Beierwaltes WH, Wieland DM, Yu T, Swanson DP, Mosley ST: Adrenal imaging agents: Rational, synthesis, formulation and metabolism. Semin Nucl Med 8:5–21, 1978.
26. Chatal JF, Charbonnel B, LeMevel BP, Guihard D: Uptake of ^{131}I-19-iodocholesterol by an adrenal cortical carcinoma and its metastases. J Clin Endocr Metab 43:248–251, 1976.

27. Seabold JE, Schteingart DE: I-131-iodocholesterol imaging in adrenal neoplasms. J Nucl Med 16:566, 1975.
28. Sarkar SD, Beierwaltes WH, Ice RD, Basmadjian GP, Hetzel KR, Kennedy WP, Mason MM: A new and superior adrenal scanning agent, NP-59. J Nucl Med 16:1038–1042, 1975.
29. Thrall JH, Frietas JE, Beierwaltes WH: Adrenal scintigraphy Semin Nuclear Med 8:23–41, 1978.
30. Winter JSD: Adrenal tumors in childhood. In: Endocrine and genetic diseases of childhood and adolescence, Gardner L, (ed) WB Sanders Co, Philadelphia, 1975, p 507–513.
31. Hutter AM Jr, Kayhoe DE: Adrenal cortical carcinoma: Results of treatment with o,p,DDD in 138 patients. Am J Med 41:581–592, 1966.
32. Schteingart DE, Cash R, Coon JW: Amino-glutethimide and metastatic adrenal cancer. JAMA 198:1007–1010, 1966.
33. Hoffman MG, Mattox VR: Treatment of adrenal cortical carcinoma with o,p,DDD. Med Clin N Am 56:999–1012, 1972.
34. Percarpio B, Knowlton AH: Radiation therapy of adrenal cortical carcinoma. Acta Rad Ther 15:288–292, 1976.
35. Tang CK, Gray GF: Adrenocortical neoplasms: Prognosis and morphology. Urology 5:691–695, 1975.
36. Heinbecker P, O'Neal LW, Ackerman LV: Functioning and non-functioning adrenal cortical tumors. Surg Gynecol Obstet 105:21–33, 1957.
37. Hough AJ, Hollifield JW, Page DL, Hartmann WH: Prognostic factors in adrenal cortical tumors. A mathematical analysis of clinical and morphologic data. Am J Clin Pathol 72:390–399, 1979.
38. Hogan TF, Gilchrist KW, Westring DW, Citrin DL: A clinical and pathologic study of adrenal cortical carcinoma. Therapeutic implications. Cancer 45:2880–2883, 1980.
39. Lewinsky BS, Grigor KM, Symington T, Neville AM: The clinical and pathologic features of 'non-hormonal' adrenocortical tumors. Report of twenty new cases and review of the literature. Cancer 33:778–790, 1974.
40. King DR, Lack EE: Adrenal cortical carcinoma. A clinical and pathologic study of 49 cases. Cancer 44:239–244, 1979.

13. Adrenocortical Neoplasia in the Pediatric Age Group. A Clinicopathologic Study of Seven Cases

LOUIS P. DEHNER and RALPH A. FRANCIOSI

When the subject of neoplasia of the adrenal gland in childhood is considered, the discussion is usually directed toward the medullary-derived tumors, i.e., neuroblastoma and its morphologic variants and pheochromocytoma. In terms of incidence, there is an appreciable disparity between the number of neuroblastomas which are diagnosed and treated in a year's period of time in comparison to the adrenal cortical tumors. Our own experience for the year of 1980 was a ratio of 10:1 in favor of neuroblastoma to cortical neoplasms in children. Thus the adrenocortical adenoma and carcinoma are relatively rare tumors in the pediatric age group [1–3]. This communication briefly describes our experience with these tumors which have been studied at the University of Minnesota as in-patients or consultations.

1. MATERIALS AND METHODS

The seven cases in this study were accumulated during a five year period. It represents a combined experience of patients from the University of Minnesota and Minneapolis Medical Center (Children's Health Center). Pathologic material was available in all cases. The clinical charts were reviewed and follow-up was obtained from the attending physician.

2. RESULTS

2.1. Clinical findings

The children ranged in age from 4 months to 10 years at the time of diagnosis (median age, 3 years). There were four females and three males. Signs and symptoms generally evolved over a period of many weeks or months and one patient (Case 4, Table 1) was considered Cushingoid since

G. Bennett Humphrey et al. (eds), Adrenal and Endocrine Tumors in Children.

Table 1. Clinical and pathologic summary of childhood adrenocortical tumors.

Case	Age/sex	Clinical findings	Laboratory values	Treatment	Pathologic findings
1	8 m/o M	Weight gain, abdominal protuberance, ? Cushingoid facies, right abdominal mass, hypertension (220/120)	Serum Na, 137; K, 3.0–3.5; Cl, 101; HCO_3, 25; serum cortisol (31 mcg/dl, PM; 37 mcg/dl, A.M.), non-suppressible	Right adrenalectomy	Circumscribed brownish mass, 7 × 7 × 7 cm, 200 gm
2	3 y/o F	Asymptomatic upper abdominal mass, polyuria and polydipsia since very early childhood, normotensive; nontender mass in left upper quadrant	Serum Na, 144; K, 2.4 Cl, 32: HCO_3, 98; aldosterone, 50–100 ng./ml., renin 18 (elevated)	Left adrenalectomy	Circumscribed multi-nodular mass, yellow 6.5 × 5.5 × 4 cm
3	14 m/o F	Clitoromegaly, pubic hair, increased bone age, abdominal mass	Elevated serum testosterone	Left adrenalectomy	Cystic and partially hemorrhagic mass, 8 × 6 × 5 cm, 125 gm
4	4 m/o M	Cushingoid features noted from birth, abdominal mass, no virilization	Elevated serum and urinary 17-hydroxy- and 17-ketosteroids	Left adrenalectomy	Encapsulated yellowish brown partially hemorrhagic mass, 4.5 × 3.3 × 2.5 cm
5	12 y/o M	Headache, weight gain (6 mo), hypertension (180/110), Cushingoid features	Normal serum electroytes elevated cortisol (16 mcq./dl, A.M.; 2019 mcg/dl, A.M.)	Right adrenalectomy	Circumscribed, reddish-purple mass, 2.5 × 8 × 1 cm
6	7 y/o F	Calcified mass in right suprarenal area detected on pre-operative abdominal X-ray. F. H. Gardner's syndrome	Normal catecholamines, post-operative 17-hydroxy and 17-ketosteroids normal	Right adrenalectomy	Encapsulated, predominantly solid greyish-pink to yellowish mass, 7.5 × 6 × 4.5 cm, 712 gm
7	10 y/o F	Hirsutism, weight gain, abdominal mass, hypertension, 3 mo.	Elevated 17-ketosteroids and serum cortisol	Left adrenalectomy and removal of tumor thrombi from renal vein and inferior vena cava	Encapasulated mutli-nodular yellowish-brown mass, 20.8 × 15 × 8.5 cm, 1350 gm

birth. The most frequently noted clinical feature was the presence of Cushingoid facies (Cases 1, 4, 5, Table 1). Two patients had the stigmata of androgenization with clitoromegaly, hirsutism and accelerated bone age (Cases 3 and 7, Table 1). The notable abnormalities on physical examination were hypertension (Cases 1, 5, 7, Table 1) and an abdominal mass in six of seven patients. Pertinent laboratory findings have been summarized in Table 1. The 17-hydroxy- and/or keto-steroids were elevated in five patients and one child (Case 2, Table 1) had hyperaldosteronism. A preoperative endocrinologic evaluation was not performed in one case (Case 6, Table 1). This patient was the only one in this study who did not have features of a functioning neoplasm. Roentgenographic findings were generally confined to the documentation of an upper abdominal mass in a suprarenal location by routine procedure or computerized axial tomography (Figure 1). Partial calcification of a right suprarenal tumor was noted in one case (Case 6, Table 1). This patient's diagnostic work-up was focused on the possibility of an adrenal medullary neoplasm. An adrenalectomy was performed in each case.

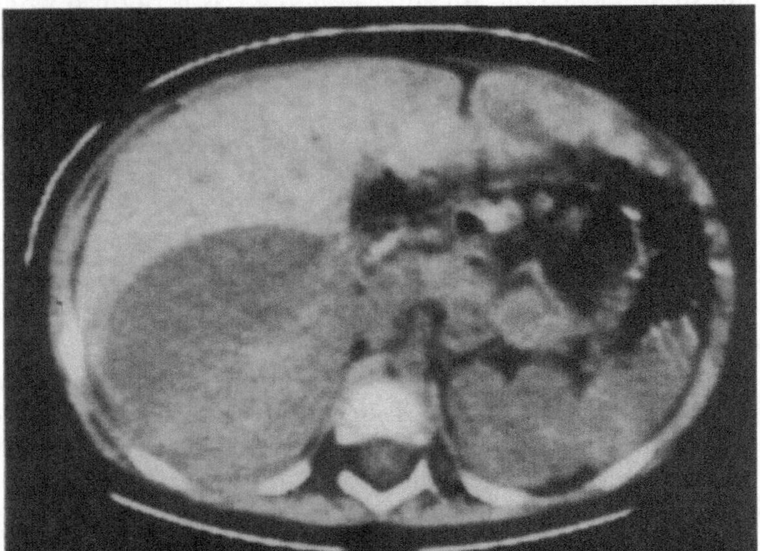

Figure 1. Large homogeneous suprarenal mass without calcification as demonstrated by CAT scan in 8-month-old boy with Cushingoid features (Case 1).

Two cases in this series warrant a more detailed review of the clinical manifestations and management. One child had an aldosteronoma (Case 2, Table 1) and the other (Case 7, Table 1), an unequivocal adrenocortical carcinoma with a prolonged survival period belying the past and present evidence of metastatic disease.

Case 2 (Table 1). The patient, a 3-year-old white female, was apparently well according to the parents at the time of an examination for routine immunizations. A pediatric nurse practitioner detected a mass in the left upper quadrant of the abdomen. The parents in retrospect had noted polyuria and polydipsia (20 glasses of fluid daily) since early childhood. She was an otherwise active, alert and well nourished child. The blood pressure was 95/60 and the only physical abnormality was the presence of a 4×4 cm firm, nontender mass in the left upper abdomen. Clinical laboratory values included a hemoglobin of 13.1 gm/dl, a normal differential count but abnormalities of serum electrolytes (Na, 144 meq/l; K, 2.4 meq/l; bicarbonate, 98 meq/l and 32 meq/l). Further studies indicated that the aldosterone levels were elevated (46-96 ng/ml). Cortisol levels before surgery failed to demonstrate any diurinal variation.

During the pre-operative period, the patient developed multiple acute episodes of severe hypertension with systolic elevations to 180 mm Hg and diastolic value in excess of 100 mm Hg. She was successfully treated with antihypertensives. The hypokalemia was also managed before surgery with potassium supplementation. An adrenalectomy was performed without difficulty and she was maintained on corticosteroids for approximately two months during the period of contralateral adrenal recovery. She remains normotensive after two years.

Case 7 (Table 1). This 10-year-old white female was well until four months before admission when she noted rapid weight gain, deepening of her voice and hirsutism. In addition to these changes, the physical examination revealed hypertension (160/100) and a large abdominal mass predominantly on the left side. The laboratory results showed an elevation of serum cortisol and urinary 17-ketosteroids. A left adrenalectomy-nephrectomy was performed. There was invasion of the left renal vein to the ostium of the inferior vena cava by tumor. Residual macroscopic tumor was not identified. The patient did well post-operatively. Abnormal laboratory values returned to normal during the recovery period. The signs of virilization have remained throughout her course.

Approximately four months later in a follow-up examination, a mass was palpated in the right lobe of the liver. Chemotherapy consisted of 5-fluorouracil and adriamycin (four courses over six weeks). A subtotal resection of the right hepatic lobe was performed seven months after the original surgery. Multiple nodules in the left lung were discovered 13 months after the initial adrenalectomy-nephrectomy. A portion of the left lower lobe was resected following a negative survey for other sites of metastatic disease. The patient was begun on ortho-para-DDD (mitogen). She has been maintained on this drug from the time of the lobectomy to the present. The period of survival is 44 months in the presence of hypertension, androgen excess, borderline renal function (creatinine clearance, 33 cc/hr) and a recurrent abdominal mass with obstruction of the inferior vena cava.

2.2. Pathologic findings and prognosis

The left adrenal was involved in four cases and the right adrenal in three. A circumscribed yellowish to brownish mass measuring from 2.5 to 20.8 cm in greatest dimension was the usual macroscopic appearance. The cut surface was infrequently homogeneous but rather focally nodular, cystic or hemorrhagic (Figure 2). Weights were recorded in four cases and these ranged from 125-1350 gm. The largest neoplasm (Case 7, Table 1) is an unequivoval adrenocortical carcinoma which was described as an encapsulated mass but vascular invasion was evident at the time of surgery. Calcification was a prominent feature in one case (Case 6, Table 1).

Histologically, the patterns varied from a trabecular and nesting arrangement to solid sheets of cells interrupted by fibrous bands or areas of hemorrhage and/or necrosis. A finding that was more impressive in the

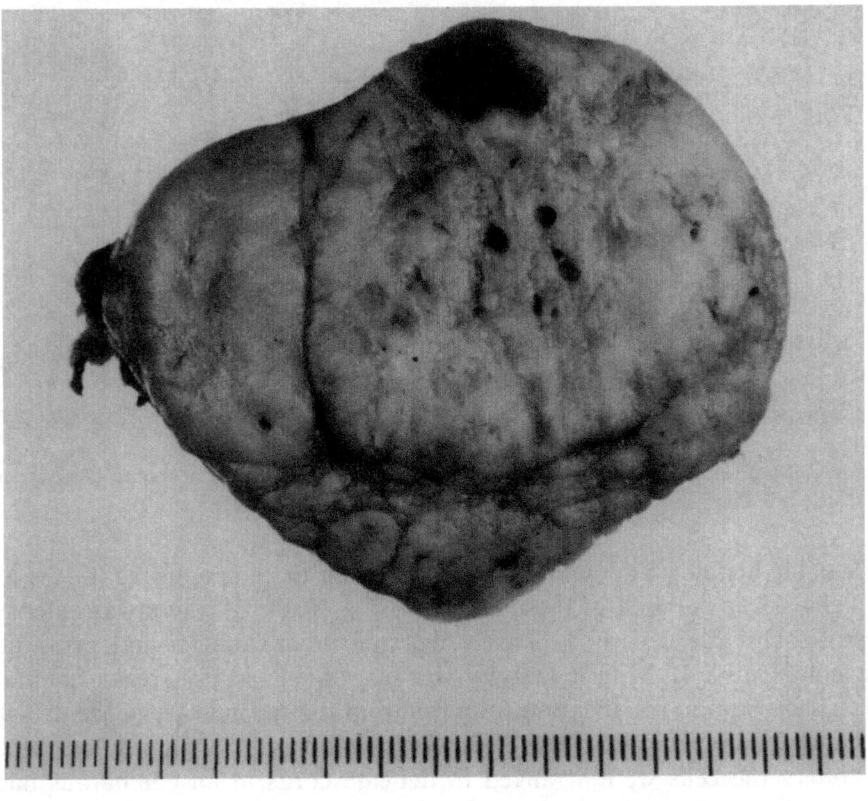

Figure 2. Focal hemorrhage and occasional cysts are noted on the cut surface of this circumscribed, yellowish-tan multinodular tumor from a child with hyperaldosteronism (Case 2).

gross examination was the circumscription or even encapsulation. The demarcation from the residual normal or atrophic cortical parenchyma was less apparent microscopically in most cases. If a fibrous capsule was identified, it was often interrupted or poorly defined. Foci of necrosis were noted in five of seven cases. The trabecular pattern in one case (Case 1, Table 1) had a pseudoglandular appearance secondary to cellular loss in the center of the nests (Figure 3). There were cytologic similarities including polygonal shape, granular, vacuolated or clear cytoplasm and some nuclear pleomorphism in all tumors which had no clinicopathologic significance .

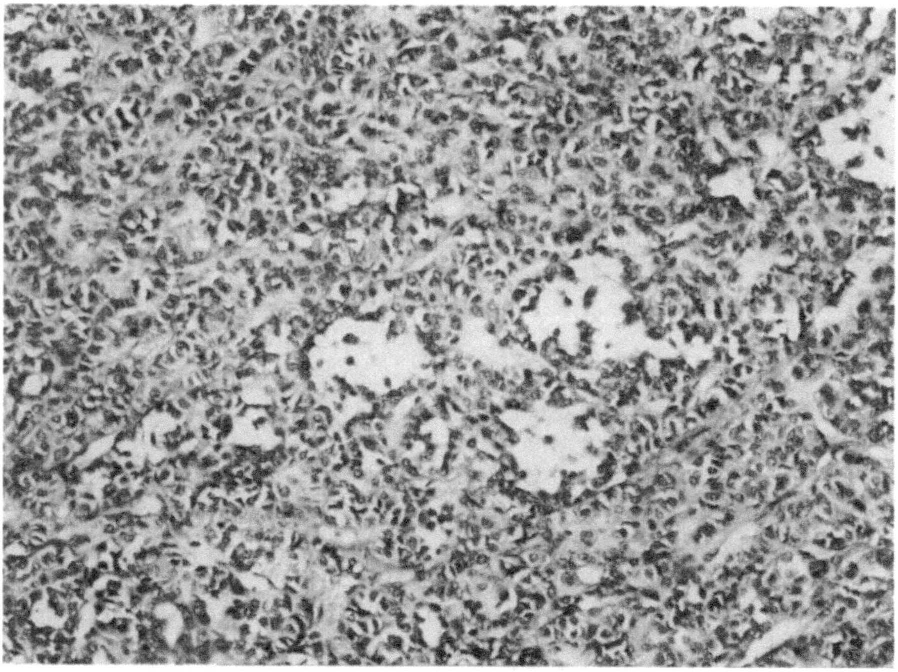

Figure 3. Focal areas with pseudoglandular appearance in a cortical adenoma (Case 1) may produce some confusion about the diagnosis (Hematoxylin and Eosin, × 160).

Notable histologic deviations were present in three neoplasms (Cases 4, 6, 7, Table 1). In the first of these cases (Case 4, Table 1), there was extensive necrosis and the cells had densely hyperchromatic nuclei and prominent nucleoli (Figure 4). Mitotic activity was inapparent. Many areas of hemorrhage, necrosis and calcification were found in the second case (Case 6, Table 1). There were foci of tumor cells with a solid growth pattern but at the periphery the cells were arranged in delicate cords in an edematous background(Figure 5). One other interesting but presumably insignificant finding was the presence of tumor cells in small vascular spaces in the fibrous cap-

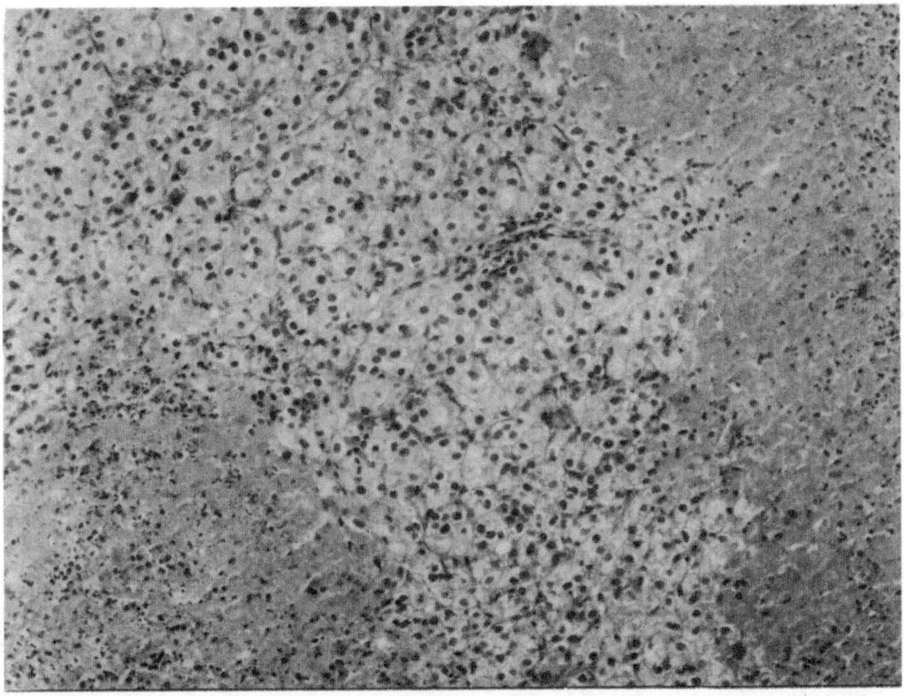

Figure 4. Some cellular pleomorphism and hyperchromatic nuclei were present in this cortical neoplasm (Case 4). Extensive areas of necrosis were noted throughout the tumor but single cell necrosis was not evident (Hematoxylin and Eosin, ×160).

sule (Figure 6). Overtly anaplastic cells were not identified but an occasional mitotic figure was evident. Vascular invasion and direct extension beyond the adrenal gland were not found in Cases 3 or 6. Cellular anaplasia, mitotic activity and direct vascular permeation were the features of Case 7 which established the diagnosis of adrenocortical carcinoma (Figure 7).

All patients in this study are alive from 3-50 months after adrenalectomy. With one exception already cited (Case 7, Table 1), the patients have done well with amelioration of symptoms following surgery. The patient with adrenocortical carcinoma is alive but with recurrent tumor. There was some concern about the prognosis in Case 6. This patient has done well after 50 months although the tumor was originally interpreted as a carcinoma.

3. DISCUSSION

The infrequency of adrenocortical neoplasia in the pediatric age group is readily apparent from the individual case studies and size of clinical series

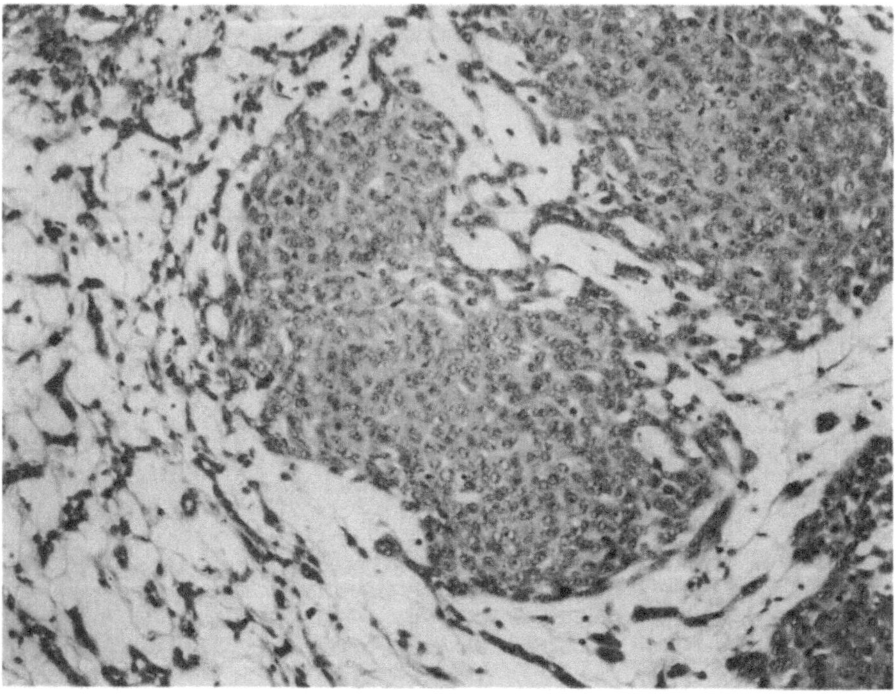

Figure 5. Solid nests of atypical acidophilic cells in an edematous background were sufficiently disturbing for an initial diagnosis of adrenocortical carcinoma (Case 6). Mitoses and single cell necrosis are inapparent (Hematoxylin and Eosin, ×160).

from the larger insitutions [2, 4–9]. Most of these tumors in children are hormonally functional but occasionally, the patient only presents with an abdominal mass such as Case 6 in this report. Cushing's syndrome and virilization are the two most common manifestations in childhood. There is an important aspect of adrenocortical neoplasia in the younger age group which is not a consideration in adults. Although not apparent in our series of seven cases, a cortical neoplasm may be one component of a complex dysontogenetic syndrome(s) with congenital hemihypertrophy, Wilms' tumor, hamartoma of soft tissues, astrocytoma, anomalies of the urinary tract, agenesis of the contralateral adrenal gland and the Beckwith-Wiedemann syndrome [10–12]. An impression from the literature and our experience is that only a minority of children with adrenocortical tumors has an associated lesion. One child in the current study had a family history of Gardner's syndrome but she does not currently have any stigmata of the disorder.

This study did not undertake the more comprehensive problem of hyperfunctional disorders of the adrenal cortex in childhood and therefore, we are

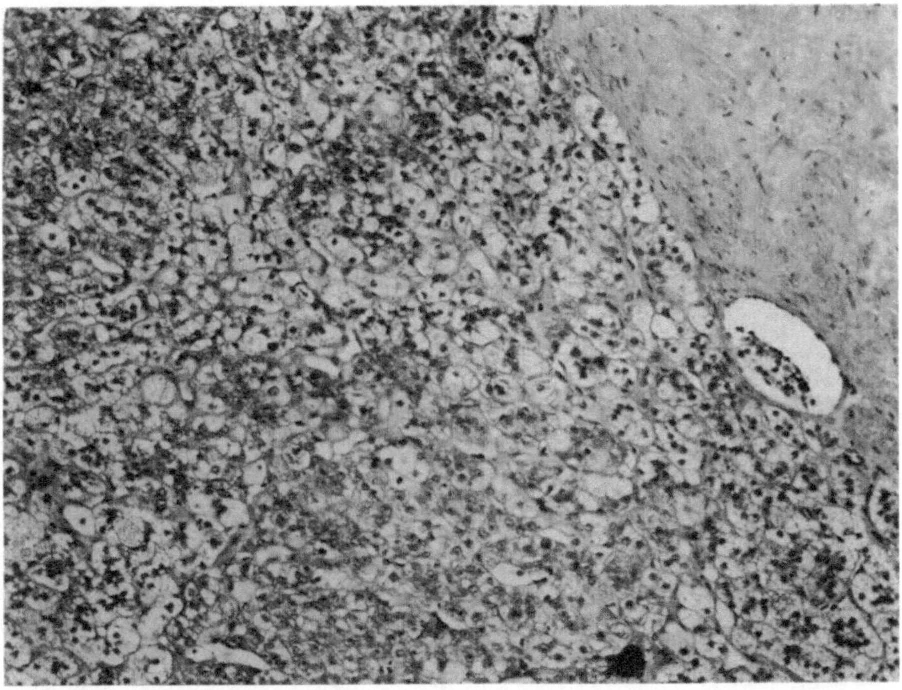

Figure 6. Aggregate of cortical cells in a small vascular structure in the dense fibrous capsule of this cortical neoplasm does not categorically imply malignant behavior (Case 4), (Hematoxylin and Eosin, × 160.

unable to state whether an adrenal cortical neoplasm is the most frequent cause of Cushing's syndrome in this age group [13, 14]. It is stated that most cases of Cushing's syndrome in the adult are secondary to abnormal secretion of corticotrophin with the consequence of bilateral cortical hyperplasia [13]. There is some ambiguity in the pediatric endocrinologic literature about the primacy of an adenoma or a carcinoma as the more common neoplasm regardless of the functional characteristics. Our very limited experience in conjunction with other recent studies would lead us to conclude that the adenoma is the more important of the two tumors. There is one obvious explanation for some of the confusion which relates to the difficulty in the unequivocal pathologic distinction between the adenoma and carcinoma when the tumor is encapsulated and confined to the adrenal gland [15, 16]. With one exception (Case 7, Table 1), the remaining patients in this study with localized tumors in the adrenal gland have done well although there were some disquieting histologic findings in three of the six cases. Prior studies have emphasized the obvious and some of the subtle pathologic differences between the adenoma and carcinoma: size (greater than 100 gm), capsular penetration, vascular invasion, necrosis, hemorr-

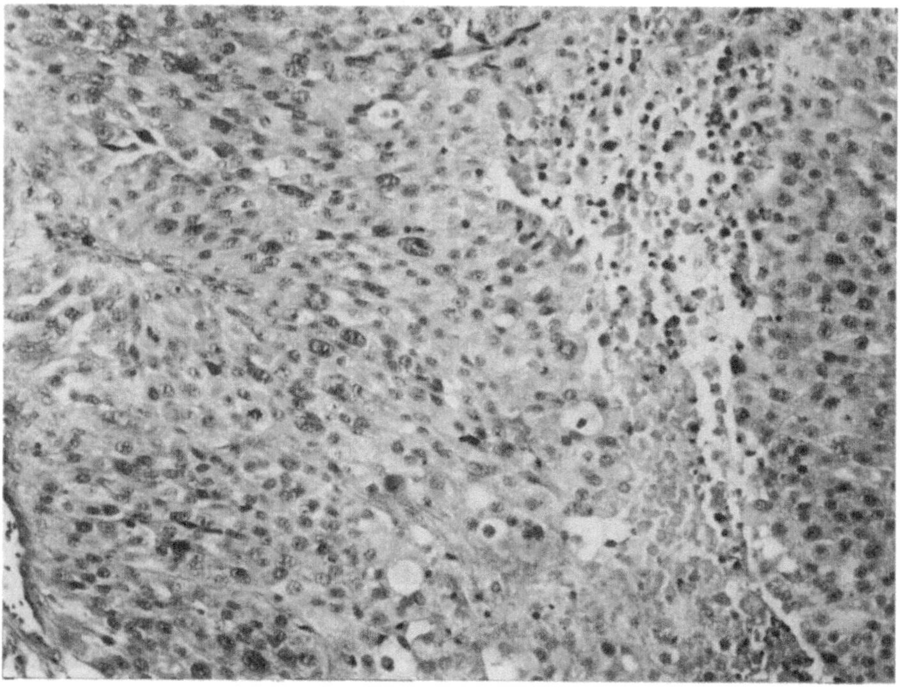

Figure 7. Adrenocortical carcinoma (Case 7) showing markedly atypical cytologic features including abundant mitotic activity and multiple foci of single cell necrosis (Hematoxylin and Eosin, ×160).

hage, trabecular versus diffuse growth pattern, broad fibrous bands, cellular anaplasia and mitotic activity [17, 18]. Overt virilization and weight loss are considered ominous clinical features [17].

An analysis of our cases indicates that none of the children experienced weight loss but rather a recorded gain in most instances. Cushing's syndrome (three cases), virilization (two cases), aldosteronism (one case) and a nonfunctional abdominal mass (one case) were the presenting features. One of the two children with virilization had an adrenal cortical carcinoma and the other child (Case 3, Table 1) has remained well after surgery although there were disturbing histologic findings in a mass confined to the adrenal gland. Some circumspection about the prognostic implications of one or another pathologic features is warranted in a series of this size. The four tumors with recorded weights were in excess of 100 gms. It was our impression that dimensions and weight are not overtly compelling parameters of benignancy or malignancy. A thorough gross examination and extensive sampling of the peripheral aspects of tumor are indicated in the situation of a very large tumor. A tumor which exceeds a kilogram as Case 7 should be viewed with obvious concern. Areas of macroscopically visible hemorrhage and necrosis are likewise less significant than the microscopic presence of a single cell necrosis. An external inspection of the mass for invasion is unquestionably a critical observation. Histopathologically, the cortical neoplasms are similar to many other endocrinologic tumors such as parathyroid adenomas, islet cell tumors of the pancreas and follicular neoplasms of the thyroid where conspicuous cytologic atypia with bizarre, hyperchromatic nuclei and sporadic mitotic activity does not immediately imply malignancy. A trabecular or nesting pattern was apparent in four cases (Cases 1, 2, 3, 5, Table 1). Diffuse sheets of acidophilic cells were present in the remaining cases (Cases 4, 6, 7, Table 1), Some cellular atypia was noted in Cases 4 and 6 but mitotic activity was virtually nonexistent in both. These patients have done well and of particular note is Case 6 with an original interpretation of adrenocortical carcinoma. There were occasional nests of tumor cells in small vascular spaces of the capsule. This finding is a disturbing one but not as ominous as involvement of arteries and veins. She has been examined at regular intervals and she has not required additional treatment, now 50 months after the adrenalectomy. Necrosis of single cells, numerous mitotic figures, invasion of major vessels, a very large size and finally hepatic and pulmonary metastases established one (14%) of our seven cases as a carcinoma. This patient's course has been remarkable in its length despite the presence of continued local abdominal disease.

Our study confirmed an already well documented fact in the literature which is the rarity of adrenocortical neoplasms in childhood. Cushing's syndrome or virilization are the commonest initial manifestations. The preoperative evaluation should characterize the major hormonal abnormalities since the levels become important in the follow-up period. Some pathologic criteria to differentiate an adenoma from a carcinoma are not absolute with the exception of gross vascular invasion and metastasis. In the borderline case, it is more judicious for the pathologist to equivocate rather than overdiagnose a neoplasm as a carcinoma. These children are best managed by periodic physical and laboratory examinations rather than some form of adjuvant therapy.

REFERENCES

1. Dehner LP: Pediatric Surgical Pathology, St. Louis, The CV Mosby Company, 1975, p 430–432.
2. Levine GW: Adrenocortical carcinoma in two children with subsequent primary tumors. Am J Dis Child 132:238–240, 1978.
3. Steward DR, Jones PHM, Jolleys A: Carcinoma of the adrenal gland in children. J Pediatr Surg 9:59–67, 1974.
4. McArthur RG, Cloutier MD, Hayles AB, Sprauge RG: Cushing's disease in children: findings in 13 cases. Mayo Clin Proc 47:318–326, 1972.

5. Ganguly A, Bergstein J, Grim CE, Yum MN, Weinberger MH: Childhood primarly aldosteronism due to an adrcnal adenoma: preoperative localization by adrenal vein catheterization. Pediatrics 65:605–609, 1980.
6. Kenny FM, Hashida Y, Askari A, Sieber WH, Fetterman GH: Virilizing tumors of the adrenal cortex. Am J Dis Child 115:445–458, 1968.
7. Kafrouni G, Oakes MD, Lurvey AN, De Quattro V: Aldosteronoma in a child with localization by adrenal vein aldosterone: collective review of the literature. J Pediatr Surg 10:917–924, 1975.
8. Kelch RP, Connors MH, Kaplan SL, Biglieri EG, Grumbach MM: A calcified aldosterone-producing tumor in a hypertensive, normokalemic prepubertal girl. J Pediatr 83:432–437, 1973.
9. Howard CP, Takahshi H, Hayles AB: Feminizing adrenal adenoma in a boy. Case report and literature review. Mayo Clin Proc 52:354–357, 1977.
10. Tank ES, Kay R: Neoplasms associated with hemihypertrophy, Beckwith-Wiedemann syndrome and aniridia. J Urol 124:266–268, 1979.
11. Fraumeni JF Jr, Miller RW: Adrenocortical neoplasms with hemihypertrophy, brain tumors, and other disorders. J Pediatr 70:129–138, 1967.
12. Sotelo-Avila C, Gonzalez-Crussi F, Fowler JW: Complete and incomplete forms of Beckwith-Wiedemann syndrome: Their oncogenic potential. J Pediatr 96:47–50, 1980.
13. Streeten DHP, Faas FH, Elders MJ, Dalakos TG, Voorhees M: Hypercortisolism in childhood: shortcomings of conventional diagnostic criteria. Pediatrics 56:798–803, 1975.
14. Cushing's syndrome in childhood. (Editorial). Lancet 2:267, 1972.
15. Kay S: Hyperplasia and neoplasia of the adrenal gland. Pathol Annu 11:103–139, 1976.
16. Neville AM, O'Hare MJ: Aspects of structure, function and pathology. In: The Adrenal Gland, VHT James (ed), New York, Raven Press, 1979, p 1–65.
17. Hough AJ, Hollifiedl JW, Page DL, Hartmann WH: Prognostic factors in adrenal cortical tumors: a mathematical analysis of clinical and morphologic data. Am J Clin Pathol 72:390–399, 1979.
18. O'Hare MJ, Monaghan P, Neville AM: The pathology of adrenocortical neoplasia: a correlated structural and functional approach to the diagnosis of malignant disease. Hum Pathol 10:137–154, 1979.

14. Adrenocortical Carcinoma in Children: Experience at the Children's Hospital of Philadelphia, 1961-1980

R. BEVERLY RANEY, Jr., ANNA T. MEADOWS and GIULIO J. D'ANGIO

Carcinomas of the adrenal cortex are exceptionally uncommon in children. There were four cases of adrenocortical carcinoma recorded in the Third National Cancer Survey, conducted a decade ago [1]. In addition, carcinomas of unidentified types were rare. Guidelines for management of these rare tumors are generally based on data obtained in adults, since there are only anecdotal reports of these diseases in the pediatric population.

The Tumor Registry at The Children's Hospital of Philadelphia contains information on 7 children diagnosed with adrenocortical carcinoma during the period 1961-1980. Their age, sex, race, clinical and pathologic features, treatment, and outcome are summarized in Table 1.

The 7 children with *adrenal tumors* ranged in age from 0.6–6 years at diagnosis. Four were female; only 1 was black. The tumors arose in the left adrenal of 4 patients and the right adrenal of 2 patients; one patient (number 2 in Table 1) had simultaneous bilateral adrenal carcinomas. No patient presented with metastases; all had grossly complete removal of tumor at unilateral (6 patients) or bilateral adrenalectomy (1 patient). The tumors from 4 patients were measured and ranged from 3 to 8 cm in widest diameter.

Associated findings at diagnosis included signs of virilization (pubic hair, increased size of phallus, and advanced bone age) in 6 patients, one of whom also had café-au-lait spots. The seventh patient presented with macroglossia and an omphalocele at birth, and was diagnosed with Beckwith-Wiedemann syndrome. Subtotal pancreatectomy was required by 2 months of age because of refractory hypoglycemia. Ultrasound examinations subsequently showed a 3 cm left adrenal mass, which was removed at 7 months of age.

Supported in part by USPHS Grants CA-14489, and CA-19372, and CA-26191.

G. Bennett Humphrey et al. (eds), Adrenal and Endocrine Tumors in Children.

Table 1. Adrenocortical carcinoma: children's Hospital of Philadelphia.

Patient number	Age (yr)	Sex/ race	Site of tumor	Associated findings	Mangement[2]	Subsequent tumor	Current status, time after Dx.[3]
1	2	F/W	R. adrenal	Virilized	R. adrenex.	Local Recur. at 7 months → partial resection +o, p - DDD	DOD, 19 months
2	5	F/W	Both adrenals	Virilized	Bilat. adrenex., Cortisone	Lung metastases at 10 months → 1200 rad, both lungs	DOD, 23 months
3	2	F/W	R. adrenal	Virilized, Cafe-au-lait	R. Adrenex.	Thalamic astro-cytoma at 31 months	Dead of second tumor, 10.1 yr
4	0.6	M/W	L. adrenal	Not virilized; Beckwith-Wiedemann Syndrome	L. Adrenex.	0	Dead of respiratory obstruction, 20 months. Autopsy: no tumor
5	4	F/B	L. adrenal	Virilized	L. Adrenex.	0	NED, 16.4 yr
6	1	M/W	L. adrenal	Virilized	L. Adrenex., Cortisone	0	NED, 16.2 yr
7	6	M/W	L. adrenal	Virilized	L. Adrenex.	0	NED, 15.3 yr

[1] F, female; W, white; M, male; B, black.
[2] R, right; L, left; Adrenex, adrenalectomy.
[3] Dx., diagnosis; DOD, dead of disease; NED, no evidence of disease.

After surgery, 2 patients received cortisone acetate, including the one who had a bilateral adrenalectomy. No anti-tumor chemotherapy or radiation therapy was administered. Two patients ultimately died of carcinoma which recurred within a year after diagnosis. Two additional patients succumbed. The patient with café-au-lait spots developed a second, intracranial neoplasm and died 7.5 years after the thalamic tumor was diagnosed; the child with Beckwith-Wiedemann syndrome expired because of respiratory obstruction and had no tumor at autopsy. Three patients are alive and well over 15 years after diagnosis.

It is obvious that this group of patients is too small for firm conclusions to be drawn regarding management of future children with these diseases.

The mainstay of treatment would appear to be surgery. The role, if any, for post-operative chemotherapy is undefined, since the rate of recurrence is low and the diseases are quite rare. Similarly, the role of post-operative radiation therapy is unclear. The young age of the patients, the proximity of the adrenal gland to other vital structures such as the kidney or liver, and the relative insensitivity of adenocarcinomas to radiation all speak against the routine use of radiation therapy for such children.

ACKNOWLEDGEMENT

The authors are very grateful for the assistance of Ms. Patricia Jarrett, Senior Tumor Registrar at The Children's Hospital of Philadelphia in the preparation of Table 1.

REFERENCE

1. Young JL Jr., Miller RW: Incidence of malignant tumors in U.S. children. J Pediatr 86:254–258, 1975.

15. Adrenocortical Carcinoma in Children

RAYMOND J. HUTCHINSON and RUTH M. HEYN

INTRODUCTION

Adrenocortical carcinoma (ACC) is an uncommon neoplasm in the pediatric age group, occurring in fewer than 15 children per year in the United States [1]. Many of these tumors are hormonally active, producing a variety of presenting manifestations [2, 3]. Features at diagnosis include an abdominal mass, facial acne, growth acceleration, deepening of the voice, growth of axillary and pubic hair, precocious genital development, and hypertension. Because of the rarity of the tumor in children, accurate survival statistics are difficult to ascertain. In a series of 49 adult patients, death due to metastatic disease occurred in 73% [4].

Diagnosis is facilitated by obtaining intravenous pyelography and ultrasonography of the abdomen. Assays of twenty-four hour urine collections for 17-ketosteroids and 17-hydroxysteroids are useful when elevated, particularly when the metabolite excretion appears independent of pituitary control after dexamethasone suppression. Definitive diagnosis is made by histopathologic examination of tumor tissue, with differentiation between benign and malignant adrenal tissue proving subtle in many instances. In addition to cytologic appearance, emphasis is placed upon mitotic activity, the presence or absence of capsular invasion, blood vessel invasion, and the presence of distant metastases [4].

PATIENTS

Three children with a diagnosis of ACC have been cared for at the University of Michigan in recent years. The clinical features of these patients at the time of diagnosis are summarized in Table 1. Two of the three were noted to be hypertensive at diagnosis or recurrence. One of the two hyper-

G. Bennett Humphrey et al. (eds), Adrenal and Endocrine Tumors in Children.

Table 1. Clinical features at diagnosis of patients with adrenocortical carcinoma.

Patient	Sex	Age	Primary	BP	17-Ketosteroids (mg/24°)	17-Hydroxysteroids ($mg/m^2/24°$)	LDH (IU/L)	Presentation
1	M	8 wks	R adrenal	260/140	15.4	26.2	2286	CVA, acne
2*	M	2 yrs	L adrenal	210/140	10.4	21.3	1500	Acne, hirsutism, precocious genital developmental, abdominal mass
3	M	6 yrs	L adrenal	115/60	53.5 (N < 2.0 mg/24°)	2.4 (N 1–5 $mg/m^2/24°$)	ND (N 124–226 IU/L)	Marked gynecomastia, acne, hirsutism, abdominal mass, increased growth

* Data at the time of recurrence.
N = normal; ND = not done; CVA = cerebrovascular accident.

tensive patients presented with a left head tilt, ptosis of the right eyelid, deviation of the eyes to the right, and bloody cerebrospinal fluid, all consistent with a cerebrovascular accident. The other two patients presented with features of precocious or aberrant sexual development and evidence of an intra-abdominal mass. One demonstrated features of both virilization and feminization. All three had elevations of 17-ketosteroids and/or 17-hydroxysteroids. Serum lactic dehydrogenase was elevated in the two patients in whom it was measured.

RESULTS

All three children had gross total removal of the primary tumor surgically. Postoperatively patient 1 received radiotherapy with 1840 rads to the whole abdomen and an additional 700 rads to the right upper quadrant. He remains free of disease 55 months from the date of the diagnosis.

Patient 2 received no other therapy postoperatively and had gross evidence of recurrent abdominal tumor 2 months later. He was treated with o,p′DDD (1,1-dichloro-2-(o-chlorophenyl)-2-(p-chlorophenyl)-ethane) orally for 2 months without evidence of tumor regression. He received 2 doses of high-dose methotrexate (8 gm/dose) without effect. Oral o,p′DDD was continued, and he was treated with 1680 rads to the whole abdomen and 2 courses of combination chemotherapy including vincristine, actinomycin D, cyclophosphamide and 5-fluorouracil. Despite this therapy he developed pulmonary metastases and expired 9 months after diagnosis.

Patient 3 was initially diagnosed as having an adrenocortical adenoma with a solitary nest of neoplastic cells in a dilated vein within the tumor mass. No further therapy was given postoperatively. All evidence of virilization and feminization subsided and he developed normally for 7 years. He then returned with complaints of hip pain and weight loss and was found to have lung and bone metastases. He failed to respond to either a course of methotrexate, chlorambucil and actinomycin D or to o,p′DDD. He expired 8 years after diagnosis and at autopsy had tumor in lungs, ribs, vertebrae, retroperitoneum and retroperitoneal nodes. The pathological tissue was identical to that of his initial tumor. This patient has been previously reported [5].

DISCUSSION

These patients illustrate the variability of clinical presentation noted with ACC. The elevation of 17-ketosteroids and/or 17-hydroxysteroids in the urine can serve as indices of tumor response to therapy and of tumor recurrence. The levels for patients 2 and 3 rose with tumor recurrence whereas they have remained normal in patient 1.

Complete surgical removal of the primary tumor is indicated for initial treatment. Pathologic evaluation should include the adequacy of surgical margins. It is important to provide appropriate steroid supplementation intraoperatively and postoperatively.

The role of aduvant therapy in the ultimate control of this highly malignant tumor has not been answered. Although subjective and objective responses have been reported with radiotherapy [4, 6], there is only one instance in which postoperative radiotherapy was associated with tumor regression [2]. An 18 month old child with removal of the primary tumor but not of the vena caval extension received 2500 rads to the abdomen and continued disease free for several years. Of the 4 children in the same series who were treated with postoperative radiotherapy to the abdomen, 3 remain well and the only patient who expired had metastatic disease at diagnosis. In another report a 5 year old girl who presented with paraplegia was found to have extradural tumor compressing the cord [7]. A laminectomy and biopsy were performed and she was treated with radiotherapy and chemotherapy (vincristine, actinomycin D and cyclophosphamide). She recovered normal motor function but documentation of the degree of tumor regression was not reported. She developed acute paraplegia twice in the following 4 months making the role of radiotherapy difficult to assess.

Documentation of the effectiveness of chemotherapy is also limited in ACC. The first use of o,p′DDD was reported in 1959, with 3 of 8 adults showing significant regression of metastatic lesions [8]. The decrease in steroid hormone excretion was well documented by these authors. A review of the use of this compound from a collective series reported a 34% objective response rate in 59 patiens with evaluable disease [9]. Long term survival, however, did not appear to be influenced by this therapy. A single documented cure of metastatic disease with the combined use of o,p′DDD and fluorouracil given for 5 months has been reported [10]. The patient expired 10 years later and at autopsy had no evidence of tumor. A further report of a 4 month old baby whose tumor was removed suggested that there was a response to actinomycin D, cyclophosphamide and 5-fluorouracil given for 13 months since transient postoperative hypertension and elevated 17-hydroxy and ketosteroids regressed while on therapy and she remained well 22 months after therapy was stopped [11].

It is obvious that the use of radiotherapy or chemotherapy as adjuvant postoperative treatment needs to be carefully evaluated. In addition to better surgical and pathological evaluation, the consistent use of a single dose of radiotherapy to the abdomen should clarify its role in local disease control. Until there is further evidence for tumor regression in response to specific chemotherapeutic regimens, the adjuvant use of chemotherapy would not appear warranted.

Finally, ACC in children is associated with significant other pecularities. Second malignancies, especially of the brain, have been reported in a number of patients with ACC [1]. In addition, ACC occurs in association with several congenital problems, including Beckwith-Wiedemann syndrome, hemihypertrophy, and genitourinary anomalies [2, 3], and it may occur in more than one family member or in association with an array of other neoplasms [1]. One of our patients, patient 3, had a twin sister with aniridia. Hence, genetic factors may operate to influence the development of ACC.

REFERENCES

1. Miller RW: Peculiarities in the occurrence of adrenal cortical carcinoma. Am J Dis Child 132:235–236, 1978.
2. Stewart DR, Morris Jones PH, Jolleys A: Carcinoma of the adrenal gland in children. J Pediatr Surg 9:59–67, 1974.
3. Zaitoon MM, Mackie GG: Adrenal cortical tumors in children. Urology 12:645–649, 1978.
4. King DR, Lack EE: Adrenal cortical carcinoma: a clinical and pathologic study of 49 cases. Cancer 44:239–244, 1979.
5. Bacon GE, Lowrey GH: Feminizing adrenal tumor in a six-year-old boy. J Clin Endocr 25:1403–1406, 1965.
6. Percarpio B, Knowlton AH: Radiation therapy of adrenal cortical carcinoma. Acta Radiol (Ther) (Stockh) 15:288–292, 1976.
7. Marsden HB, Morris Jones P, Lees PD, Hann IM: Late functioning adrenocortical carcinoma in a 5-year-old girl. Arch Dis Child 53:341–342, 1978.
8. Bergenstal DM, Lipsett MB, Moy RH, Hertz R: Regression of adrenal cancer and suppression of adrenal function in man by o,p′DDD. Trans Assoc Am Physicians 72:341–350, 1959.
9. Hutter AM Jr, Kayhoe DE: Adrenal cortical carcinoma: results of treatment with o,p′DDD in 138 patients. Am J Med 41:581–592, 1966.
10. Ostuni JA, Roginsky MS: Metastatic adrenal cortical carcinoma: documented cure with combined chemotherapy. Arch Intern Med 135:1257–1258, 1975.
11. Visconti EB, Peters RW, Cangir A, Zorn GL Jr, Fisher S: Unusual case of adrenal cortical carcinoma in a female infant. Arch Dis Child 53:342–344, 1978.

16. Adrenal Cortical Carcinoma and Multiple Endocrine Neoplasia

BARBARA CUSHING and A. JOSEPH BROUGH

Tumors of the endocrine system in the pediatric age group are a very small percentage of the total number of malignancies. Of these, germ cell tumors, some with encocrine function, and papillary or follicular thyroid carcinomas, associated with prior radiation exposure, are the most common. Tumors of the adrenal cortex and multiple endocrine neoplasia (MEN) are exceedingly rare. The following chapter discusses the four cases presenting to Children's Hospital of Michigan from 1963 to 1981.

Adrenal cortical carcinoma (ACC) frequently presents with clinical and laboratory evidence of increased steroid hormone production [1] and has a peak occurrence in early childhood [2]. Differentiation between benign and malignant ACC appears related to absence of metastases at diagnosis, size of tumor, and histologic criteria of cellular pleomorphism, whether differentiated or anaplastic [3]. We have experience of only one case of MEN in childhood.

Table 1. Rare endocrine tumors, Children's Hospital of Michigan (1963–1980).

Age	Sex	Race	Hormone activity	Therapy	Status
Adrenal Cortical Carcinoma					
7 mo	F	Caucasian	Yes	Surgery	NID
7 mo	F	Caucasian	No	Surgery, RT	NID
17 mo	F	Caucasian	Yes	Surgery, o,p'-DDD	Died
Multiple Endocrine Neoplasia					
11 yr	M	Caucasian	–	Surgery	–

G. Bennett Humphrey et al. (eds), Adrenal and Endocrine Tumors in Children.

ADRENOCORTICAL CARCINOMA

Case 1: Seven month old female presented with features of Cushing's disease: moonface, buffalo hump, hirsuitism, glucosuria, without virilization. Blood pressure was within normal range. Weight was above the 97th percentile and height was 25th percentile. On intravenous pyelogram a left adrenal mass was visualized. A 24 hour urine collection for 17 ketosteroids was 4.0 mg (normal less than 0.5 mg). Cortisol levels were not measured. At exploratory laparatomy a 5.5 cm diameter, well-encapsulated tumor was found in the left adrenal gland. The histology was moderately well differentiated adrenocortical carcinoma with cellular pleomorphism. There was no distinct evidence of vascular invasion; the presence of small numbers of neoplastic cells arranged within the thin capsule was considered evidence for capsular invasion. No metastatic disease within the abdomen was found. Clinically, the tumor behaved as a benign adenoma, with no further recurrence after surgical removal.

Case 2: Seven month old female presented in congestive heart failure with tachypnea, tachycardia, bilateral rales, hepatosplenomegaly and a large left flank mass extending to the inguinal ligament. Chest x-ray was compatible with pulmonary edema. Hemoglogin 2.8 gm %. The infant's weight and height fell below the 3rd percentile. Intravenous pyelogram visualized a right suprarenal mass with calcification. The inferior vena cava was obstructed due to extrinsic compression. Exploratory laparotomy was done for presumed neuroblastoma: a large tumor was encountered filling the right upper quadrant and extending to the pelvis, overriding vena cava and aorta. The decision was made to biopsy and treat with radiation and chemotherapy prior to an attempt at surgical resection. The histology was not neuroblastoma, but adrenocortical carcinoma with masses of cells having an epithelial configuration and containing bizarre nuclei and eosinophilic cytoplasm. Necrosis and hemorrhage were present as were capsular and venous invasion. Twelve days later the baby was re-explored and the right kidney and suprarenal mass were removed in continuity; the adrenal mass measured 9 × 7 × 4 cm, was necrotic, partially encapsulated and sharply separated from the kidney. An endocrine work-up confirmed a non-functioning tumor.

Post-operatively, she received three courses of radiotherapy to the tumor bed: 1660, 1333 and 1328 roentgens. She has had no recurrent disease. At age ten, a severe lumbar kyphosis was corrected surgically.

Case 3: Seventeen month old girl presented with a less than one month history of virilization: acne, pubic hair, and clitoral enlargement. A left upper quandrant mass was palpable. She was hypertensive. On IVP a large mass was visualized in the left adrenal area. Endocrinologic evaluation included a normal bone age, 24 hour 17 ketosteroids 10.8 mg (normal 0.5), 17 hydroxycorticosteroids 1.1 mg (normal) and dehydroepiandrosterone as assayed by the Allen blue test 51.0 μg (normal 4.0). At exploratory laparatomy, the tumor was not well encapsulated and invaded the superior pole of the kidney and adrenal vein. A 10 cm tumor was resected. Histology was characteristic of adrenocortical carcinoma with marked cellular pleomorphism, containing areas of necrosis and hemorrhage. A small remnant of residual, atrophic adrenal gland was found. Tumor cells were present within the capsule and vascular invasion was present.

Nineteen months later 17 ketosteroids were again markedly elevated. On IVP calcification was present in the area of the right adrenal and the left kidney was displaced downward. At laparatomy, recurrence was found in the inferior vena cava at the level of the renal veins and was resected. Three months later, tumor recurred in the vena cava from the right common iliac vein to the right atrium. Mitotane (o,p′-DDD) was begun with no clinical response.

In summary, all three patients were females ranging from 7 to 17 months at diagnosis. Two were endocrinologically functioning, one with Cushing's disease and the other with virilization. None of the three had metastatic disease at presentation, and tumor was completely resected. All three had typical histologic features of adrenal cortical carcinoma. Vascular invasion and/or capsular infiltration (considered evidence of malignancy) were present in all three. One child had no further therapy and no recurrence; one child received radiation to the tumor bed with no recurrence; one child had recurrent and ultimately fatal disease.

MULTIPLE ENDOCRINE NEOPLASIA

Only one child has been evaluated in this institution in the past ten years for this disorder; he represented a MEN, Type III (or IIB). At 7 years of age a plexiform neurofibroma was removed from the upper lip. The lesion had been present since age 3 and over the past two years small white papular lesions appeared on the tip of the tongue. At age eleven the patient was re-admitted with multiple papillary lesions on the upper lip, tongue, and buccal mucosa, suggestive of multiple mucosal neuroma syndrome. Small, discrete cervical nodes were present, thyroid was normal on palpation. Serum calcitonin was less than 336 pq/ml (elevated). Remainder of thyroid and adrenal work-up was normal. (Urinary catecholamine excretion was low.) A thyroidectomy was done because of the high incidence of carcinoma, and microscopically medullary carcinoma was present in a 3 mm nodule in the right lobe. The patient has not developed pheochromocytoma or neurologic abnormalities but has a unicord habitus with long, thin face and high arched palate.

COMMENTS ON FUTURE MANAGEMENT

Despite the extremely rare occurrence of these endocrine tumors in a pediatric oncology referral population, recognition of the diagnosis and integrated multi-modal management may be successful. Data relating to management of ACC from adult series indicates that early diagnosis, complete surgical resection, tumor size, and histologic characteristics favoring adenomas, differentiated or anaplastic carcinomas are essential to both management and survival. It appears that with complete surgical resection and absence of metastases with differentiated histology, one would follow closely for recurrence. For residual tumor palliative irradiation has been successful in 50% of adults [1] and perhaps was curative in one of our patients. We would give tumor bed irradiation for residual disease, however techniques and dosages would differ from our previous patient. Mitotane (o,p′-DDD) to suppress functioning residual ACC appears to have clinical results when given early [4, 5]. Antineoplastic agents have not shown encouraging results, however, may have some effect on the anaplastic, non-functioning carcinoma [1, 3].

REFERENCES

1. King DR, Lack EE: Adrenal cortical carcinoma. A clinical and pathologic study of 49 cases. Cancer 44:239–244, 1979.
2. Hough AJ, Hollifield JW, Page DL, Hartmann WH: Prognostic factors in adrenal cortical tumors. A mathematical analysis of clinical and morphologic data. Am J Clin Pathol 72:390–399, 1979.
3. Hogan TF, Gilchrist KW, Westring DW, Citrin DL: A clinical and pathological study of adrenocortical carcinoma. Therapeutic implications. Cancer 45:2880–2883, 1980.
4. Lubitz JA, Freeman L, Okun R: Mitotane use in inoperable adrenal cortical carcinoma. JAMA 223:1109–1112, 1973.
5. Harrison JH, Mahoney EM, Bennett AH: Tumors of the adrenal cortex. Cancer 32:1227–1235, 1973.

17. Experience with Adrenal Cortical Carcinoma in Children

ELAINE R. MORGAN, EDWARD S. BAUM and PATRICE M. WEST

Cancers of the adrenal cortex most commonly present with virilization or as Cushing's syndrome, depending on whether they secrete androgens or cortisol [1, 2]. Very rarely, tumors of the adrenal cortex in children may cause feminization or aldosterone secretion [3, 4]. Tumor size is quite variable at the time of diagnosis, since many are detected when they are quite small because of the excessive hormone secretion [5]. Although metastasis is rare, it can occur in association with malignant lesions.

In addition to isolated neoplasias of endocrine tissue, such as those described above, several interesting syndromes, termed multiple endocrine neoplasias (MEN), have been described. Like the other endocrine carcinomas, these are rarely diagnosed in children. However, they may be familial, and in certain instances various manifestations of the syndrome may occur asynchronously with some symptoms being detected in childhood and others not occurring until adulthood.

At the present time, three types of MEN have been described. Type 1 consists of involvement of the pancreatic islet cells, pituitary, and parathyroid glands [6, 7]. Type 2 consists of pheochromocytomas, medullary thyroid carcinomas and parathyroid tumors [7, 8]. Type 3 (alternately called IIb by some authors) is characterized by mucosal neuromas, pheochromocytomas and medullary thyroid carcinomas with or without the presence of marfanoid habitus [9, 10]. Gastrointestinal manifestations and mucosal lesions frequently present early in life [11].

Adrenal cortical tumors are most commonly treated by surgery alone [6]. There is little information about other modalities of therapy in this tumor type. Similarly, patients having one or more manifestations of the MEN syndromes are most commonly treated with surgical removal of the malignant tissue [6–10]. This frequently requires total removal of the gland in the case of medullary thyroid carcinoma or parathyroid carcinoma [7–9].

Most of the information concerning treatment of these lesions comes

G. Bennett Humphrey et al. (eds), Adrenal and Endocrine Tumors in Children.

Table 1. Clinical experience with adrenal cortical carcinoma.

Pt.	Date Dx.	Sex	Age at Dx.	Diagnosis	Presenting symptoms	F Hx	Rx	Comments
DA	1979	M	6 years	MEN 2B (medullary thyroid ca)	↑ T_4 on screening	$\bar{0}$	Total Thyroidectomy	Ganglioneuromatosis diagnosed at age 2 yrs. NED with persistent diarrhea
LT	1955	19 mos.	Carcinoma, rt adrenal Cortex	Virilization	Sibling (see BT)	Adrenalectomy, Post op XRT	NED	
BT	1957	M	3 years	Carcinoma, rt adrenal cortex	Virilization	Sibling (see LT)	Adrenalectomy, Post op XRT	NED
NMcK	1980	F	2 years	Adrenocortical carcinoma	Virilization	$\bar{0}$	Surgery, removal right adrenal gland + encapsulated mass	
MW	1980	F	16 mos.	Adrenocortical carcinoma	Virilization LUQ mass on ultrasound	$\bar{0}$	Surgery removal left adrenal gland + mass	

from experience with adults, which may or may not be applicable to the rare cases of endocrine neoplasia which present in childhood.

We have reviewed the tumor board records concerning all children who have presented with one of the above mentioned malignancies in the past years at Children's Memorial Hospital and the University of Chicago. The information concerning age at diagnosis, type of malignancy, family history, therapy and outcome are summarized in the accompanying table. Only two of our 5 patients had a positive family history for endocrine neoplasis (BT and LT, siblings with adrenal carcinoma).

As will be noted from the table, all patients are alive and well with no subsequent neoplasia. Total surgical resection of the tumor was accomplished in these patients.

REFERENCES

1. Cahill GF, Melecow MM, Darby HH: Adrenal Cortical Tumors: The Types of Non-Hormonal and Hormonal Tumors. Surg Gynecol Obstet 74:281–305, 1942.
2. Fraumine JF, Miller RW: Adrenal Cortical Neoplasias and Hemihypertrophy, Brain Tumors and Other Disorders. J Pediatr 70:129–138, 1967.
3. Higgins GH, Brounlee WE, Monty FH: Feminizing Tumors on the Adrenal Cortex. Am Surg 22:56-79, 1956.
4. Cavell B, Sandegard E, Hakfelt B: Primary Aldosteronism Due to an Adrenal Adenoma in the Three Year Old Child. Acta Paediatr Scand 53:205–212, 1964.
5. Clayton GW: Tumors of the Endocrine Glands. In: Clinical Pediatric Oncology, Mosby CV, 1977 (2nd edition), p 525–540.
6. Johnson GJ, Summerskill, Anderson VE, Keating FR: Clinical and Genetic Investigation of a Large Kindred with Multiple Endocrine Adenomatosis. N Engl J Med 277:1379–1385, 1967.
7. Steiner AL, Goodman AD, Powers SR: Study of a Kindred with Pheochromocytoma, Medullary Thyroid Carcinoma, Hyperparathyroidism and Cushing Disease, Multiple Endocrine Neoplasia, Type 2. Med 47:371–409, 1968.
8. Block MA: A Component of an Interesting Endocrine Syndrome. CA-A Cancer Journal for Clinicians 19:74–79, 1969.
9. Khaire MRA, Dexter RN, Burgynski NJ, Johnston CC: Mucosal Neuroma, Pheochromocytoma, and Medullary Thyroid Carcinoma. Med 54:89–112, 1975.
10. Carney JA, Go VLW, Sizemore GW, Hayles AB: Alimentary Tract Ganglioneuromatosis: A Major Component of the syndrome of Multiple Endocrine Neoplasia, Type 2B. N Engl J Med 295:1287–1291, 1976.
11. Grosfield JL, Clatworthy HW, Hamoudi AB: Pancreatic Malignancy in Childhood. Arch Surg 101:370–375, 1970.

18. Cancer of the Adrenal Gland in Children: Experience at the M.D. Anderson Hospital and Tumor Institute

NORMAN JAFFE and AYTEN CANGIR

Adrenal cortical carcinoma is a rare neoplasm in infancy. Most cases present with Cushing's syndrome, hirsuitism, precocious puberty, or rarely inappropriate ADH secretion. Associated congenital anomalies and concurrent central nervous system and hepatic tumors have also been documented. Occasionally, the tumor may be non-functioning. Three cases have been seen at the M.D. Anderson Hospital and Tumor Institute with a variety of presentations and outcome.

One patient presented at the age of 5 months with a history of a term delivery to a 27 year old gravida II, primiparous mother [1]. At three months, transient bloody stools appeared but resolved after a change in the milk formula. At four and a half months, a left abdominal mass was noted with a two week history of weight loss, irritability and increasing abdominal girth. A tender left abdominal mass filling the entire side of the abdomen was detected. The blood pressure was 140/90.

Surgical exploration revealed a $10 \times 18 \times 10$ cm hemorrhagic mass occupying the entire left retroperitoneum, encasing the left kidney and invading the mesocolon and splenic flexure. It was removed. Microscopic examination showed massive tumor necrosis with marked vascularity and extensive hemorrhage. Viable portions of the tumor were arranged in sheets and columns of cells around dilated ectatic veins. The cytoplasm of many of the cells contained droplets of neutral lipid. Marked nuclear and cytoplasmic gigantism was also present. There were numerous abnormal mitotic figures.

Biochemical examination revealed transient elevations of 24 hr 17-hydroxy and 21-oxosteroids which normalized during treatment. The latter comprised Actinomycin-D, Cyclophosphamide and 5-fluorouracil. Chemo-

Supported in part by Grant No. CA 03713 from the National Institute of Health.

G. Bennett Humphrey et al. (eds), Adrenal and Endocrine Tumors in Children.

therapy continued for five consecutive days at three weekly intervals for $13\frac{1}{2}$ months. The duration of treatment was based upon the length of pregnancy, plus time at diagnosis. At the time of the report, the patient was well 21 months after completion of the chemotherapy with no evidence of primary or metastatic tumor. Ortho, para DDD (1, 1-dichloro-2-(o-chlorophenyl)-2-(p-chlorophenyl)-ethane, or mitotaine, an isomer of DDD was not used. The agent causes hemorrhagic necrosis in the dog adrenal cortex and in view of the patient's age, difficulties were anticipated with its side-effects.

The second patient was an eleven year old girl who was referred to the M.D. Anderson Hospital and Tumor Institute after incidental discovery of a calcified right suprarenal mass on radiographic examination. The latter had been obtained during the course of investigation for a gangrenous appendix which was removed. There was no evidence of Cushing's syndrome, precocious puberty or virulism. A twenty-four hour urinary VMA, catecholamines and HVA were within normal limits.

The suprarenal gland was removed after convalescence from appendectomy and a diagnosis of adrenal cortical carcinoma was advanced. There was no evidence of metastatic disease and since there were no metabolic disturbances, adjuvant therapy was not administered. She has remained alive and well for the past 11 years.

The microscopic features of this tumor were variable. In some areas it was epithelial and showed a relationship with adrenal cortical tissue. In others it was less well differentiated with a somewhat mesenchymal pattern. Electron microscopy demonstrated closely opposed cytoplasmic membranes and numerous small cell contacts. There was a smooth endoplasmic reticulum and occasional lipid bodies. These features supported the light microscopic interpretation of adrenal cortical carcinoma.

The third patient was a $13\frac{1}{2}$ year old female. She was well until approximately six months prior to admission when she gained 40 pounds in weight. She also developed increased dryness of the skin, an acneform eruption, dry brittle hair, dependent edema, striae, bruising and a blue tinge to the skin. Radiographic examination of the abdomen revealed a calcified adrenal cortex. The chest radiograph revealed pulmonary metastases. The cortisone level was elevated at 477 ng.

The hypertension and hypercortisonemia decreased with the administration of metapyrone. This was also accompanied by a decrease in the acneform eruption and facial flushing. A right adrenalectomy was performed. Pathological examination of the adrenal gland confirmed the diagnosis of adrenal cortical carcinoma. Treatment with ortho para DDD and later a combination of adriamycin, cyclophosphamide, vincristine and 5-fluorouracil was instituted. Both chemotherapeutic programs failed to achieve a response and the patient died five months after admission.

REFERENCES

1. Visconti EB, Peters RW, Cangir A, Zorn GL Jr, Fisher S: Unusual case of Adrenal Cortical Carcinoma in a female infant. Arch Dis Child 53:342–344, 1978.

19. Carcinoma of the Adrenal Gland in Children – A Study of 12 Patients

HELEN S.L. CHAN

INTRODUCTION

The adrenal gland is an uncommon site for tumors in the pediatric age group. The majority of these tumors are neuroblastomas. Carcinomas and adenomas represent less than 4% of all adrenal tumors [1]. Between 1943 and 1981, a total of 12 cases of carcinoma and 5 cases of adenoma were seen at the Hospital for Sick Children, Toronto. All these children had functioning adrenocortical tumors.

Less than 50% of adult patients presenting with adrenocortical carcinoma are suitable candidates for curative cancer surgery [2, 3]. Of this group, MacFarlane reported a 65% 3-year survival. In patients whose tumors have not been completely resected, less than a third showed temporary tumor regression when treated with o,p′-DDD (1,1-dichloro-2-(o-chlorophenyl)-2-(p-chlorophenyl)-ethane; mitotane) [4, 5]. Other than one pediatric report of the benefit of post-operative radiation therapy [1], most authors consider adrenocortical carcinoma to be a radioresistant tumor [6].

The following report describes our approach in treating patients with surgically unresected or metastatic disease with a combination of radiation therapy and chemotherapy using o,p′-DDD and 5-Fluorouracil.

PATIENTS

The clinical features of twelve patients with adrenocortical carcinoma at the time of diagnosis are summarized in Table 1. All patients presented with virilization or precocious puberty, hypertension and abdominal masses. Two children (Patients 1 and 2) also appeared cushingnoid. No patients had features of feminization.

All patients tested had increased 24-hour urinary 17-ketosteroids which were not suppressed by dexamethasone, increased plasma testosterone and

G. Bennett Humphrey et al. (eds), Adrenal and Endocrine Tumors in Children.

Table 1. Clinical features at diagnosis of patients with adrenocortical carcinoma.

Patient	Year	Sex	Age (yrs)	Adrenal	Duration of symptoms	Virilized	Abd. mass	Others	↑ 17-KS	↑ C	↑ T	↑ A
1	1943	F	2	R	4 months	+	+	–	ND	ND	ND	ND
2	1950	M	4½	L	2½ years	+	+	Polycythemic	+	ND	ND	ND
3	1954	F	1	R	11 months	+	+	–	+	ND	ND	ND
4	1956	F	4	L	2 months	+	+	–	+	ND	ND	ND
5	1959	F	11	L	11 years	+	+	–	+	ND	ND	ND
6	1963	F	1	L	5 months	+	+	–	+	ND	ND	ND
7	1976	F	2½	R	1 year	+	+	–	+	+	+	+
8	1978	M	9½	L	6 months	+	+	Hypokalemic alkalosis	+	+	+	+
9	1979	M	2½	L	6 months	+	+	–	+	+	+	+
10	1980	F	9½	R	6 months	+	+	Liver & lung metastases	+	+	+	+
11	1980	F	1½	R	2 months	+	+	–	+	+	+	+
12	1981	F	11½	L	1 year	+	+	Hypokalemia, lung metastases	+	+	+	+

17-KS = urinary 17-ketosteroids; C = plasma cortisol; T = plasma testosterone; A = plasma androstenedione; ND = not done.

androstenedione, and increased plasma cortisol with loss of diurnal variation. We also utilized ultrasonography, computerized axial tomography before and after contrast enhancement, intravenous pyelography and angiography to localize the primary tumor. Computerized axial tomography, ^{99m}technetium-sulfur colloid liver scan and ^{99m}technetium-polyphosphate bone scan were used to diagnose lung, liver, brain and bone metastases.

Table 2. Treatment and outcome of patients with adrenocortical carcinoma.

Patient	Status	Duration of survival	Cause of death	Surgery	Radiation	Chemotherapy
1	Dead	2 days	Adrenal failure	CR	–	–
2	Dead	19 yrs	2nd tumor – malignant neurilemmona	PR	Abdominal	–
3	Dead	11 months	Local recurrence & lung metastases	CR	–	–
4	Dead	2 months	Lung metastases & local recurrence	PR	–	–
5	Dead	7 months	Lung metastases & local recurrence	B	Abdominal	o,p′-DDD for lung metastases 3 months later
6	Dead	1 yr	Lung & spinal metastases	CR	Right flank for recurrence 3 months later	o,p′-DDD for recurrence 3 months later
7	Alive, NED	5+ yrs	–	PR	Abdominal	o,p′-DDD for 6 months
8	Alive, NED	3+ yrs	–	CR*	–	–
9	Alive, NED	1½+ yrs	–	CR	–	–
10	Alive	1¼+ yrs	–	PR	Pulmonary	o,p′-DDD for 1 yr, 5-FU for 1¼+ yrs
11	Alive, NED	8+ months	–	CR*	–	o,p′-DDD & 5-FU for 6 months
12	Alive	4+ months	–	B	Pulmonary & abdominal	o,p′-DDD & 5-FU for 4+ months

NED = no evidence of disease; CR = complete resection; PR = partial resection; B = biopsy; * = vascular invasion seen within the tumor; 5-FU = 5-Fluorouracil.

RESULTS

The treatment and outcome of the twelve patients with adrenocortical carcinoma are summarized in Table 2. Six children with adrenocortical carcinoma have died of their disease or of complications.

Of five patients with complete resection of tumor, two (Patients 8 and 9) are alive and well at 1½ and 3 years, respectively, without further treatment. One child (Patient 1) who did not receive cortisone coverage died of adrenal failure shortly after surgery. The fourth child (Patient 3) died of local recurrence and pulmonary metastases 11 months after surgery. The last child (Patient 6) had complete resection of her left adrenal tumor including a mesocolon metastasis, but developed a right flank recurrence 3 months later. She did not respond to radiation therapy or o,p′-DDD and died one year later.

In the remaining seven children, the tumors were only biopsied or partially resected. One child (Patient 4) had no further treatment and died of disease after 2 months. Another child (Patient 5) had abdominal radiation after her tumor was biopsied. She developed pulmonary metastases 3 months later, did not respond to o,p′-DDD, and died 7 months later. A third boy (Patient 2) had abdominal radiation (1750 rads in 17 fractions over 19 days) after partial resection of tumor. He was well and free of recurrences for 19 years but died of a second tumor, a malignant neurilemmona of the cauda equina. The fourth child (Patient 7) had abdominal radiation (2500 rads in 20 fractions over 4 weeks) after partial resection of tumor which had invaded the adrenal vein, hepatic vein and inferior vena cava. She received a six months course of o,p′-DDD which had to be discontinued because of ataxia. She is alive and well at 5 years. Patient 10 had multiple pulmonary metastases at diagnosis and after partial resection of her right adrenal tumor, she received bilateral pulmonary radiation (2000 rads in 20 fractions over 4 weeks), o,p′-DDD and 5-Fluorouracil. Her pulmonary metastases and hormonal findings regressed completely but recurred after 8 months. She is still alive with pulmonary and brain metastases. Of the 2 recently treated patients, one girl (Patient 11) was given a six-month prophylactic course of o,p′-DDD and 5-Fluorouracil because of evidence of vascular invasion within her tumor and she is alive and well at 8 months. The last girl (Patient 12) had an inoperable tumor and pulmonary metastases. She received pulmonary radiation 1500 rads in 15 fractions over 3 weeks and abdominal radiation 2000 rads in 20 fractions over 4 weeks and 4 months of o,p′-DDD and 5-Fluorouracil. Her disease has shown more than 50% regression as measured by computerized axial tomography.

The dosage of o,p′-DDD and 5-Fluorouracil used and the side effects encountered are summarized in Table 3. 5-Fluorouracil produced few side

Table 3. Chemotherapeutic agents used in treatment of adrenocortical carcinoma and their side effects.

Agent & route	Dosage	Side effects	Patients treated	Patients affected
5-Fluorouracil, intravenous	1 gm/m^2 every 2 wks	Neutropenia	3	1
		Gastrointestinal		0
		Alopecia		0
o,p′-DDD, oral	3–6 gm/day	Gastrointestinal	6	6
		Neurological		3
		Lethargy		4
		Hypotension		1
		Rash		2
		Gynecomastia		2
		Adrenal failure		2

effects but many patients experienced toxicity with o,p′-DDD [4]. In addition, two patients (Patient 10 and 11) developed unexplained gynecomastia and transient vaginal spotting without increase in serum estradiol. The dosage of pulmonary radiation ranged between 1500 rads in 15 fractions over 3 weeks and 2000 rads in 20 fractions over four weeks. For abdominal radiation, patients generally received between 2000 rads to 2500 rads in 20 fractions over four weeks. Patients treated with a combination of radiation and chemotherapy tolerated the treatment well.

DISCUSSION

Past experience showed that the survival of adults with adrenocortical carcinoma is extremely poor unless the tumor had been completely resected [2]. Radiation did not seem to improve their prognosis [3]. While o,p′-DDD did improve the quality and duration of survival of patients with functioning adrenal tumors, only a minority of patients showed an objective tumor response and few, if any, were cured [4, 5] Chemotherapeutic agents like methotrexate, vincristine and cyclophosphamide were relatively ineffective in treatment of adrenocortical carcinoma [7], but there is a previous report of a patient with metastatic disease cured with a combination of o,p′-DDD and 5-Fluorouracil [8].

Our experience, and that of Stewart and coworkers [1], suggested that abdominal radiation can cure some children with partially resected adrenocortical carcinoma. One boy (Patient 2) survived 19 years after abdominal radiation following partial resection of tumor but died of a second malignancy. Another girl (Patient 7) is well and disease-free 5 years after abdominal radiation and a 6-month course of o,p′-DDD following partial resection of tumor. Recently, we have adopted a combined approach of radiation therapy and chemotherapy (o,p′-DDD and 5-Fluorouracil) in treatment of patients with unresectable disease, with metastases, and with partially resected tumors. The combination did not appear to be more toxic than o,p′-DDD alone. The significance of vascular invasion seen within tumor which had been completely resected is uncertain. Patient 8 who did not receive further treatment is alive and disease-free at 3 years while Patient 11 who received a 6-months course of o,p′-DDD and 5-Fluorouracil has only been followed for 8 months.

In summary, 12 patients with adrenocortical carcinoma have been described. Six patients are alive and four have no evidence of disease. Based on our experience, we advocate the use of combination radiation therapy and chemotherapy in treatment of all patients who did not have completely resected tumors.

ACKNOWLEDGEMENT

The author is grateful to Dr. Alvin Zipursky for reviewing the manuscript.

REFERENCES

1. Stewart DR, Morris Jones PH, Jolleys A: Carcinoma of the adrenal gland in children. J Pediatr Surg 9(1):59–67, 1974.
2. MacFarlane DA: Cancer of the adrenal cortex. Ann Royal Coll Surg 23:155–186, 1958.
3. Lipsett MB, Hertz R, Ross GT: Clinical and pathophysiologic aspects of adrenocortical carcinoma. Am J Med 35:374–383, 1963.
4. Hutter AM Jr, Kayhoe DE: Adrenal cortical carcinoma: results of treatment with o,p′-DDD in 138 patients. Am J Med 41:581–592, 1966.
5. Hoffman DL, Mattox VR: Treatment of adrenocortical carcinoma with o,p′-DDD. In: The Medical Clinics of North America, Randall RV (ed), WB Saunders Company 56(4):999–1012, 1972.
6. Hutter AM Jr, Kayhoe DE: Adrenal cortical carcinoma: clinical features of 138 patients. Am J Med 41:572–580, 1966.
7. Lewinsky BS, Grigor KM, Symington T, Neville AM: The clinical and pathological features of 'non-hormonal' adrenocortical tumors. Cancer 33(3):778–790, 1974.
8. Ostuni JA, Roginsky MS: Metastatic adrenal cortical carcinoma: documented cure with combined chemotherapy. Arch Intern Med 135:1257–1258, 1975.

20. Childhood Multiple Endocrine Neoplasia (MEN) Medullary Thyroid Carcinoma, Pheochromocytoma and Adrenal Cortical Carcinoma: MCH Experience

MARION S. STERNBACH, JOHN D. MILLER and LOUISE CHEVALIER

INTRODUCTION

Multiple Endocrine Neoplasia (MEN) or Adenomatoses usually occur as familial disorders, characteristically presenting as amine or peptide producing tumors. These are pediatric neoplasias are classified in three groups. MEM Type I (or Wermer's Syndrome) is characterized by pituitary, parathyroid and pancreatic tumors. MEN Type II (IIa or Sipple's Syndrome) consists of medullary thyroid carcinoma (MTC), pheochromocytoma and parathyroid disease; while MEN III (or IIb) includes multiple mucosal neuromas (MMN) in addition to the MTC and pheochromocytoma. This paper summarizes the 30 year experience of the Montreal Children's Hospital with MEN, isolated MTC and pheochromocytoma. In this review we have included patients with adrenal cortical tumors; however, these neoplasias are not associated with the MEN Syndromes.

MATERIALS AND METHODS

Patients' charts, pathology and investigations were retrospectively reviewed and summarized.

RESULTS

Five patients with medullary thyroid carcinoma were identified and are listed with the pertinent data in Table 1. Three patients had the syndrome of multiple mucosal neuromas. All patients were female and over eight years of age at the time of diagnosis. The two patients with isolated medullary thyroid carcinomas, not associated with the MMN Syndrome, pre-

G. Bennett Humphrey et al. (eds), Adrenal and Endocrine Tumors in Children.

Table 1. Medullary thyroid carcinomas.

Patient No.	Year Dx.	Age at Dx.	Sex	Presenting thyroid findings	Tumor location: Lobes Rt.	Lt.	Metastases	Surgery	Associated neoplasia
I	1973	8 4/12	F	Firm (3×2 cm) right lobe nodule (cold on ^{131}I Scan)	+	–	to one anterior cervical node	Modified total thyroidectomy	None
II	1975	12 11/12	F	Firm (1.5×4 cm) left lobe nodule (cold on ^{131}I Scan)		+		Modified total thyroidectomy	None
III M.M.N.	1966	18	F	Firm small left lobe nodule (cold on ^{131}I Scan)	+	+		Total thyroid-ectomy	Pheochromocy-toma
IV M.M.N.	1972	13 9/12	F	Firm (1.5×1 cm) right lobe nodule	+	+	No	Total thyroid-ectomy	Left adrenal pheochromo-cytoma (1978)
V M.M.N.	1972	10 6/12	F	Firm (1×1 cm) left lobe nodule	–	+	No	Total thyroid-ectomy	None

Table Ia. Medullary thyroid carcinomas (continued).

	Laboratory follow-up					
			Catecholamines			
No.	Calcium	Phosphorus	Urinary	Plasma	Calcitonin	Outcome
I	N	N	N	-	N	Well
II	N	N	N	-	N	Well
III	N	N				Lost to follow-up
IV	N	N	↑*	↑*	↑*	Well at present
V	N	N	N	N	↑*	Well at present

* Elevated prior to the diagnosis of pheochromocytoma.
≠ Persistently elevated pentagastrin stimulated calcitonin levels.

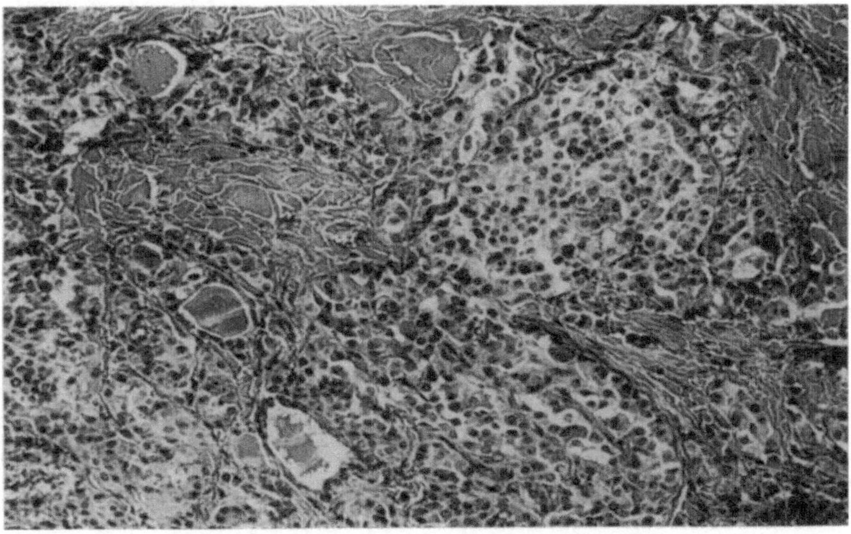

Figure 1. Medullary carcinoma of thyroid HYE, 322×.

sented with a thyroid nodule. An ^{131}I Scan in both cases showed no radioactive uptake by the nodule. Two of the patients with the MMN Syndrome had been followed in our clinic prior to the finding of the thyroid nodule, while Patient III presented with a slipped femoral epiphysis and was found at that time to have a thyroid nodule and features of MMN Syndrome. The site of the tumor was the right thyroid lobe in one case, the left in two, and bilateral in the remaining two.

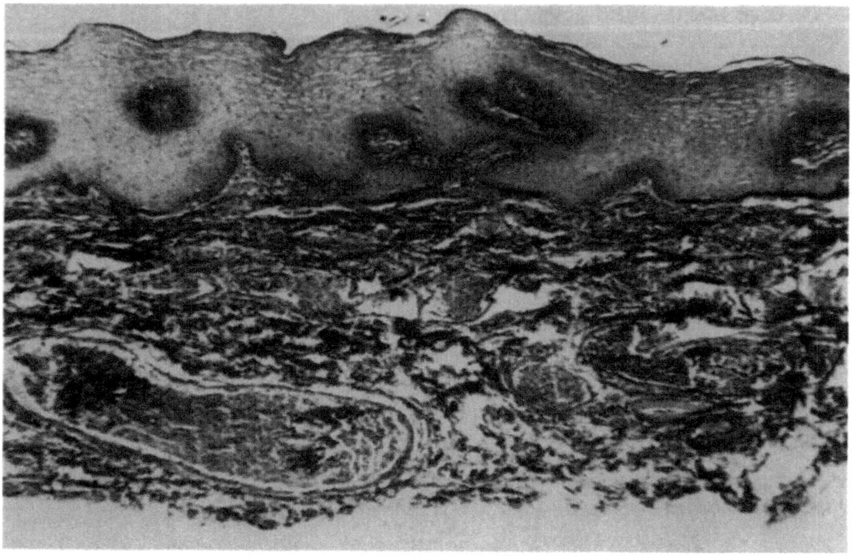

Figure 2. Oral mucosal neuroma in the multiple mucosal neuroma syndrome HYE. 195×.

Initial therapy included either a total or modified total thyroidectomy in all patients. Local metastasis to a cervical lymph node was present in Patient I only. Multifocal disease and C-cell hyperplasia were found on histological examination in patients III and IV. On surgical exploration of the abdomen there was no evidence of a controlateral adrenal tumor in the same two patients. No patients have shown laboratory or radiologic evidence of lung, liver, or bony metastases at diagnosis or in subsequent follow up. Serum calcium and phosphorus levels have been normal in all patients. Basal serum calcitonin and either calcium or pentagastrin stimulated calcitonin levels were normal in the two patients with isolated medullary carcinoma, but were elevated at the time of diagnosis in Patients IV and V with MMN Syndrome.

Patients III and IV have had pheochromocytoma. Patient IV had elevated serum calcitonin levels prior to the diagnosis of the left adrenal pheochromocytoma. Patient V presently has elevated pentagastrin stimulated calcitonin levels, but shows no metastases from the MTC or evidence of pheochromocytoma.

Careful yearly follow-up with serum calcitonin levels after pentagastrin stimulation has been attempted in all patients. Where possible, all family members have been examined and have no clinical evidence of thyroid disease, MMN Syndrome or elevated calcitonin levels. All patients had initial surgery and no further treatment. Unfortunately Patient III has been lost

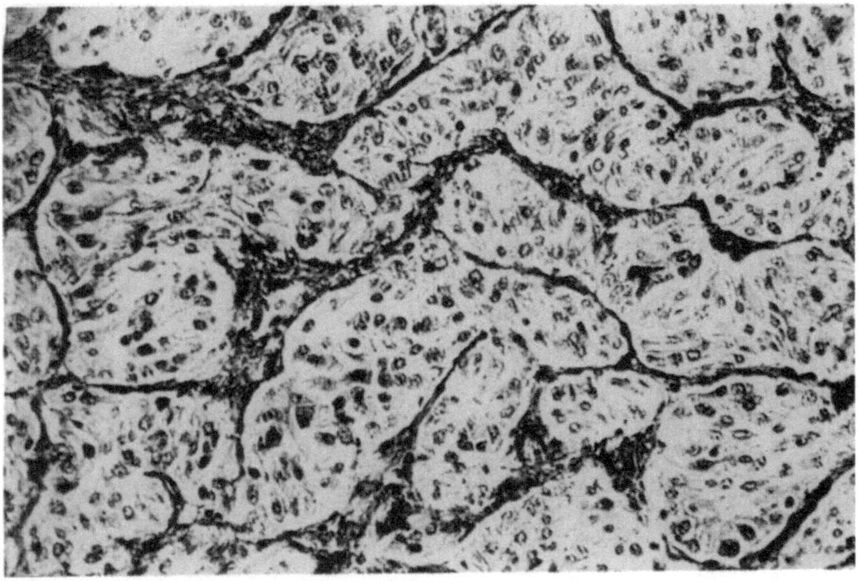

Figure 3. Pheochromocytoma of adrenal HYG 856× HYE

to follow-up; the remainder are well at least eight years following diagnosis.

Table 2 summarizes our experience with isolated adrenal medullary and cortical tumors. One patient with a right pheochromocytoma has been recently treated. He presented at age seven years with a six month history of night sweats, flushing, headaches and constipation. At the time of his initial hospital admission, the pulse rate was 140/min, the BP was 240/140 mmHg; bilateral papilledema and cotton wool exudates were present. Marked elevation of plasma and urinary catecholamines were found as noted in Table 2. An I.V.P. and abdominal computed tomography demonstrated a right supra-renal mass. His initial management included intra-venous phentolamine followed by phenoxybenzamine hydrochloride. Propranolol decreased the tachycardia and sodium nitroprusside controlled the acute paroxysms of hypertension during the ten days prior to surgery. A multi-focal right adrenal medullary pheochromocytoma (6 cms in size) was surgically removed. The left adrenal gland, explored at surgery, was found to be normal. The patient made an uneventful recovery and has been normotensive since surgery. Serum calcium and pentagastrin stimulated calcitonin levels have been normal. There is no family history of endocrine neoplasia. Investigations of the immediate family have been normal.

Three patients with adrenal cortical carcinoma have been evaluated. Patient II presented with precocious adrenarche. At diagnosis, urinary 17-ketosteroids, serum testosterone and dihydroepiandrosterone sulfate

Table 2. Adrenal tumors.

Patient No.	Year Dx.	Age at Dx.	Sex	Presenting symptoms	Tumor location			Pathology	Surgery and Rx.	Associated Neoplasia
					Rt.	Lt.	Metastases			
I	1980	7 2/12	M	Six month history of headache, flushing, constipation	+			6 cm multifocal pheochromocytoma	Rt. Adrenalectomy Exploration of lt. gland	-
II	1976	1 6/12	F	Two month history of clitoral enlargement and pubic hair		+		Well encapsulated adrenal cortical carcinoma (ultra structurally of zona reticularis origin)	Lt. adrenalectomy	-
III	1976	1 8/12	M	Beckwith's Syndrome diagnosed at age 2 months. IVP revealed supra renal mass (left)		+		Adrenal cortical carcinoma with vascular infiltration	Lt. adrenalectomy with radiotherapy	-
IV	1970	5 6/12	F	Left breast enlargement, hepatomegaly and large adrenal mass	+		To liver, lungs and bone	Adrenal cortical carcinoma	Tumor biopsy, radiotherapy, cyclophosphamide and 5 FU	

Table 2b. Adrenal tumors (continued)

	Laboratory findings at diagnosis										
	Catecholamines*				Steroids**						
	Plasma NEP	EP	D	Urine VMA	1. AM Cortisol	2. DHEAS	3. Test	4. 17 Keto	5. Preg	6. 17 OHS	Outcome and other
I	35.5	0.97	0.28	10.2	9.	–	–	2.64	–		Alive and well. Serum Ca and pentagastrin stimulated calcitonin levels are normal
II	–	–	–		28.0	250	425	11.7	0.15		Bone age 2½–3 years at diagnosis. Alive and well
III	–	–	–	2.6	14.	–	–	0.4	–		Bone age 20 months at diagnosis. Alive and well
IV	–	–	–	2.9	25.	–	–	0.6	0.15	1.4	Died within 5 months of diagnosis

* NEP = Norepinephrine (N = 0.1–0.25 ng/ml)
EP = Epinephrine (N = 0.05–0.15 ng/ml)
D = Dopamine (N = 0–0.05 ng/ml)
VMA = Vanillylmandelic acid (N = 0.1–4.8 mg/24 h)

** 1. Cortisol (N = 10 ± 2 μgm/dl)
2. DHEAS – Dihydroepiandrosterone Sulfate (N<50 μg/dl)
3. Test – Testosterone (N<100 ng/dl)
4. 17 Keto – 17 Ketosteroids (N 0–4 mg/24 h)
5. Preg – Pregnanetriol (N 0–1 mg/24 h)
6. 17 OHS – 17 Hydroxysteroids (0–3 mg/24 h)

(D.H.E.A.S.) were elevated. The initial I.V.P. and ultrasound suggested a left adrenal mass which was confirmed during surgical excision. Patient III was known to have Beckwith's Syndrome and the calcified adrenal mass was noted on I.V.P. No tumor hormonal production was demonstrated. Because of the vascular invasion by the tumor, the child was treated with local radiotherapy (2500 R) after surgery. Both patients have done well. Patient V presented with left breast enlargement, abdominal distension and hepatomegaly. Since extensive metastases were present at diagnosis, only palliative treatment was considered, and the child expired within five months of diagnosis. Although the presentation of premature thelarche suggested excess estrogen, incubated tumor tissue did not produce estrone, estradiol or estriol. These findings, however, do not preclude previous tumor estrogen production nor synthesis of steroids that were undetectable by conventional assays at the time of the child's diagnosis.

DISCUSSION

Multiple endocrine neoplasias are rare tumors and we have treated only children with documented MEN III (IIb).

The three major components of this syndrome are neuromas, medullary

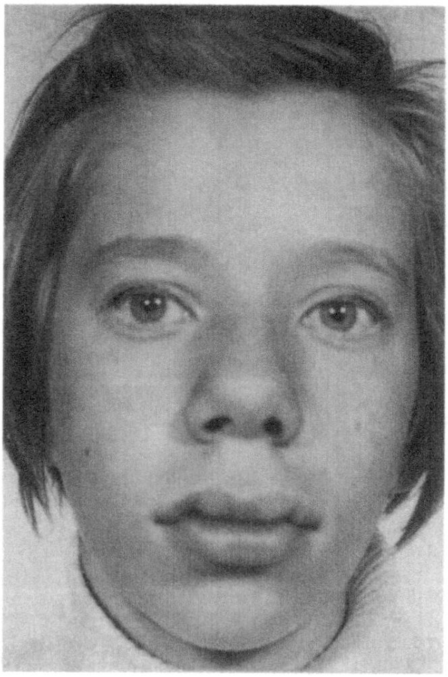

Figure 4.

thyroid carcinoma and pheochromocytoma. These patients often have a distinctive physical appearance consisting of mucosal neuromas, thick lips, soft tissue prognathism, everted eyelids, and slender build with poor development of body musculature (see Figure 4). Inheritance may be on an autosomal dominant basis; however many patients including the three described here appear to be from sporadic mutations [1, 5]. Because of the high predisposition to medullary thyroid carcinoma, patients with the MMN Syndrome must be followed closely post diagnosis. Our patients appear to have had a more indolent course than the evolutions described with MMN in the literature [1, 5].

MTC derives from the parafollicular C cells of the thyroid gland, which normally produce calcitonin. These cells are TSH independent and do not incorporate radioiodine. With the help of immuno-histochemical methods (immuno-peroxidase and specific antisera against calcitonin) it has become possible to detect very early precarcinomatous proliferation of these C cells as nodular aggregates within the thyroid follicles. Patients with MTC may have watery diarrhea and flushing secondary to carcinoma production of serotonin, prostaglandins and the enzymes, histaminase and aromatic L-amino acid decarboxylase. As found in our cases, medullary thyroid carcinoma is most often bilateral and multicentric. Total thyroidectomy is therefore indicated followed by full thyroxine replacement. Serum calcitonin concentrations and screening tests for pheochromocytoma and parathyroid disease are indicated in following patients with MTC or MMN.

Two of our three patients with pheochromocytoma have the MMN Syndrome. The third child and his family show no evidence of MEN. Pheochromocytomas are rare tumors in adults and even rarer in childhood. They originate most frequently from the adrenal medulla (the right more often than the left), but may arise anywhere in the chromafin system, along the sympathetic chain from the neck to the abdomen and pelvis [1, 4]. Pheochromocytoma may be multiple or bilateral in MEN Type II or III. Malignant pheochromocytoma is found in 8–10% of adults [1], but is rare in children. There is a 3:2 male to female preponderance. The clinical manifestations are so varied. that diagnosis may be difficult and delayed. Symptoms are triggered by the release of epinephrine and norepinephrine by the tumor. Classically, headaches, paroxysms of hypertension, produse sweating, palpitations, pallor, weakness and blurred vision occur during intermittent attacks. Nausea, vomiting, abdominal pain, poor weight gain and failure to thrive may be additonal features. The diagnosis is confirmed after clinical suspicion, by the presence of elevated catecholamines-vanillylmandelic acid (VMA), norepinephrine, epinephrine, normetanephrine or metanephrine in the urine and epinephrine, norepinephrine and dopamine in the plasma. In addition to intravenous pyelography, the CT Scan is a useful non-invasive method in localizing pheochromocytoma. It has identified correctly the same tumors visualized by selective arteriography [3, 4].

The primary therapy is surgical excision with adequate preparation to prevent bouts of hypertension [1, 4]. A long-acting alpha adrenergic blocking agent, phenoxybenzamine (Dibenziline), is given orally every 12 hours. Phentolamine (Regitine), a short-acting alpha blocker, may be used intravenously. Sodium nitroprusside, a powerful vasodilator, with a rapid onset but short duration of action, is effective in controlling acute paroxysms of hypertension. Occasionally Propranolol may be required for blocking beta receptor stimulation.

Adrenal cortical tumors are not found in the MEN Syndromes. These neoplasms often produce excess or abnormal steroids, not peptides or amines. Adrenal tumors, either adenomas or carcinomas, are more common in younger children. Virilizing tumors present with clitoral enlargement in girls, penile enlargement in boys with persistence of immature testes, pubic and axillary hair, and accelerated linear growth.

Adrenal tumors may be the etiology of Cushing's Syndrome, with its clinical manifestations of obesity, growth retardation, and hypertension. Feminizing adrenal tumors are very rare; they cause isosexual precocity in girls and usually gynecomastia in boys. Beckwith-Wiedemann Syndrome, (Patient III, Table 2), hemihypertrophy, urinary tract anomalies, brain tumors, and cutaneous lesions have been associated with adrenocortical carcinoma [6].

Laboratory findings in a virilizing tumor, as in Patient II, would include elevated urinary 17-ketosteroids, plasma D.H.E.A.S. and testosterone. One would expect raised plasma estrogens in a feminizing tumor. I.V.P., ultrasound, abdominal computed tomography, and photoscanning with ^{131}I-19-iodocholesterol may be helpful in localizing the tumor. Therapy is surgical with pre- and post-operative glucocorticoid therapy. In most instances the contralateral gland is atrophic as a result of suppression by high circulating levels of steroids produced by the tumor. Adrenal carcinoma usually does not metastasize early, but if mestastases do occur, the lungs, liver and regional nodes are the usual affected organs.

Our experience with several rare childhood endocrine tumors has been described. Diagnosis is dependent on clinical features, radiological investigation, and plasma and urinary hormonal evaluation. For the majority of these tumors, surgery and careful follow-up would be the recommended disposition.

ACKNOWLEDGEMENTS

The authors thank Dr. H. Guyda, Director of Endocrinology and Dr. R. Bolande, Department of Pathology, at the Montreal Children's Hospital. The secretarial assistance of Miss Karen Berg was greatly appreciated.

REFERENCES

1. Voorhess ML: Disorders of the Adrenal Medulla and Multiple Endocrine Adenomatoses. Pediatr Clin North Am 26 (1):209–222, 1979.
2. Alberts WM, McMeekin JO, George JM: Mixed Multiple Neoplasia Syndromes. JAMA 244 (11):1236–1237, 1980.
3. Ganguly A, Henry DP, Yune HY, Pratt JH, Grim CE, Donohue JP, Weinberger MH: Diagnosis and localization of pheochromocytoma. Detection by measurement of urinary norepinephrine excretion during sleep, plasma norepinephrine concentration and computerized axial tomography (CT Scan). Am J Med 67:21–26, 1979.
4. Stringel G, Ein SH, Creighton R, Daneman D, Howard N, Filler RM: Pheochromocytoma in Children – An Update. J Ped Surg 15 (4):496–500, 1980.
5. Brown RS, Colle E, Tashjian AH: The syndrome of multiple mucosal neuromas and medullary thyroid carcinoma in childhood. J Pediatr 86:77–83, 1975.
6. Fraumeni JF, Miller RW: Adrenocortical neoplasm with hemihypertrophy, brain tumor and other disorders. J Pediatr 70:129–138, 1967.

21. Multiple Endocrine Neoplasia Type 2b: Experience at Villejuif Mucosal ganglioneuromatosis medullary thyroid carcinoma and pheochromocytoma

PH. ROUGIER, B. CAILLOU, C. PARMENTIER and J. LEMERLE

Multiple endocrine neoplasia, type 2b (MEN 2b) is a disorder characterized by medullary thyroid carcinoma (MTC), pheochromocytoma, ganglioneuromatosis, dysmorphy with connective tissue and skeletal abnormalities. Since 1967 five European patients with MEN 2b have been treated at Institut Gustave-Roussy and their principal characteristics are summarized in Table 1.

PATIENTS

Patient No. 1 had severe gastro-intestinal symptoms with many fecal impactions as early as six years of age. There were seven surgical procedures which finally resulted in a total colectomy at 13 years of age and the establishment of an ileostomy. Histologically diffuse ganglioneuromatosis of the submucosa and myenteric plexus of the large colon was present. Thyroid disease was suspected at 13 years of age because of dysphonia. A partial thyroidectomy and modified cervical node dissection were performed. The MTC was only partially resected due to extensive local infiltration. This young girl died suddenly two weeks after surgery during an episode of extensive vomiting. The etiology of the vomiting may have related to the intestinal ganglioneuromatosis.

Patient No. 2 was a 15-year-old girl who presented with cervical lymphadenopathy. At the first evaluation we found pulmonary and bone metastases. She had been dysmorphic since birth, which included well-known characteristics of MEN 2b: hypertrophied lips, tongue neuromas and Marfan's habitus. The first thyroid related anomaly noted at 12 years of age was cervical enlargement.

Patient No. 3 was symptomatic early in life. There were multiple episodes of constipation and fecal impactions. Two surgical procedures were neces-

G. Bennett Humphrey et al. (eds), Adrenal and Endocrine Tumors in Children.

CHARACTERISTICS	CASE 1*	2*	3**	4	5
SEX	F	F	F	M	F
MTC					
-age at diagnosis	13	15	2.5	6	12
-thyroid extension	unilateral	unilateral	bilateral	bilateral	bilateral
-cervical nodes	unilateral	unilateral	bilateral	bilateral	bilateral
-invasion of neck structures	extensive	yes	no	no	no
-distant metastasis	0	lung-bones	0	0	0
-treatment	PT + MCND	biopsy	TT + MCND + RT	TT + MCND	TT + MCND
-CT post treatment	-	380	3 65	36	2 4
-CEA post treatment	-	-	7	39	45
-Survival (year)	0 (DCD)	0.5 (DCD)	3.5	2	2
Pheochromocytoma	ND	?	0	0	?
-HVA (μmol 24h) N 44		45	3	6.4 μmol ml	30
-VMA (μmol 24h) N 25		120	3 3	5.2 μmol ml	24
-Ad / -N Ad } N 8 nmol 1		-	-	} 35	} 2.4
Dysmorphy	yes	yes	yes	yes	yes
-hypertrophied lips	+	+	+	+	+
-eversion of upper eyelids	-	-	-	-	+
Mucosal neuromas (age:year)	no	yes 15	no	yes 2.5	yes 4
-lips	-	-	-	-	+
-tongue	-	+	-	+	+
-angle of mouth	-	-	-	-	+
-buccal mucosa-jaw	-	-	-	-	+
Musculo-skeletal abnormalities					
-marfanoid habitus	-	+	0	+	0
-poor muscle bulk	+	+	0	+	0
-hyperlaxity	ND	ND	-	+	+
-dental caries	ND	ND	-	+	+
-osseous abnormality		pes cavus	pes cavus		kyphosis
Gastro-intestinal symptoms	extensive	yes	extensive	yes	yes
age at onset	at birth	15	1	0.5	1
-constipation	+	-	+	+	+
-fecal impaction	+	-	+	-	-
-neurogangliomatosis	+	-	+	?	?
-diarrhea	-	+	+	-	-
-bladder dysfunction	-	-	-	yes, at 2.5 yr	-
Familial disease	ND	-	-	-	-
age at examination at IGR (year)	15	13	2	6	15
Weight in kg	33	36	11.6	-2 SD	43
Size in cm	158	159	80	N	156

Principal characteristics of five cases: Medullary thyroid carcinoma : MEN II B

Abbreviation:

MTC medullary thyroid carcinoma PT partial thyroidectomy. TT Total thyroidectomy.

MCND modified cervical neck dissection. RT cervical radiotherapy. CT calcitonin (normal range · 0 25 ng/ml).

CEA carcinoembryonic antigen (normal range · 5ng/ml). HVA homo vanilic acid in urine (normal range · 44 μmole.).

VMA vanil mandelique acid in urine (normal range · 25 μmolg/24h). AD + NAD epinephrine + norephinephrine (normal 8 nmole ml)

ND not detected *already published LEVY et col 1970. **partly published NAVARRO and col 1979

TABLE I

sary and ended in a colostomy at two years of age. Histologically, the ganglioneuromatosis was continuous from the jejunum to the rectum with maximal involvement in the colon. This girl received two years of continuous parenteral nutrition, which resulted in an excellent nutritional status when she came to thyroid surgery. The only dysmorphic feature at that time was hypertrophy of the lips. Serial serum calcitonins (CT) were elevated at four years of age. At that time the thyroid gland was normal to palpation. She underwent a total thyroidectomy. The thyroid was bilaterally involved with multifocal lesions associated with a diffuse hyperplasia of C cells. One unilateral lymph node was involved as well. CT levels did not return to normal after surgery and cervical radiotherapy. Therapy was poorly tolerated due to cervical edema. Three years after this aggressive treatment regimen, she is well without evidence of residual disease in spite of high CT levels, but quite normal carcinoembryonic antigen (CEA) level. This patient is being followed annually and being evaluated for pheochromocytoma.

Patient No. 4 was a few months old when urinary tract difficulties and constipation were noted. At four years a rectal biopsy demonstrated ganglioneuromatosis. At the same time he required urinary catheterization for urine retention. At that time the dysmorphic features were very prominent with hypertrophy of the lips, tongue neuromas, gingival hypertrophy, extensive dental caries, and severe amyotrophia. At six years of age, a thyroid nodule and cervical adenopathy were discovered. Total thyroidectomy and bilateral lymph node dissection were not curative since this patient has high CT and CEA levels. Small cervical lymph nodes were palpable and presumably contained metastatic tumor. Three points seem very important in his case:

(a) Cachexia with a -2 standard deviation in weight, amyotrophia and weakness.

(b) Urinary troubles which require continuous urinary catheterization with infectious complications. Surgical exploration demonstrated a significant thickening of the bladder wall and histology revealed bladder ganglioneuromatosis with foci of microscopic tumor. Venous sampling during selective catheterization demonstrated an elevated CT gradient at the level of the bladder. It is possible that CT is secreted partially by the bladder neuromatosis. This bladder complication is very rarely noted in MEN, type 2b. Pharmacological agents (atropine and sympathomimetics) have been ineffective.

(c) After total thyroidectomy, an episode of laryngeal dyspnea occurred which required intubation and assisted ventilation for two days. The only gross abnormality was laryngeal edema, but the possibility of laryngeal ganglioneuromatosis is raised.

Patient No. 5 had a club foot and congenital dislocation of the hip which were present at birth. At four years of age, small nodules on the gingivae and tongue were noted. They became bigger and multiple on the lips, tongue, jaw and oral mucosa. An ogival palate was noted and hypertrophied lips and eversion of the upper eyelids developed completing the typical clinical aspects of MEN 2b. At ten years of age, a biopsy of a submucosal oral nodule confirmed the diagnosis of mucosal neuromas, and a complete investigation discovered thyroid nodules with high CT levels suggesting a medullary thyroid carcinoma (MTC). At 12 years of age, CT levels were elevated at which time thyroid nodules were palpable. A total thyroidectomy was performed. After surgery the CT levels remained elevated. No metastasis could be demonstrated, but selective venous sampling during catheterization demonstrated bilateral cervical gradients. At 13 years of age, reexploration with a modified radical neck dissection resected metastases to the lymph nodes bilaterally. This procedure was also complicated by laryngeal dyspnea. At present she is in a very good clinical state, with normal mental development. Two questions remain:

(a) Her catecholamines are at the upper levels of normal, suggesting a developing pheochromocytoma.

(b) She continues to have clinically significant constipation. Barium enema and rectal biopsy are normal, but we suspect intestinal neuromatosis.

DISCUSSION AND IMPLICATIONS

(1) Apparently we have observed five cases of sporadic MEN 2b, but in three of these cases, familial investigations were incomplete. The investigation of CT after stimulation with pentagastrin for close relatives is mandatory because approximately 50% of MEN 2b are familial.

(2) The aggressive nature of MTC in MEN 2b is evident in our cases as it is in the literature. Our first two cases had extensive involvement and died rapidly. Even early diagnosis as in case No. 3 with agressive treatment resulted in persistent elevations of CT and presumed small foci of neoplastic tissue. The MTC in MEN 2b has a poorer prognosis than in sporadic forms and other familial forms without polyadenomatosis.

(3) The MTC can be bilateral and multifocal. In our three cases, lymph nodes were involved so we feel that a total thyroidectomy plus bilateral sub clavicular lymph node biopsies are justified. If the lymph nodes are involved, then modified radical neck dissection is indicated. The possibility of post operative laryngeal dyspnea must be appreciated and prevented. Preoperative laryngeal examination is important. Cervical radiotherapy should be considered when surgical treatment is unsatisfactory as was done in our third case.

(4) We have not observed pheochromocytomas in these five cases, but we have two patients with catecholamines at the upper limits of normal. In both cases radiological evaluation is normal. If catecholamines become elevated, exploratory laparatomy will be done. In MEN 2b, pheochromocytomas are aggressive but seldom malignant. They can occur bilaterally, generally five to ten years after the occurrence of MTC. It is therefore important to evaluate catecholamines annually. In our experience, measurement of metanephrine and normetanephrine are the best tumor markers.

(5) Neuromatosis was clinically significant in three of our cases. In two (No. 1 and No. 3), intestinal involvement led to colostomy in one case and total colectomy in another after multiple surgical interventions. In the third case (No. 4), the major problem was urinary tract involvement with neuro-

matosis which has been very difficult to manage. In patients 4 and 5, the intestinal manifestations are moderate, but is is known that these lesions can be progressive, and therefore intestinal function will be followed throughout their life.

(6) Dysmorphy is characteristic. In one case (No. 3) with hypertrophy of the lips, screening for MTC was emphasized and treatment started before clinical evidence of thyroid disease.

Two additional signs seem important to us: (a) the importance of dental caries in two cases; (b) the importance of amyotrophia which explains the weakness and the diagnostic difficulties. Hypertrophy of lips and submucosal oral neuromas are evocative of MEN 2b, thus requiring annual evaluation of CT. Total thyroidectomy is indicated in all cases with abnormal CT values. In the same manner, when urinary catecholamines are elevated, a laparotomy and surgical excision of pheochromocytomas is indicated. Digestive neuromatosis should be evaluated in all patients with the above mentioned dysmorphic syndromes.

REFERENCES

Levy M, Habib R, Lyon G, Schweissguth O, Lemerle J, Royer P: Neuromatose et épithélioma à stroma angloide de la thyroide chez l'enfant. Arch Fr Ped 27:561–583, 1970.

Navarro F, Weisgerber G, Sonsino E, Rivron M, Pons G, Polonouski C: Nueroapudomatose de type Steiner révélée par une pseudo maladie de Hirshprung. Nouv Presse Med 8:1413–1415, 1979.

22. Overview on the Management of Adrenocortical Carcinoma (ACC)

G. BENNETT HUMPHREY, THEODORE PYSHER, JOHN HOLCOMBE, MILTON GROSS, HELEN CHAN, BARBARA CUSHING, GIULIO J. D'ANGIO, PHILIP SCHEIN, JEAN LEMERLE, J.A. CARNEY and BEVERLY RANEY, Jr.

INTRODUCTION

The case material included in this volume includes 72 carcinomas, 30 adenomas and 12 cases diagnosed as 'tumor'; this includes 22 cases analyzed in depth by Weatherby and Carney in their review of pathology [1]. The largest collection of cases and the most detailed clinical analysis is from France. LeFevre and co-workers were able to review 42 children treated between 1958 and 1980 [2].

This is not the largest collection of adrenocortical carcinoma (ACC). Hutter and Kayhoe have reported an analysis of 138 adults and children, and Hayles and co-workers reported 12 of their own pediatric cases and analyzed data on 222 children taken from the literature [3, 4]. This overview will emphasize unique observations based on this collection of cases and discuss current difficulties in management. Whenever possible, recommendations for management of future patients will be made.

CLINICAL PRESENTATION

The predominant clinical syndromes at the time of diagnosis are nicely tabulated by Weatherby and Carney and LeFevre and co-authors [1, 2]. A mixture of syndromes is the most common presentation, but Cushing's disease and virilization are also common; feminization and aldosteronism are rare. For adenomas, the male to female ratio is 1:10, and the age distribution is relatively even (Figure 1). For carcinoma, the overall male to female ratio is 1:1.7 for the 72 cases taken as a whole (Figure 2). However, the age distribution is not equal and two groups are suggested: an infantile group with a peak incidence in the first year of life with a decreasing incidence to age 7 (61 cases), and an adolescent group in which age is evenly distributed

G. Bennett Humphrey et al. (eds), Adrenal and Endocrine Tumors in Children.

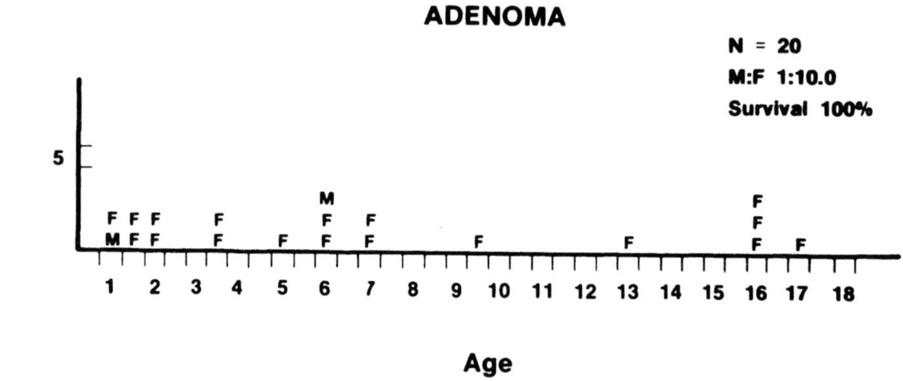

Figure 1. Age and sex distribution of 20 cases of adrenal cortical adenoma. F = female, M = male.

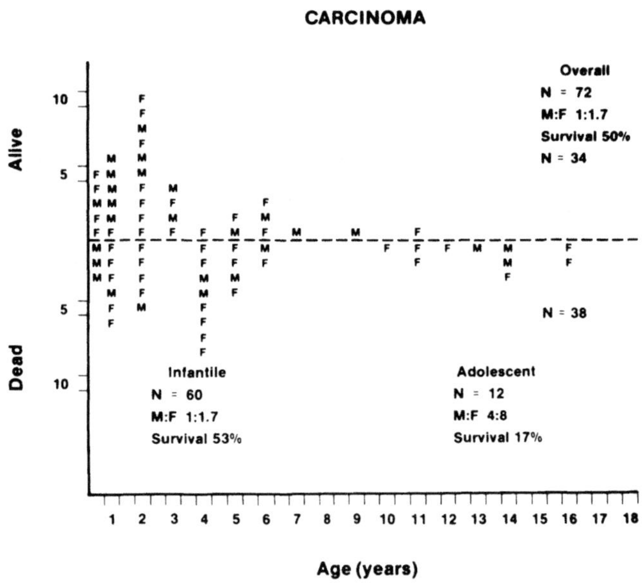

Figure 2. Age and sex distribution of 72 cases of ACC. F = female, M = male. Cases above dashed line (Alive) were reported as longer term survivors or in rare cases die of an unrelated cause. Cases below line were dead or in a few cases were alive with active disease and presumably have died since the report was submitted.

between the ages of 9 and 16 years (11 cases). For the infantile group, the male to female ratio is 1:1.7. There are four males and seven females in the adolescent group presented.

The endocrine side effects of ACC are similar to what is already reported in the literature. The suggestion that ACC is not one disease, but rather two diseases with different age distributions, has not previously been emphasized but has been noted in other series [5–7]. For example, Hough and co-workers alluded to this in their analysis of 138 cases which were tabulated by decade [5]. They noted two peaks; one in childhood and the second during middle age. The data in this volume suggests that cases of childhood ACC in patients seven years of age and younger belong in an infantile group. The adolescent group is presumed to be one extreme of ACC of the adulthood type with its peak incidence in the fourth decade. For infantile ACC, one wonders if an oncogenic agent plays a role in the etiology of this tumor. The suggestion of an infantile and adult form of ACC has interesting implications, as will be discussed under pathology and prognosis.

PREOPERATIVE AND OPERATIVE MANAGEMENT

The preoperative evaluation and diagnostic procedures available to the clinician in evaluating a child with possible ACC are well outlined by Gross and co-authors [8]. Surgical management is reviewed by Tunnell [9]. LeFevre and co-authors relate some interesting experience with preoperative and postoperative op′DDD and radiotherapy [2]. In four cases, op′DDD was used after incomplete resection and resulted in one subsequent complete resection and long-term survival. In one out of 11 cases, radiotherapy resulted in tumor reduction and subsequent complete resection of a previously unresectable tumor. That case is also a long-term survivor.

The multiplicity of tests of localization for adrenal tumors has rendered the evaluation of these patients somewhat easier. Unfortunately, there is insufficient data to allow a comprehensive comparison of the sensitivities and specificities of these studies; but a few guidelines do emerge in the localization of adrenal lesions. As radiation exposure is an important consideration, the evaluation of diseases in childhood ultrasound and/or the newer generation CT scanners would be reasonable alternatives for localization once an adequate biochemical diagnosis has been established. Certainly CT has demonstrated efficacy in the localization of all types of adrenal tumors, and if one test were available CT would probably represent the best first alternative for localization studies. If radiation exposure or availability of CT were a problem then ultrasound would be an alternative choice for tumor localization. It must, however, be remembered that the spatial resolution achieved by CT is greater than that achieved by ultrasound.

Adrenal scintigraphy remains an investigational procedure and although it can provide information concerning both function and anatomy of adrenal lesions, its lack of availability and stringent criteria for performance make it less important a modality of localization than either CT or ultrasound.

In those instances where detailed anatomic or vascular evaluation must be made, angiography is the only modality that provides the necessary spatial resolution for this form of localization analysis.

An evaluation of an adrenal tumor must be individualized. It is important for the clinician to realize that individual medical centers differ in their ability to perform these studies. Moreover, each clinician must be familiar with the limitations/contraindications of these modalities and the individual institutional experience be considered when selecting a particular diagnostic/localization scheme.

The experience with preoperative op′DDD or postoperative op′DDD in unresectable cases is limited and therefore no conclusions can be drawn. However, in inoperable cases, a trial of op′DDD might be of value followed by a second surgical attempt at complete excision. LeFevre and co-workers also have a unique experience in an inoperable case that responded to radiotherapy with subsequent resection [2]. This too might be considered in an inoperable case which does not respond to op′DDD, even though radiotherapy is considered to be of little value in ACC.

PATHOLOGY

A variety of different pathological criteria are reported in this volume. In some institutions, the general principles of pathology (invasion of blood vessels, metastatic rate, etc.) are applied and all cases are classified as either adenoma or carcinoma. In other institutions, this same application results in a third indeterminate category which is called 'tumor'. Some institutions are using the criteria developed by Hough and co-workers [5] which is based on both parametric and nonparametric statistical analysis of histological and nonhistological features. These criteria were developed from a retrospective study, and all survivors had been under observation for five years or longer. In this study, there were five malignant tumors and one benign tumor in children 10 years of age and younger, and one benign tumor and two malignant tumors in children in the second decade of life. The remaining 32 cases were adults. Eleven characteristics were evaluated. The most significant were weight loss, broad fibrous bands traversing the tumor, and a diffuse growth pattern. Weatherby and Carney's classification in this volume was an invited review to establish criteria for childhood ACC and is drawn from an evaluation of three adolescents and six infantile cases [1]. Finally, the French investigators have drawn attention to tumor weight as an important criteria for the determination of outcome [2].

The designation of an indeterminant category of 'tumor' may be justified at present and will be used in the future at two institutions. One institution stated that the criteria of Hough and co-workers will be used in the future. None of the institutions other than the Mayo Clinic had access to Weatherby and Carney's criteria and, thus, none of the respondants to our questionnaire on the future management of ACC commented that they would be using these criteria in the future. The criteria of Weatherby and Carney are weighted towards the infantile group. It would be of interest to compare the pathology of infantile cases to adolescent cases as a separate study. If these are different tumor groups, then there may also be a difference in their pathology. For example, Hough and co-workers, in their analysis of a largely adult population, emphasized the prognostic significance of fibrous bands traversing the tumors. Weatherby and Carney, in their criteria, do not emphasize this histological feature. Thus, one might expect fibrous bands to be a pathological feature of adolescent cases and not infantile cases.

PROGNOSIS

The overall survival for ACC in childhood is 50%, based on the 72 cases collected in this volume. The prognostic significance of tumor weight is discussed by LeFevre and co-authors who also place prognostic significance on the ease or difficulty of surgery (ease = good prognosis, difficulty = poor prognosis) [2]. Holcombe and co-workers review the prognostic significance of Hayes and co-workers' original discussion of the ratio of tumor weight to body weight [10].

When the data are analysed in terms of an infantile and an adolescent group, the survival rates are 53% and 17% respectively. This supports the concept that ACC in childhood is made up of two different malignancies. Complete data (age, survival and tumor weight) were obtained on 51 cases of ACC (Figure 3). Many of the reports in this volume do not contain tumor weight, but this was obtained by telephone requests. In the infantile group of 40 cases, the overall survival was 55% (22/40). However, survival for those 18 cases whose tumors weighed less than 170 grams was 74%, and those tumors weighing greater than 170 grams was only 36%, suggesting that in the infantile group tumor weight has prognostic significance. There are not enough cases in the adolescent group to allow comment. There are too many exceptions in all groups to allow tumor weight to be used as a single pathological criterion of malignancy. The figure of 170 grams is arbitrary, and either 150 or 200 could have been used.

Using a tumor weight-body weight ratio, Hayles and co-workers reported fewer metastases in children whose ratio was less than 0.7 grams of tumor per 100 grams of body weight [4]. We have attempted to evaluate the data presented in Figure 3 in this manner. The child's actual weight was not

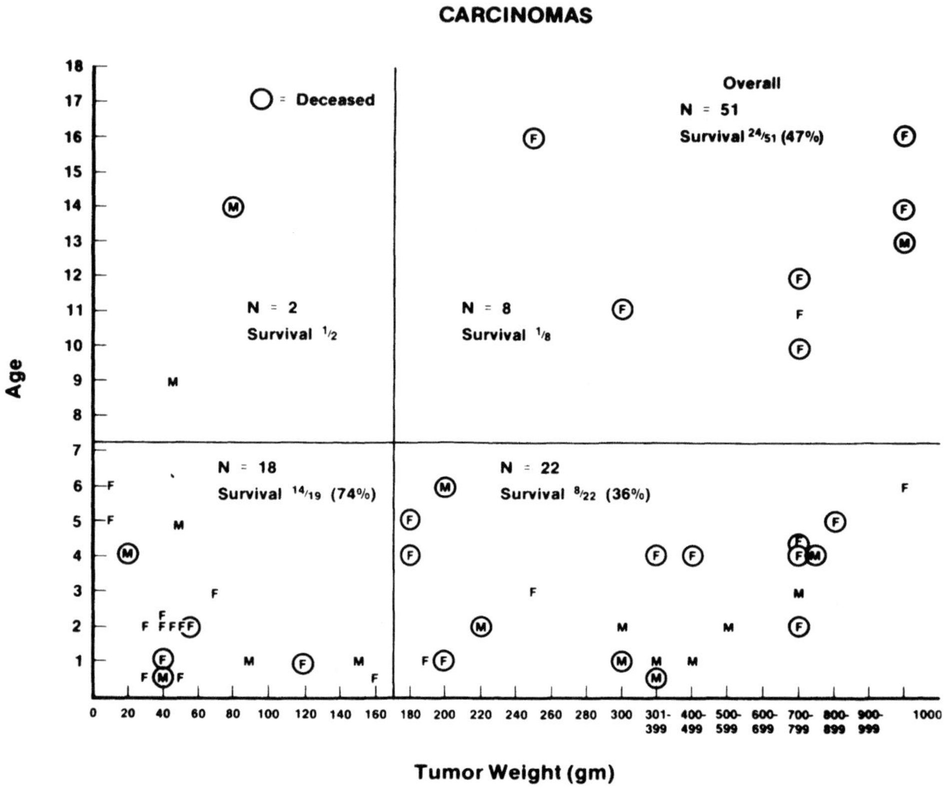

Figure 3. Scattergram of age and tumor weight. F = female, M = male. Circled O cases are diseased.

used, but the 50th percentile for each age was obtained from standard growth charts. A similar scattergram was constructed for tumor weight–body weight ratio. When 150 grams gross tumor weight and a tumor–body weight ratio of 0.7 were used to divide the case material into good and bad prognostic groups, the distribution of the case material in the two groups was identical. Thus, we do not feel that determining tumor–body weight ratios increases the predictability of metastases or a fatal outcome.

The ease or difficulty of surgery is a very subjective measure, however, we hope that criteria can be established that can quantitate this and that information will be recorded for future analysis.

NON-FUNCTIONING TUMORS

There are six patients who presented with non-functioning tumors or with only an abdominal mass. The tumor weight is known in five of these cases.

They are generally large: 80, 158, 300, 470 and 712 grams. Two of the three adolescents are dead. The three younger children were all one year of age or less; one of these three is dead.

A review of 41 adults and 1 child with non-functioning ACC demonstrated a shorter median survival for functioning tumors than non-functioning tumors [11]. Our case material is unfortunately small and does not allow any conclusions to be drawn. One might expect that a non-functioning tumor could achieve a greater tumor mass before becoming clinically apparent and therefore might have a greater chance of metastasizing.

METASTASIS

The natural history and metastatic nature of ACC is well tabulated by LeFevre and co-workers [2]. Most of the recurrences or metastases will occur within two years, however, late metastases or recurrence at nine years have been reported.

In the future, any retrospective pathological study which includes survivors should be drawn from case material that has been under observation for a minimum of five years and preferably ten years.

SECOND MALIGNANCIES AND ASSOCIATED PROBLEMS

In one case reported from Philadelphia, a two-year-old white female developed a thalamic astrocytoma after the diagnosis of ACC [12]. ACC is also reported in one child with Beckwith syndrome [12].

The thalamic astrocytoma is probably not a random event. In an analysis of 62 children with ACC, Fraumeni and Miller found two who developed astrocytomas (an 8-year-old male and a 4-year-old male) [13]. Other anomalies such as Beckwith-Wiedemann syndrome, hemihypertrophy, etc. also were found. Second malignancies appear to be less common in children than in adults. In a review of 41 adults, a second primary cancer was noted in 22.4% of cases [11].

TREATMENT

The vast majority of cases reported in this volume underwent complete surgical excision of the tumor. Radiation therapy was used in a minor portion of patients. The preoperative use of op′DDD or radiotherapy or their use in unresectable tumors by LeFevre and co-workers has already been mentioned [2]. These same investigators report the use of op′DDD in 7 cases for the treatment of recurrent or metastatic disease resulting in two long-term survivors. For those patients not responding to op′DDD, there is no consistent use nor success with standard anti-cancer chemotherapeutic agents.

Surgical excision is obviously the treatment of choice. Our radiation therapy consultant (D'Angio) feels that radiation therapy is not routinely indicated in childhood ACC because of proximity to vital structures and the fact that a dose of known therapeutic effectiveness remains to be established. Adjuvant chemotherapy cannot be recommended in any case. For recurrent or metastatic disease, most of the respondents were not very enthusiastic about using op'DDD in ACC. However, until a standard chemotherapeutic agent achieves equal success, a trial of op'DDD is probably warranted in cases of local recurrence or metastases. LeFevre and co-workers reported a rather unique experience using op'DDD in childhood ACC [2]. Hogan and co-workers report one complete response and cite four additional cures from the literature [14]. One of our respondents favored the use of op'DDD plus 5-Fluorouracil at 1 g/m^2 every two weeks as the treatment of choice for metastatic disease. This is based on a cure of a 17-year-old female who received this combination in 1966. The same patient died of a narcotic overdose, and her autopsy (in 1975) demonstrated no residual tumor [15]. Our consultant (P. Schein) feels that 5-Fu has not been demonstrated to have any activity as a single agent and therefore sees no reason to combine it with op'DDD.

There does not seem to be any effective cancer chemotherapy for ACC. Multiple drug therapy has been used on occasion, but there have been no reported therapeutic successes. We would therefore recommend that single agents be used at maximum dose in an attempt to identify active agents that might be combined in the future. Clinical investigators are encouraged to use doxorubicin alone or Cis-platinum alone or Cytoxan alone at maximum doses. Haq and co-workers have evaluated 27 trials of various chemotherapeutic agents given to 12 adults with metastatic ACC; they conclude that alkylating agents and doxorubicin appear to have antitumor activity [16]. The editorial office of *Pediatric Oncology* will attempt to serve as a data bank for successful or unsuccessful trials, and those pediatric oncologists who treat metastatic ACC are encouraged to send an informal letter summarizing their experience or their flow sheets to our editorial offices: Editorial Offices, Pediatric Oncology, care of G. Bennett Humphrey, Oklahoma Children's Memorial Hospital, P.O. Box 26307, Oklahoma City, OK 73126. Any results obtained will then be shared with those clinicians who are required to treat a child with metastatic or recurrent ACC.

CONCLUSIONS

For the immediate future, we believe that infantile ACC should be separated clinically from adolescent ACC since the former has a better prognosis. A review of the pathology of ACC in childhood is presented in this volume, which we hope will be used to evaluate pediatric case material in the future in conjuntion with other published criteria. For adolescent or infantile cases whose tumor mass exceeds 170 grams, we feel the prognosis should be guarded and that frequent and complete postoperative evaluation is recommended for two years. Radiation therapy is generally not recommended. For recurrent or metastatic disease, a trial of op'DDD is probably warranted. Very few complete remissions are anticipated, and patients who do not respond to op'DDD should be treated with single agent chemotherapy so that active agents can be identified for future combination chemotherapy.

REFERENCES

1. Weatherby RP, Carney JA: Pathologic features of childhood adrenocortical tumors. In: This volume.
2. LeFevre M, Gerard-Marchant R, Gubler JP, Chaussain JL, Lemerle J: Adrenal cortical carcinoma in children. 42 patients treated from 1958 to 1980 at Villejuif. In: This volume.
3. Hutter AM, Kayhoe DE: Adrenal cortical carcinoma. Results of treatment with op'DDD in 138 patients. Am J Med 41:581–592, 1966.
4. Hayles AB, Hahn HB, Sprague RG, Bahn RC, Priestley JT: Hormone-secreting tumors of the adrenal cortex in children. Pediatrics 37(1):19–25, 1966.
5. Hough AJ, Hollifield JW, Page DL, Hartmann WH: Prognostic factors in adrenal cortical tumors. A mathematical analysis of clinical and morphologic data. Am J Clin Pathol 72:390–399, 1979.
6. Lipsett MB, Hertz R, Ross GT: Clinical and pathophysiologic aspects of adrenocortical carcinoma. Am J Med 35:374–383, 1963.
7. Lewinsky BS, Grigor KM, Symington T, Neville AM: The clinical and pathologic features of 'non-hormonal' adrenocortical tumors. Report of twenty new cases and review of the literature. Cancer 33:778–790, 1974.
8. Gross MD, Bowerman RA, Mori KW, Cho KJ: The role of ultrasonography, computed tomography, scintigraphy and angiography in the localization of adrenal disease. In: This volume.
9. Tunell WP: The surgical management of tumors of the adrenal gland. In: This volume.
10. Holcombe JH, Pysher TJ, Kirkland RT: Functioning adrenocortical tumors in childhood. In: This volume.
11. Didolkar MS, Bescher RA, Elias EG, Moore RH: Natural history of adrenal cortical carcinoma: A clinicopathologic study of 42 patients. Cancer 47:2153–2161, 1981.
12. Raney RB, Meadows AT, D'Angio GJ: Adrenocortical carcinoma in children: Experience at the Children's Hospital of Philadelphia, 1961-1980. In: This volume.
13. Fraumeni JF, Miller RW: Adrenocortical neoplasms with hemihypertrophy, brain tumors, and other disorders. J Pediatr 70(1):129–138, 1967.
14. Hogan TF, Citrin DL, Johnson BM, Nakamura S, Davis TE, Borden EC: o,p'-DDD (mi-

totane) therapy of adrenal cortical carcinoma. Observations on drug dosage, toxicity, and steroid replacement. Cancer 42:2177–2181, 1978.
15. Ostuni JA, Roginsky MS: Metastatic adrenal cortical carcinoma. Documented cure with combined chemotherapy. Arch Intern Med 135:1257–1258, 1975.
16. Haf MM, Legha SS, Samaan NA, Bodey GP, Burgess MA: Cytotoxic chemotherapy in adrenal cortical carcinoma. Cancer Treat Rep 64:909–913, 1980.

23. Overview of the Multiple Endocrine Neoplasia Syndromes in Infancy and Childhood

G. BENNETT HUMPHREY, THEODORE PYSHER, JOHN HOLCOMBE, J. JAMES ROWSEY, TERRY E. BURRIS, JEAN LEMERLE, STUART D. WILSON, J.A. CARNEY and R. NEIL SCHIMKE

The multiple endocrine neoplasia (MEN) syndromes raise several issues of interest to the pediatrician-oncologist. These include the management of functional endocrine neoplasias, the diagnosis of associated endocrine lesions and the screening of asymptomatic relatives in these familial cancer syndromes. When dealing with these neoplasias, a pediatric endocrinologist and an adult endocrinologist need to be added to the traditional oncology team.

MEN TYPE I

The minimal criteria for the diagnosis would include the presence of endocrine tumors or hyperplasia in two or more of the potentially affected glands (parathyroid, pituitary, pancreas, adrenal). Hyperplasia must be functional, not just anatomic. If there is no obvious family history, the diagnosis is probable but not definite since apparent nonsyndromal endocrine tumor associations have been described. Multifocality lends additional support to the diagnosis of an hereditary endocrinopathy in questionable cases. Alternatively, the diagnosis should be considered firm in a patient with a tumor and/or hyperplasia of one of the glands comprising this syndrome and the presence of a positive family history.

Recommended screening for MEN type tumors would include yearly appraisals of serum calcium, phosphorus and gastrin levels in first degree relatives. Other studies could be undertaken as indicated by the appropriate complaints or physical findings; in other words, if a patient had complaints indicative of ulcer, hypoglycemia, amenorrhea and so forth. More extensive yearly evaluation is probably not cost effective.

It has been recommended that screening begin at 15 years of age; however, as children have been symptomatic as early as 10 years of age, screen-

G. Bennett Humphrey et al. (eds), Adrenal and Endocrine Tumors in Children.

ing should probably begin during the first decade of life [1, 2]. The medical and surgical management of MEN is discussed in this volume by Schimke [3]. The surgical management of MEN has been discussed in great detail by Wilson [1]. That review contains a very useful management flow chart. MEN I patients may experience their first episode of bleeding or ulceration secondary to gastrin secretion from a pancreatic tumor i.e., Zollinger-Ellison Syndrome (ZES) following any type of surgery or stress. Friesen and co-workers recommend that cimetidine therapy should be started in asymptomatic MEN individuals who must undergo elective surgery or curative surgery for MEN associated neoplasias [4]. A common example would be parathyroid surgery for mild hyperparathyroidism in an MEN individual. Surgery for ZES has been discussed in a review on the management of pancreatic malignancies and that review as well as some of the original literature are recommended to readers [5–7]. The ZES has poorer prognosis in patients with MEN type I than in sporadic cases.

Presentation of this syndrome during childhood is rare but does occur [2]. None of the case material in this volume includes a child symptomatic from MEN type I.

MEN TYPE II

The minimal criteria for the diagnosis would include the presence of multifocal medullary thyroid carcinoma with a positive family history of such or of relatives with pheochromocytoma and/or hyperparathyroidism in individuals who do not have a pathognomonic facies or body habitus. In clinically unaffected relatives of an affected proband elevated serum baseline calcitonin levels in the absence of any other obvious source (for example, small cell lung carcinoma) would be diagnostic of medullary thyroid carcinoma. If baseline calcitonin levels are normal in relatives, an exaggerated response to calcium-pentagastrin infusion is indicative of C-cell hyperplasia and provides justification for early surgery.

Recommended screening for MEN type II would include yearly calcium-pentagastrin provocative screening for medullary thyroid carcinoma. Yearly measurement of serum calcium, phosphorus and urinary VMA levels should be performed under controlled circumstances. The latter test could be performed sooner if there is any evidence of hypertension as determined by the family physician. It has been recommended that screening begin between the ages of 5 and 8 for children at risk [8]. The need for early surgery for medullary thyroid carcinoma (MTC) has been stressed by Schimke and by the case reports in this volume [10–12]. The possibility of a pheochromocytoma must be vigorously evaluated before thyroid surgery or before any surgical procedure, otherwise there may be a catastrophic event [13]. Presentation of this syndrome is rare during childhood but two cases are described by Sternlicht and co-authors.

MEN TYPE III

The minimal criteria for the diagnosis would include the same tumors as MEN type II and the additional clinical features of a peculiar facies with mucosal neuromas and a marfanoid habitus. Other physical findings have been summarized by Schimke [3]. Recently it has been reported that opthalmologists have a unique opportunity to identify cases of MEN type III [14]. The most characteristic finding is a greatly thickened corneal nerve. Other findings include corneal and eyelid neuromas, and keratoconjunctivitis sicca [15]. The corneal nerve anomaly is present in children as young as 2 years of age and is possibly present at birth [15, 16].

Screening for MTC is possibly risky in these patients because the malignancy tends to appear very early and to be highly malignant. When the pathognomonic facies and body habitus are present, Schimke would recommend total thyroidectomy, even when the calcitonin level is normal. Thereafter, patients should have an annual urinary VMA screening test performed.

The management of these cases would include early thyroidectomy and, as already stated, the same concern about pheochromocytoma probably applies to patients with MEN type III as has been suggested for MEN type II [13]. Recurrence of MTC is three times more common in MEN III than in MEN II and therefore after thyroidectomy, patients should be evaluated frequently for recurrence.

Rougier and colleagues have observed some unusual complications with MEN type III presenting during childhood [11]. Their experience with colon neurogangliomatosis is unusual but has been previously described. Their experience with the urinary neurogangliomatosis is unique and should be reviewed by any physician who is involved with children presumed or known to have MEN type III.

These two latter syndromes, MEN type II and III, probably occur with equal frequency, but the material in this volume would suggest MEN type III is more likely to be symptomatic during childhood than MEN type II [17]. This is also suggested in Schimke's review [3].

REFERENCES

1. Wilson SD: Wermer's syndrome: Multiple endocrine adenopathy, type I. In: Surgical endocrinology, Friesen SR (ed), J.B. Lippincott Co., 1978, p 265–283.

2. Snyder N III, Scurry MT, Deiss WP Jr: Five families with multiple endocrine adenomatosis. Ann Intern Med 76:53–58, 1972.
3. Schimke RN: In this volume.
4. Friesen SR, Hermreck AS, Brackett CE, Schimke RN: Cimetidine in the management of synchronous crises of MEA I. World J Surg 4:123–129, 1980.
5. Wilson SD: Ulcerogenic tumors of the pancreas: The Zollinger-Ellison syndrome. In: The pancreas, Carey LC (ed), CV Mosby Co., 1973, 295–318.
6. Pysher T, Humphrey GB, Wilson SD, Schein PS, Donaldson SS, Bukowski RM, Kissane J: Overview of childhood pancreatic tumors. In: Pediatric oncology, Volume 2.
7. Wilson SD, Schulte WJ, Meade RC: Longevity studies following total gastrectomy in children with the Zollinger-Ellison syndrome. Arch Surg 103:108–115, 1971.
8. Freitas JE, Sisson JC, Freier DT, Thompson NW: MEN type IIa syndrome: Dilemmas in modern management. Semin Nucl Med 8(1):73–78, 1978.
9. Fox PS, Hofmann JW, DeCosse JJ, Wilson SD: The influence of total gastrectomy on survival in malignant Zollinger-Ellison tumors. Ann Surg 180(4):558–566, 1974.
10. Cushing B, Brough AJ: In this volume.
11. Rougier P, Caillou B, Parmentier C, Lemerle J: In this volume.
12. Sternbach MS, Miller JD, Chevalier L: In this volume.
13. Sternbach MS, Miller JD, Chevalier L: Sipple families. Lancet 939–940, April 30, 1977.
14. Riley FC, Robertson DM: Ocular histopathology in multiple endocrine neoplasia type 2b. Am J Ophthalmol 91:57–64, 1981.
15. Robertson DM, Sizemore GW, Gordon H: Thickened corneal nerves as a manifestation of multiple endocrine neoplasia. Trans Am Acad Ophthalmol Otolaryngol 79:772, 1975.
16. Rowsey JJ, Burris TE: Personal communication.
17. Chong GC, Beahrs OH, Sizemore GW, Woolner LH: Medullary carcinoma of the thyroid gland. Cancer 35:695–704, 1975.

Subject Index

GPSR Compliance

The European Union's (EU) General Product Safety Regulation (GPSR) is a set of rules that requires consumer products to be safe and our obligations to ensure this.

If you have any concerns about our products, you can contact us on ProductSafety@springernature.com

In case Publisher is established outside the EU, the EU authorized representative is:

Springer Nature Customer Service Center GmbH
Europaplatz 3
69115 Heidelberg, Germany

Batch number: 10620143

Printed by Printforce, the Netherlands